The Inner World of Medical Students

The Inner World
of Medical Students
Listening to Their Voices in Poetry

Johanna Shapiro PhD

Professor, Department of Family Medicine
Director, Program in Medical Humanities and Arts
University of California, Irvine School of Medicine

Foreword by
Howard F Stein PhD

Professor and Special Assistant to the Chair
Department of Family and Preventive Medicine
University of Oklahoma Health Sciences Center

Radcliffe Publishing
Oxford • New York

Radcliffe Publishing Ltd
18 Marcham Road
Abingdon
Oxon OX14 1AA
United Kingdom

www.radcliffe-oxford.com
Electronic catalogue and worldwide online ordering facility.

British Library Cataloguing in Publication Data

A catalogue record for this book is available from the British Library.

ISBN-13: 978 185775 752 1

Typeset by Pindar NZ, Auckland, New Zealand
Printed and bound by Cadmus Communications, USA

Contents

Foreword

Why the poetry of medicine and medical students? Why the need for this book?

Countless teachers and practitioners of American biomedicine have long insisted on a dichotomy between "real medicine" or "hard science" and "soft stuff" such as the social sciences and humanities. In this view, "real medicine" is biology, and everything else is either mere "background" or superfluous information. There, are, however, many ways of knowing in medicine and life, and we all are impoverished to the degree that human tissue is the only worthwhile type of knowledge that is valued. Poetry, story, visual art, and music bring onto center stage the doctor and patient as experiencing subjects, the "who" that is always a part of the "what" of medicine.

This is the opposite of the common disparagement of personal and social viewpoints as "merely subjective," in supposed contrast with the "objectivity" that is medicine's gold standard. The humanities offer different but equally worthwhile kinds of facts, and raise different but equally legitimate kinds of questions, from those of "hard science." Ironically, the inclusion or exclusion of personal and social factors affects the collection of some of the most important clinical facts that physicians need to make diagnoses and treatment plans. "Soft" is in fact quite "hard"! Poetry can help physicians to create new space in their minds, to explore new clinical possibilities, and thereby enhance both their relationships with patients and their families, and their biomedical practice. This brings me to the author and subject of this book.

Dr. Johanna Shapiro is one of the most vital and lucid voices in the medical humanities within American biomedicine. *The Inner World of Medical Students* represents the culmination of over two decades of her thinking, teaching, writing, research, and publishing in the medical humanities.

Historically, this field underwent a rebirth in the mid-1980s. It emerged as a much needed corrective to the objectifying clinical "gaze" that had transformed the patient into an animate "thing" that harbored disease or injury – a scientific tradition that had likewise made the physician into an anonymous, scientific technician. Through physicians' renewed emphasis on clinical narrative, story, poetry, and visual art, the patient began to come alive as an experiencing subject. Moreover, practicing physicians also began to write accounts of their experience of becoming a physician and of medical practice.

Much of the foundation of the medical humanities lies "in the work of great writers and writer-physicians." This book goes one step further. For years, in her own teaching, Dr. Shapiro has invited physicians-in-the-making to record and document their journey, and she has devoted considerable effort to listening to the stories that they, and students from many other medical schools, tell through their poetry. In *The Inner World of Medical Students* is to be found both insight into and wisdom about the inner worlds of patient and medical student – as well as their intersubjective or relational world. Clearly, much of the "inner" world of medical students is an emotional precipitate of their relationships with others – patients, fellow students, residents, faculty physicians, nurses, family members, etc.

Dr. Shapiro has contributed abundantly to the literature of medical humanities. Her most innovative contribution is, I believe, the attention that she has given to the lived worlds of the medical students whom she teaches. She takes seriously the human voice of her medical students, specifically the experience of what it is like to become a physician. My guess is that subsequently, when they are physicians, these students will be more likely to want to listen – and be emotionally capable of listening – to their patients, because as medical students they were so attentively listened to by Dr. Shapiro. What starts out as a class exercise turns into a rare opportunity to put into words the feelings, images, and thoughts that students might not have even known they were experiencing. The writing and the subsequent discussion of their poems in class becomes more than a cognitive exercise. I think that it is somewhat therapeutic as well.

I hasten to add that Dr. Shapiro's "data" – that is, medical students' poems – come from multiple sources (from her own students over a 10-year period, and also the published poems of medical students at other institutions). This fact gives further weight to the generalizability of Dr. Shapiro's interpretations.

A healing environment is sorely needed in medical school – for students. One recurrent meta-theme in this book is that many poems are about resistance to, or even protest against, the degrading, brutalizing, life-sucking relationships and overall structure of medical education. Building upon the work of Arthur Frank, Dr. Shapiro offers and abundantly illustrates a typology of narrative themes into which her students' poems can be classified – chaos, restitution, quest, witnessing, journey, and transcendent. Here, medical students' poetry of resistance is a kind of Ariadne's thread through the Minotaur's labyrinth of medical education, and through the myriad poems contained in this book. Their poems offer me a little hope that the common trajectory in medical school from compassion to scorn toward patients might be interrupted and altered. This book is a kind of reclamation of voice in the midst of silencing of personal voice. It is quietly political, even "anti-colonial," in the sense that biomedicine and its training "colonize" both patient and doctor. The "inner" world of medical students says much about the "outer" world.

This brings me to the question of the value of developing and applying narrative typologies in relation to the poetry. All science – in which I wish to include the humanities, at least in some respects – relies on creating typologies with which to organize the swirling array of material or data. Here poetry constitutes a form of data. I think that one can understand and appreciate poetry more, rather than less, by asking questions such as "What kind of poem (and poet) is this?" and "How does this poem relate to others?" The comparative method can enrich rather than impoverish our comprehension of a poem. A thought-provoking interpretive framework can connect poems and deepen our appreciation of an individual poem. "Classification" should not be a dirty word in relation to the medical humanities. Let me briefly illustrate this point. I think that all the many kinds of poems, from restitutional to transcendent, stand at the edge of the cliff of chaos. None of the others is so firm that it cannot be under threat of being undone by anxiety about infirmity, loss, and death.

I think that it is significant for the emotional architecture of the book that the first voice we hear is not that of Dr. Shapiro, but one of her students, in a poem. Except for the detailed analysis of the first poem, Dr. Shapiro's subsequent interpretations are brief and cogent, and invite the reader to think and feel more. She gives both the students and the reader new space within which they can explore meaning and feeling. Refreshingly, this book is not author-centered, which is to say interpretation-centered. The author is as much witness as guide. She is always inquisitive, always respectful, and never intrusive. She makes exquisite "music" without ever drawing attention to her virtuosity. Only at the book's end does she situate herself in her own and her students' narrative.

Medical students are in some ways in a unique position in our society, for they are at the frontline in being socialized to face and address issues of illness, suffering, and death – issues that most of us would rather avoid and delegate to physicians as "their role." Thus their poetry reflects not only their concerns as they make their way through life's journey, but also in some ways our own concerns. How do we relate to those who are suffering and in pain, both others and our own? Even as Dr. Shapiro enters deeply into medical students' poetry, she is also, through her incisive commentary and gentle guidance, holding up a mirror to our own lives as we struggle to address many of the same questions.

I cannot think of anyone in medical education who would not benefit from reading *The Inner World of Medical Students*. Although this book is about medical students, their experiences and relationships, it is not only for those who teach medical students. I could imagine it being read by pre-med students who would like to know "what it is like" to be at medical school. I could equally imagine it being read by residency faculty who should be interested in what their future interns and residents are thinking about. It urgently needs to be read by deans, department chairs, and faculty who make medical school policy and curricula. Finally, in a larger sense, the issues addressed in this book speak to all of us as we struggle to make sense of life, seek deeper, more authentic, and compassionate ways to relate to each other, and search for meaning in the face of illness, suffering, and death. This book deserves a long and fruitful life.

Howard F Stein PhD
Professor and Special Assistant to the Chair
Department of Family and Preventive Medicine
University of Oklahoma Health Sciences Center
Oklahoma City, OK, USA
January 2009

About the Author

Johanna Shapiro received her PhD from Stanford University. She is currently a professor in the Department of Family Medicine, University of California Irvine School of Medicine. Trained as a clinical psychologist, her main area of academic interest has focused on various aspects of the doctor–patient relationship, including physician interactions with "difficult," stigmatized, and culturally diverse patient populations. She has authored or co-authored over 100 refereed publications. Dr. Shapiro is also Director of Medical Humanities and Arts for the UC Irvine School of Medicine, and in this capacity she develops and evaluates the humanities- and arts-based curriculum across all four years of medical school. She is feature editor of the *Family Medicine* column, "Literature and the Arts in Medical Education," and faculty co-advisor to the medical student-initiated *Plexus: UCI-COM Journal of Arts and Humanities*. She has also published original poetry in the *Journal of the American Medical Association, Journal of Medical Humanities, The Healing Muse, Blood and Thunder, Hospital Drive, International Journal of Healthcare and Humanities, Families, Systems, and Health* and *Journal of Family Practice*.

Acknowledgments

I wish to express my deep thanks and appreciation to the following individuals, without whom this book could never have been written. The mistakes and shortcomings of this text are entirely my own, but whatever insights it might contain and whatever light it might shed are largely due to the support, encouragement, and inspiration of these people:

UCI School of Medicine students:

Sayeh Beheshti, a gifted writer, poet, and future psychiatrist.

Jena Berg, responsible for conceptualizing the UCI School of Medicine elective in humanities research, which has successfully enrolled 18 students over the past 8 years.

Sarah Blaschko, who proved that poetry and urology are not incompatible.

Sheila Chan, an exceptional pianist, poet, and artist who is an equally impressive neurologist.

Melinda Glines and Lorena Hillman, who cheered me on in the early days and always showed uncommon devotion to humane patient care.

Meghann Kaiser, a brilliant student and future surgeon whose view into the heart of medicine is always incisive and penetrating.

Brian McMichael, a supremely discerning physician-poet who fearlessly witnesses to both the shortcomings and the possibilities of medicine.

Sarah Mourra, a remarkable student and luminous poet who gave me the privilege of participating in so many aspects of her life.

Grainne Mulholland, a true humanist physician, who helped to conceive and provided the leadership to bring to fruition the very first issue of *Plexus*.

Sheela Reddy, who because of her courage in coming to know herself can now compassionately guide patients to know themselves.

Elena Rios-Ruiz, who took the risk of emotionally engaging with the sickest pediatric patients and their families.

Gail Ryan, an extraordinarily talented and perceptive artist, and a compassionate, caring psychiatrist.

Aparche Yang, the very first student to enroll when the UCI School of Medicine literature and medicine elective was first offered in 1999.

UCI Department of Family Medicine: Past and present chairs, especially Joe Scherger, MD, MPH, who supported and encouraged the always interesting unfolding of my professional path; past and present colleagues, especially Elizabeth Morrison, MD, MS, and Desiree Lie, MD, MS, whose friendship and collegiality made such a difference along the way; and Dolores Medina-Sasina, whose dedication in tracking down long-vanished former students enabled so many of these poems to appear in this work.

UC Irvine School of Medicine: So many colleagues who sustained and advanced my work in medical humanities, especially Alberto Manetta, MD, and Lloyd Rucker, MD, who believed in the vision at its initial and uncertain inception; Robert Leonard, PhD, who instantly grasped the connection between anatomy and humanities, and has never wavered in his commitment and humanism; Penny Murata, MD, who faithfully and creatively incorporated the humanities to help students to reflect on the pediatric clerkship; Felicia Cohn, PhD, a brilliant ethicist with whom I shared so many rewarding reflective sessions; Jerome Tobis, MD, who consistently promoted the humanities in physical medicine and rehabilitation; Donna Baker, LCSW, for her steadfast awareness of the value of the arts in working with cancer patients; Ann Abrams, LCSW, who believed in readers' theater as a way to help geriatric patients and medical students to learn about each other; Merry Grasska, FNP, who welcomed poetry into the training of family nurse practitioners; Marianne Ross, PhD, who so generously shared the path of healer's art with me; and my professional soul-mate Daniel Robitshek, MD, who provided such invaluable intellectual and spiritual companionship along the way.

UC Irvine: Liane Brouillette, PhD, always willing to build cross-disciplinary bridges and challenge disciplinary boundaries; and Kristen Monroe, PhD, an extraordinarily compassionate person and renowned ethics scholar who embodies on a daily basis the essence of her academic work.

My family medicine colleagues throughout the country:

Bruce Birnberg, MSW, and Robin Winter, MD, who have done so much to help to realize a meaningful role for the medical humanities in family medicine.

John Frey, MD, the epitome of the thoughtful, compassionate, and wise family physician-scholar.

Paul Gross, MD, who invited me along on his journey to create the e-journal *Pulse* as a new way to give voice to everyone affected by sickness and healing.

Deborah Kasman, MD, MA, a dedicated, courageous, intrepid woman warrior.

Lucille Marchand, RN, MD, whose tender heart carries her fearlessly into the dark corners and then invariably illuminates them.

Susan McDaniels, PhD, and Jeanne Klee, who generously solicited my voice into the poetic conversation of the journal *Families, Systems, and Health*.

Jo Marie Reilly, MD, a wonderful mentee who has become an even more wonderful mentor.

Pamela Schaff, MD, PhD, an inspiring teacher, dedicated physician, and gifted writer.

Barry Weiss, MD, and Jan Cartwright from the journal *Family Medicine*, who were indispensable in bringing to fruition the column Literature and the Arts in Medical Education, and who were always there to provide guidance and back-up.

Caroline Wellbery, MD, PhD, who has not swerved from her aspiration to create a humane, healing practice of medicine, and who has often been willing to pursue this vision single-handedly.

My cherished colleague and friend Howard Stein, PhD, whose encyclopedic knowledge, scholarly productivity, enormous heart, and profound wisdom – Jewish and otherwise – has both awed and inspired me, whose poetry has moved me to tears with its beauty and honesty, and with whom I have been blessed to be in dialogue about matters great and small for 30 years.

... and other colleagues:

Felice Aull, PhD, whose intellectual virtuosity awes and whose kindness sustains.

Jill Beck, PhD, for her brilliant cross-disciplinary mind, her passion for the arts, and her ability to grasp so deeply their relationship to medicine.

Rita Charon, MD, PhD, a ground-breaking visionary blessed with an exceptional mind and a compassionate heart who took time to encourage this work.

Jack Coulehan, MD, MPH, my personal model of the consummate physician-poet (and ethicist, epidemiologist, and medical humanist), with whom I shared a wild intellectual ride.

Cortney Davis, RN, and Judy Schaefer, RN, colleagues who have honed my gratitude toward the nursing profession, and whose radiant poetry continues to uplift me.

Audrey Shafer, MD, a most remarkable physician, poet, and human being.

Delese Wear, PhD, a constant role model in terms of intellectual integrity and pure, passionate writing.

My international colleagues:

Pablo Blasco, MD, and his SOBRAMFA (Brazilian Society for Family Medicine) team in Brazil, who have supported, inspired, and believed in my efforts at all times, in all places.

Arielle Kliffer, PhD, France, for her beautiful laugh and no-holds-barred spirit.

Silvia Quadrelli, Argentina, for her enthusiasm and insights into the link between the movies and doctoring.

Ravi Shankar, PhD, Nepal, who proved that medical humanities can flourish even in a remote mountain kingdom.

My thanks to the following individuals for their kindness in helping me to collect poetry samples:

Catherine Belling, PhD, and Jack Coulehan, MD, MPH, *Contexts*, State University of New York – StonyBrook, School of Medicine.

Karen Carlson, *SCOPE*, Southern Illinois University School of Medicine.

Rita Charon, MD, PhD, and Tara McGann, *Reflexions*, Columbia University Medical Center.

Marcia Childress, PhD, *Veritas*, University of Virginia School of Medicine.

Sheila Crow, MA, *Blood and Thunder*, University of Oklahoma.

Frank Edwards, MD, *Loose Associations*, University of Rochester School of Medicine.

Anne Hunsaker-Hawkins, PhD, *Wild Onions*, Pennsylvania State University College of Medicine.

Amila Husic and Anas Abou-Ismail, *Paint the Walls*, Weill Cornell Medical College in Qatar.

Claire Langran, *Lifelines*, Dartmouth Medical School.

Scott Perrin, *The Legible Script*, University of South Florida College of Medicine.

Suzanne Poirier, PhD, and Mike Gill, *Body Electric*, University of Illinois, College of Medicine – Chicago.

Cynthia Shea, *Meme*, Johns Hopkins School of Medicine.

Nina Stoyan-Rosenzweig, PhD, *Panacea*, University of Florida College of Medicine.

George Trone and Howard Spiro, MD, *Yale Journal for Humanities in Medicine*, Yale University School of Medicine.

To:

My students (both those who write poetry and those who do not!) who have made my career in medical education rich, rewarding, and challenging

and

My family:

My parents, Benedict and Nancy Freedman, who have always loved me so deeply and have urged me on . . .

My brother, Michael Freedman, who is the smartest person I know and can always help me find a reason to laugh . . .

My sister, Deborah Jackson, who has stood beside me in the face of the unthinkable, and shared joy, tears, and above all song . . .

My daughter, Shauna, whose mind and heart inspire me, and who, by writing her own academic text, goaded me to keep writing . . .

My daughter, Jena, who is the best juggler I know, and whose love and admiration are unswerving, even when I don't deserve them . . .

My son, Josh, my intellectual maverick, who challenged me to write this book "if I really wanted to" . . .

My grandsons, James, Liam, Nathan, and Jackson, who embody the joy of life . . .

and my husband, soul-mate, companion, partner, team-mate, guide, and teacher, Deane, who is the wisest person I know, who knows me better than I know myself, and who has always helped me to find my voice, and to be the best person personally and professionally that I can be.

1 Medical Education as a Rite of Passage

Thoughts on George Harrison's Death By: Jena Berg, MSIII
Originally appeared in Plexus 2003, *UC Irvine School of Medicine*

Mid-lecture the ENT surgeon pointed to a slide.
It was half-head, half-recognizable.
I'd say disfigured but that implies some figured starting place
Half serious he said, "Most people who get head and neck cancer
sort of get what they deserve."
Hardened by many heads, he was ready to take on
the next terminal case with a swagger.

His bravado implied: this unfortunate head hadn't led
the clean life of a surgeon.
I imagine perhaps it had once crossed his path
in the pre-dawn hour:
the surgeon with clean trimmed nails en route to work
the head staggering home
from bars and smoky trysts.
Or maybe it had sat at home
up all night, learning the sitar.

This poem, referencing the iconic Beatle George Harrison who died from head and neck cancer, exemplifies some of what we can learn from a study of medical student poetry. It describes a situation that is apparently a straightforward lecture, but is in fact a complex encounter between physician, student, and patient. The medical student, sitting in a lecture hall, is almost invisible. She appears only twice, once noting her difficulty in describing the head in the slide, and once imagining a fantastical encounter between surgeon and head. The surgeon, on the other hand, dominates the poem. He is in charge of the lecture. He feels free to make off-the-cuff judgments about the patient; and swaggers from case to case. The patient is presumably dead, and his very presence (through the slide) is completely regulated by the physician's aims and goals.

Yet the poem demonstrates the counter-hegemonic purposes to which poetry can be put. The apparently irrelevant student is also the narrator of the poem. Thus, although she neither controlled nor had any meaningful input into the lecture, she exercises *complete* control of the *story* of what happened in that lecture. In the singular act of writing a poem, the student regains her voice and can express her anger and disappointment at the surgeon as well as her solidarity with the patient. By creating the poem, the student finds a way to comment on the ethicality of the presentation, to empathize with the patient, and to puncture the arrogance and superiority of the doctor. In a brilliant use of synecdoche, the poet continues the dehumanizing approach of the surgeon, but subverts it for her own purposes, much as the gay community reclaimed the term "queer" and people with disabilities took back the word "cripple."

The poem becomes a way of not simply ignoring a fleeting moment of insensitivity, a passing remark that was not at all "the point" of the surgeon's lecture. Instead, the powerless student reclaims power by saying, "I *heard* that comment. It *mattered* to me. I side not with you in your arrogance but with the vulnerable, suffering patient." Therefore the poem is a way for the student to manifest resistance to the dominant story the surgeon wishes to tell about his own competence and superiority, and about the patient's culpability. It is a way for the student to reclaim her own voice, her own moral judgment, her own empathy and humility in the face of the patient's suffering.

Without writing the poem, the student might easily have let the awkward moment go. Instead, she used it to empower herself, and to witness the emotional detachment and patient blaming of the surgeon, as well as the intrinsic worth of the patient. Without reading the poem, the rest of us (medical educators, doctors, other students, patients and future patients) would not have the opportunity to peer into this window to become aware of this student's moral quandary and her efforts at resolution.

BACKGROUND

There are 129 accredited medical schools in the USA. Many of these schools self-publish literary/arts journals containing original creative work of medical students (and sometimes of faculty, staff, residents, and patients as well). A certain percentage of this creative work takes the form of poetry written by medical students. Yet, despite the existence of such journals, we know next to nothing about this poetry. Why do some students write poetry? What issues does such poetry address? What narrative forms do these poems take? What themes do they explore? Perhaps most importantly, what can we learn about this future generation of physicians from an examination of their poetry? To date no systematic analysis has been undertaken regarding what can be learned about medical students and medical education from medical student poetry. It is my hope that a book which provides a comprehensive view of medical student poetry and the meanings that we can glean from this work will be a valuable resource for medical educators, medical humanities scholars, and medical students alike.

In this book, I make the case that an important source of data about some of what is right – and what is wrong – about medical education can be obtained through the study of students' personal writings, particularly their poetry. Certainly only a small minority of medical students write poetry, so it is impossible to generalize that the views they express are representative or typical of medical students generally. Nevertheless, it is often claimed that art reflects society back to itself better than society can otherwise see. If this is true, then it is possible that medical student poetry is a particularly clear and insightful crystallization of issues that might otherwise remain inchoate and unexpressed in the unconscious of large numbers of medical students. Poirier[1] argues that what distinguishes medical student writers from non-writers is not that they have different experiences, but that the former group reflects in writing on these experiences. Preliminary support for this proposition comes from a study in which first-year medical students who chose *not* to complete creative projects as a way of reflecting on their experience nevertheless stated that they learned something about their experience by viewing the creative works of their peers.[2]

The purpose of this book is therefore to provide a content analysis and grounded theory interpretations of a subset ($n = 589$) of medical student poems in the public domain or produced as part of medical school courses to enable interested medical educators, scholars, and laypersons to better understand various aspects of medical student life and training from the unique vantage point of their poetry. Specifically, this analysis may further understanding of where the process of socialization into medicine is failing students and, overall, what their concerns, worries, and insights are during this period of their training. The book may also serve to illuminate through the fresh eyes of students who are new to the practice of medicine common issues regarding doctoring and the doctor–patient relationship that are of great relevance for more experienced physicians whose attitudes and clinical behavior may have become stunted and stultified. Finally, this book examines fundamental, universal concerns for us all, filtered through the lens of medical school, such as establishing an identity, facing mortality and suffering, and seeking connectedness with others, and therefore is relevant to general readers as well. The intent of the analysis undertaken is not merely descriptive, but is also prescriptive in that it provides indications of what kinds of meta-issues medical education needs to address differently, and better.

In the remainder of this chapter, I shall first review the concept of medical education as a rite of passage, and some of the limitations in the way that this ritual succeeds in helping medical students to make the transition from layperson to physician. In the next chapter I shall turn to the functions that writing can serve for medical students, including the role that various narrative typologies can play in their development. I also acknowledge that writing is not a panacea for student distress and confusion, and briefly explore some of its limitations. From here, Chapter 3 will engage in a discussion specifically focusing on the reason for studying medical student poetry in particular, a description of my methodology, and a qualitative dissection of poetry as data.

MEDICAL EDUCATION AS A RITE OF PASSAGE

Reflections of a Pruned Medical Student By: Allison Hill
Originally appeared in Plexus *2008. UC Irvine School of Medicine*

A passerby may wonder
Why wistful I may be
Why envy haunts my vision
When I view the willow tree.

A passerby may marvel
And admire my molded form.
My every branch and twig and leaf
Has learned how to conform.

My sculptured shape is chiseled
By shears too sharp to see
For pruning is the price I paid
For this topiary me.

Meandering through scented shops
Lounging by the pool
Watching goofy sitcoms
And trying to look cool

Crosswords and sudokus
Magazines and jokes
These were clipped and hauled away
By the garden training folks.

I don't begrudge the clipping.
It was my choice, to be sure.
But when the wind blows through the willow
I feel its freedom's lure.

This poem reflects on the rite of passage that transforms the bright undergraduate premedical student into a physician. Here the author uses a classic rhyme scheme (abcb) and a traditional meter (a kind of modified iambic trimeter), as well as a consistent metaphor (a sculpted shrub) to describe her experiences in medical school. All of these conventional forms serve to emphasize how the student feels herself to be bound and constrained by the conventions of medicine.

The layperson (the casual passerby) might find much to admire in the carefully sculpted lines of this "topiary" medical student. However, the student herself knows all too well just how "sharp" were the pruning shears that chopped away all of the "unnecessary" aspects of her life. She experiences envy and longing when she contemplates the freedom of the willow tree – so spontaneous and natural, so much *itself*. The narrator laments all that she has lost – seemingly trivial things, but things that help to define the uniqueness of one's life and which add both joy and silliness. Topiary is impressive as an aesthetic accomplishment, but it is also artificial, ornamental, and sometimes vaguely ridiculous. The comparison suggests that the student believes these qualities are equally applicable to her. She ruefully acknowledges that submitting to the pruning process was her "choice," but she feels the pull of freedom, and wonders at all that she has lost.

Medical education is indeed a rite of passage, an intense and grueling process by which an ordinary (albeit highly intelligent) young adult is transformed into a physician. Less eloquently, it has sometimes been compared to military boot camp in its effort to transform people into physicians through the deconstruction and subsequent rebuilding of the individual.[3] Hawkins, drawing on the work of Joseph Campbell,[4] noted that rites of passage generally have three components:[5]

1 separation from the world, where the individual is chosen for a privileged but challenging experience
2 transition or marginality, where the individual traverses an alien world with few elements of ordinary reality
3 incorporation, in which the individual returns to normal existence, reassuming relationships, rights, and responsibilities after having been profoundly changed as a result of these unusual and demanding experiences.

Medical school embodies this process. Students selected to attend medical school are the result of a long and rigorous procedure, based primarily on academic and intellectual achievement measured by grades, particularly in the basic sciences, and performance in arduous examinations (MCATS). The profession of medicine itself is still endowed with attributes of status, privilege, and power. Therefore the sense of chosenness readily translates into feelings of specialness and sometimes entitlement. Medical students are aware that they represent an elite social group.

Separation

However, the selection process is followed by separation and testing. In this regard, medical school, which offers such richness and promise, is also full of loss. There is literal loss for students who are geographically removed from family and friends. There are many emotional and psychological losses as well. Paradoxically, having reached the "top of the heap" through their acceptance into medical school, once they have matriculated, students find themselves back at the bottom. They are *all* gifted, *all* bright, *all* elite. Perhaps most challenging of all, students often feel that they must relinquish crucial aspects of their identity. On a superficial level, they may discover that they no longer have the time to indulge cherished hobbies or to take care of their own bodies, even as they absorb massive amounts of information about the bodies of others. They relinquish their soccer balls and their violins, they become accustomed to subsisting on junk food and little sleep, accustomed to becoming strangers to the outdoors and the natural world. On a deeper level, they may internalize the message that actual parts of who they are – perhaps their sensitivity or their tender-heartedness – no longer have a place in their professional persona.

Liminality

At this point, the student begins a journey into marginality and liminality in an alien and often apparently unreal world. Huge numbers of hours are spent on demanding course-work involving intense study and memorization. Students no longer have easy access to friends and family. Their new world is competitive and focused on success. This world has a strange, often initially incomprehensible language, its own attire (white coats) and accessories (stethoscopes, reflex hammers, otoscopes), its own contained environment (hospital and clinics), and its own customs (exams, "pimping" of students, long hours without sleep). In short, students have entered an unfamiliar, rigorous and sometimes overwhelming culture in which they are neither doctors nor patients. This sense of being caught between worlds is puzzling, confusing, and often demoralizing, but it also gives students a unique perspective on their experience.

Incorporation

The eventual goal of a rite of passage is incorporation, or the integration of the person back into society, bringing new wisdom, insights, and skills in the service of suffering and oppressed others. In the case of medicine, students receive the imprimatur of expertise through the granting of a medical diploma. They are then expected to use their special knowledge for the good of society, specifically for those who become their patients. Like a shaman,[6] they are forever changed by their initiation experience, by the trials and tribulations that they have confronted and overcome. These changes are expected to make them wiser, more compassionate, more skilled professionals who can successfully fulfill this function.

SHORTCOMINGS IN THE CURRENT RITE OF MEDICAL PASSAGE

The rite of passage that students undergo in medical education is intended to prepare them for new roles, first as physicians in training and eventually as physicians. However, many scholars and medical educators have questioned whether it is the appropriate and necessary rite of passage, or whether it has limitations and shortcomings that can also damage students and fail to prepare them adequately for the societal roles they are destined to play. For example, the training of medical students may be unbalanced in terms of the vast panoply of left- and right-brain skills that most physicians will actually need in clinical practice. Because of understandable needs to train its acolytes so thoroughly in the sciences, medicine runs the risk of taking whole persons and teaching them to use only half of their abilities as they approach the task of doctoring. Medicine is neither wrong nor bad in its educational priorities, but it is so powerful, hegemonic, and self-serving that it is often unresponsive to alternative points of view that might make it a more comprehensive and relevant rite of passage.[7]

Overemphasis on logico-scientific thinking and problem solving

In the educational system's zeal to provide strong scientifically based training, it may end up substituting "measurable, reductionistic, scientific skills for skills that are linguistic, empathic, and interpretive"[8,9] by conveying that the latter are soft and unscientific. Medical training attempts to order the world by relying on knowledge that can be obtained by reductionism, objectivity, and essentialism, as well as logical, rational thinking, and relationships that can be controlled by hierarchy, authority, and power. This leads to models of understanding and relationship that are excessively formulaic, rule-bound, and lacking in human connection.

Therefore, in a practice discipline that in fact requires *all* forms of knowledge to be accessible, including both logico-scientific and narrative knowledge,[10] students come to distrust the very capacities that can help them to process both their own educational experiences and the patient's experiences of illness, as well as to make emotional connections with patients. Medical students are trained to rely excessively on mechanistic ways of thinking about the body, to think in terms of universal generalities instead of idiosyncratic particulars, and to analyze through paradigms rather than through narrative. They have little opportunity to engage in bodies of knowledge other than the bioscientific, yet it is through other bodies of knowledge that issues of compassion, communication, and social responsibility are engaged and critical thinking about oneself, medicine, and society can occur.[11]

Neglect of medicine as a moral enterprise

Although medicine presents itself as a science rooted in empiricism and positivism, in fact clinical medicine, as a profession that practices on living human beings, cannot be anything other than a moral enterprise.[12,13] Yet despite valiant efforts to incorporate bioethics into medical curricula, by and large medical training discourages the analysis and expression of values, the pursuit of meaning and purpose, and the in-depth analysis of moral dilemmas, concepts that seem too abstract and not capable of being fully determined through an empirical approach. Medicine defined purely as a technical science cannot sustain learners through their training and beyond, when they must encounter the messy and anguished real lives of patients.

In fact, some scholars worry that not only does medical education not prepare students for fully grappling with the moral dimension of medicine, but also it runs the risk of confusing, demoralizing, and even morally corrupting medical students by asking them to observe or even participate in attitudes and behaviors that are ethically dubious. This leaves them with pervasive feelings of anxiety and guilt that are triggered by uncertainty and powerlessness, coupled with perceived responsibility for the resultant negative outcomes.[14] The medical sociologist Arthur Frank[15] claims that physicians often feel that something crucial to who they are as people is being destroyed by the way they must practice medicine.

Overemphasis on control

Students are often taught that being in control is a crucial aspect of their future role as physicians. The biomedical model enables the clinician to maintain control through the ability to make accurate predictions and achieved desired outcomes. As Suchman points out, control is also maintained through the structuring of relationships (hierarchical), the kinds of knowledge that are deemed desirable (objective, reductionist, essentialist, and instrumental), and the kinds of thinking that are used (rational, logical, and linear). When things are perceived as being out of control, physicians (and physicians in training) are left with feelings of impotence and shame, and fear that their inadequacy will be uncovered.[16] Despite the reality that uncertainty and lack of control are an important thread in medicine, very little attention is given to preparing physicians to act with grace and compassion in these situations.

Devaluing of personal identity

Frank has commented on the way in which medicine "hails" its members.[17] By this he means the process whereby medicine selects bodies and minds to fill certain pre-imagined slots (including both doctors and patients). In terms of medical students, "hailing" bestows status and power on medical students, identifying them as future members of an influential and powerful professional aristocracy. However, it also demands a heavy price – in order to become acceptable, one's identity must be smoothed to fit into this socially prescribed and over-determined role. Medicine speaks in the voice of the expert, the authority, and it uses its language to encourage, even coerce, people into thinking of themselves as what the institution requires them to be.

To some extent, just as modernist medicine "colonizes" the body of the patient as its territory,[18] medical education attempts to "colonize" the student. Medical sociologists point out how medicine "takes over" the patient's body as well as many aspects of the patient's life in exchange for care or cure (or, in the case of students, achievement of a highly desired goal). These imposed narratives[19] tend to stifle volitional, personal voices, so that patients (or students) try to suppress, regulate, and control their own narratives.[20] Students are encouraged to adopt rigidly defined professional identities that limit uniqueness and restrict their ability to explore or value other aspects of their personality.[21] Just as the chart "flattens" the patient, and reduces the three-dimensional person to a two-dimensional caricature, so the medical education process can do the same thing to students.[22] Institutions, including that of medicine, find it easier to manage members who think of themselves as isolated and passive.[23] It is in the interests of institutions to shut out the expression of difference, of suffering. Yet non-recognition of the person can be a form of oppression. In this way, medical education lays claim to the person of the student in exchange for transforming them into a physician. Students are encouraged to believe that they will be able to succeed while avoiding themselves – indeed, that success is in part dependent on this avoidance.[13] Students may resist this colonization, but ambivalently. They don't want to lose themselves, but they also long to become accepted and esteemed members of this closed, mysterious society.

Discounting of personal, particularistic experience

Medicine inculcates its trainees in "preformulation,"[13] or the objectification of experience into predetermined categories and interpretations. Thus the processing of experience becomes medicalized.[24] Medical education distances students from their own felt experience,[25] and encourages them to see patients not as unique individuals, but filtered through the *expectations* that have been instilled as part of their instruction. By the time they graduate from medical school, students have exchanged a natural facility for eliciting and appreciating particular patients' stories for learned expertise in constructing a medical history.[26] Experience becomes formulaic and loses its dynamism and organicity. "The thing itself" – the *person* of both patient and student – is all too easily lost.

Disqualification of narratives in medical education

One of the most consistent effects of the power embodied in medical training is its tendency to discount and prohibit local and alternative forms of knowledge. Who gets to tell the story and what can be told reflect and establish power relationships within the larger culture.[27] The goal of medical education is homogenization, and its desire is to suppress exceptional experience. Little[28] has pointed out that any "discourse community" (people who share common ideologies and common ways of speaking about things) can colonize its members to create a "monoglossic" way of speaking that shuts out the multiplicity of voices, nuances, and different perspectives. Normative pressures tend to suppress all that is unruly and difficult to order. Once committed to a discourse community, one gains a sense of privilege and security, but also an obligation to support and sustain its narrative premises.

Like most socially constructed narratives, medicine encourages stories for both patients and physicians that are tidy, neat, and predictable.[29] Patients cooperate with their physicians and get better. Students study diligently, score well on examinations, and learn to ply their trade saving lives and creating general happiness. When these stories deviate too significantly from patients' and students' lived experience, a crisis can result. This dissonance can result in moral erosion, cynicism, anxiety, and guilt for students. In effect, medical education can sometimes result in a kind of "narrative wreckage"[29] for students. Their old stories about who they are and what they are doing no longer fit their circumstances or experiences. Yet they are bereft of any guidance about how to reconstruct more healing, more meaningful stories. Except for a lucky few, the skills of narrative medicine,[30,31] the ability to make sense of and be moved by the patient's story, are inaccessible or unfamiliar. In the formal medical narrative, such as is found in the chart note or case presentation, the voice of the physician remains non-personified, and the fatter the chart grows, the more the patient's voice disappears.[32] The aspiration is complete objectivity, where subjectivity on the part of the patient or the student has been eliminated. Because students are allowed only a certain kind of technical, objectified language with which to process information and communicate with patients, their language becomes impoverished and restricted. Students may conclude that it is wrong to talk in a personal voice, and they may try to suppress, regulate, and control not only their formal interactions within medicine, but also their personal narratives. They may lose the capacity to reflect on and understand their own experiences with emotional engagement and nuance.

Encouraging distance between medical students and patients

The rite of passage that medical students undergo is intended to return them to the world at least in part in a mode of service, specifically service to patients. One of the great ironies of medical education is that, upon entering medical school, students are much closer to and more strongly identified with patients than with physicians, whereas upon graduation they have become identified much more with physicians. Marcus[33] concludes that first-year medical students relate strongly to patients, while in the third (clinical) year of medical education, they are motivated to counter-identify with patients, and instead are drawn to the ideal doctor – healthy, invulnerable, calm, skilled, effective, not overwhelmed, and having powerful knowledge and skills.

It is at this point that a barrier towards patients starts to form. Students are busily engaged in developing fluency in a new vocabulary, a new body of knowledge, and a new way of thinking and making clinical judgments about health and illness. In part, of course, this is a necessary and desirable part of the socialization process. Appropriately, students do not want to "grow up" to be patients, but to be doctors. Being a physician is a desirable goal, replete with status, power, authority, and control, whereas being a patient is a fate (never an aspiration!) to be avoided. Over the course of training, physicians and patients seem more and more to inhabit different worlds, and there is little question which world the medical student wants to be part of. This is not to say, of course, that students should want to be patients – this would indeed be a morbid desire. However, students must not become so afraid of patients that they feel repulsed or threatened by them and keep them at arm's length. Yet little in medical education helps students to understand the ways in which their experiences and those of their patients have important parallels as well as points of divergence, an insight that could be useful clinically.

In fact, patient and student emotional experiences are not just parallel, but intertwined. Patients' vulnerability and suffering remind students of their own vulnerability and suffering. Students can either choose to preserve and learn from their identification, and thus their emotional connection with patients, through "a mutual experience of joining that results in a sensation of wholeness",[34] or they can defend themselves by trying to preserve their own "clean and proper bodies"[35] in the face of the surrounding pain and degradation. Suffering affects not only the patient, but is also threatening to the "well," and results in the urge to demarcate sick from well. Students, who are already enduring their own form of suffering, fear that the patients' suffering will overwhelm them. Without the proper guidance, this discomfort and sense of unease may remain and become translated into problematic or less than ideal patient care. Yet the rite of passage designed in medical education ignores and does not make constructive use of these similarities to further student understanding. The result is that when students look at patients, they see suffering. When they look at physicians, they do not see suffering (except in the case of residents, who from the students' perspective embody the worst of both the patient and the doctor world in that they have authority and responsibility, yet still seem miserable and resentful) – although it may be there, but it is never shared, especially not "down the food chain" – and they see what they imagine is an escape from their present distress. They cannot wait to get there!

REFERENCES

1 Poirier S. Medical education and the embodied physician. *Literature and Medicine* 2006; **25**: 522–52.

2 Shapiro J, Nguyen V, Mourra S, *et al.* The use of creative projects in a gross anatomy class. *Journal for Learning Through the Arts: a Research Journal on Arts Integration in Schools and Communities* 2006; **2**:Article 20; http://repositories.cdlib.org/clta/lta/

3 DasGupta S. Reading bodies, writing bodies: self-reflection and cultural criticism in a narrative medicine curriculum. *Literature and Medicine* 2003; **22**: 241–56.

4 Cousineau P (ed.). *The Hero's Journey: Joseph Campbell on his life and work.* New York: Harper and Row; 1990.

5 Hawkins AH. Pathography and the enabling myths: the process of healing. In: Anderson CM, MacCurdy MM (eds). *Writing and Healing: Toward an informed practice.* Urbana, IL: National Council of Teachers of English; 2000.

6 De Benedetto MAC, Blasco P, Troll T. Even a little magic. *Canadian Family Physician* 2008; **54**: 1146–7.

7 Lewis BE. Prozac and the post-human politics of cyborgs. *Journal of Medical Humanities* 2003; **24**: 49–63.

8 Greenhalgh T, Horowitz B. Why study narrative? In: Greenhalgh T, Hurwitz B (eds). *Narrative-Based Medicine: Dialogue and discourse in clinical practice.* London: BMJ Books; 1998. pp. 3–16.

9 Saunders J. Validating the facts of experience in medicine. In: Evans M, Finlay IG (eds). *Medical Humanities.* London: BMJ Books; 2001. pp. 223–35.

10 Bruner J. The narrative construction of reality. *Critical Inquiry* 1991; **18**: 1–21.

11 Wear D, Castellani B. The development of professionalism: curriculum matters. *Academic Medicine* 2000; **75**: 602–11.

12 Pellegrino ED, Thomasma DC. *The Virtues in Medical Practice.* New York: Oxford University Press; 1993.

13 Martinez R. Walker Percy and medicine: the struggle for recovery in medical education. In: Elliott C, Lantos J (eds). *The Last Physician: Walker Percy and the moral life in medicine.* Durham, NC: Duke University Press; 1999. pp. 81–95.

14 Kasman D, Fryer-Edwards K, Braddock CH 3rd. Educating for professionalism: trainees' emotional experiences on IM and pediatrics inpatient wards. *Academic Medicine* 2003; **78**: 730–41.

15 Frank AW. Asking the right question about pain: narrative and phronesis. *Literature and Medicine* 2004; **23**: 209–25.

16 Suchman AL. Story, medicine, and healthcare. *Advances in Mind-Body Medicine* 2000; **16**: 193–8.

17 Frank AW. Enhancing illness stories: when, what, and why. In: Nelson HL (ed.). *Stories and Their Limits: Narrative approaches to bioethics.* New York: Routledge; 1997. pp. 31–49.

18 Frank AW. *The Wounded Storyteller: Body, illness, and ethics.* Chicago: University of Chicago Press; 1995.

19 Helfrich C, Kielhofner G. Volitional narratives and the meaning of therapy. *American Journal of Occupational Therapy* 1994; **48**: 319–26.

20 Marta J. Toward a bioethics for the twenty-first century: a Ricouerian poststructuralist narrative hermeneutic approach to informed consent. In: Nelson HL (ed.). *Stories and Their Limits: Narrative approaches to bioethics.* New York: Routledge; 1997. pp. 198–212.

21 Kaiser R. Fixing identity by denying uniqueness: an analysis of professional identity in medicine. *Journal of Medical Humanities* 2002; **23**: 95–105.

22 Hunter KM. *Doctors' Stories: The narrative structure of medical knowledge.* New Jersey: Princeton University Press; 1999 (revised edition).

23 Stanley P. The patient's voice: a cry in solitude or a call for community. *Literature and Medicine* 2004; **23**: 346–63.

24 Good BJ, Good MJD. "Fiction" and "historicity" in doctors' stories: social and narrative dimensions of learning medicine. In: Mattingly C, Garro LC (eds). *Narrative and the Cultural Construction of Illness and Healing.* Berkeley, CA: University of California Press; 2000. pp. 50–69.

25 McEntyre MC. Getting from how to why: a pause for reflection on professional life. *Academic Medicine* 1997; **72**: 1051–5.

26 Greenhalgh T, Hurwitz B. Why study narrative? *BMJ* 1999; **318**: 48–50.

27 Ochs E, Capps L. Narrating the self. *Annual Review of Anthropology* 1996; **25**: 19–43.

28 Little M, Jordens C, Sayers E. Discourse communities and the discourse of experience. *Health* 2003; **7**: 73–86.

29 Drew S. The Delta factor: storying survival and the disjuncture between public narratives and personal stories of life after cancer. *Storytelling, Self, Society* 2005; **1**: 76–102.

30 Charon R. Reading, writing, and doctoring: literature and medicine. *American Journal of the Medical Sciences* 2000; **319**: 285–91.

31 Charon R. The patient–physician relationship. Narrative medicine: a model for empathy, reflection, profession, and trust. *JAMA* 2001; **286**: 1897–902.

32 Carson RC. The hyphenated space: liminality in the doctor–patient relationship. In: Charon T, Montello M (eds). *Stories Matter: The role of narrative in medical ethics.* New York: Routledge; 2002. pp. 171–82.

33 Marcus ER. Empathy, humanism, and the professionalism of medical education. *Academic Medicine* 1999; **74**: 1211–15.

34 Suchman AL, Matthews DA. What makes the patient–doctor relationship therapeutic? Exploring the connexional dimension of medical care. *Annals of Internal Medicine* 1988; **108**: 125–30.

35 Kristeva J. *Powers of Horror: An essay on abjection.* New York: Columbia University Press; 1982.

2   Functions of Writing for Medical Students

It has been observed that medical discourse is monological, largely omitting the patient's voice.[1] Another relatively neglected voice is that of the medical student, especially as they attempt to reflect on and make sense of the process of medical education. Medical training in general tends to silence personal voice,[2-4] and students as low-status members of the hierarchy are especially vulnerable to this suppression. As has been pointed out, medical students occupy a liminal position between fully fledged physicians and laypersons.[5] For this reason, they may be perceived as unimportant or irrelevant, having a transitional and transitory role in the medical hierarchy. Often they are not included in their own stories.

Yet medical students are both moved and troubled by various aspects of the professional culture in which they are involved.[6] They often express considerable difficulty in adapting to medical culture.[7] In their medical training, students learn to tell one kind of story – the case presentation of the patient – using a highly technical vocabulary and a prescribed format based on clinical reasoning which emphasize formulaic, uniform presentation through an impersonal, passive voice that obscures the identity of the teller.[4,8] In the training environment, as noted, experience becomes medicalized. Students lose the ability to reflect on what is happening to them from a human perspective, and to explore the dissonance that they endure as they try to connect their personal values with their clinical training.[9] Personal stories represent one way in which students can examine their experience and see more deeply into its possible meanings.[10,11]

Medical educators, medical humanities scholars, and medical students themselves all have an interest in developing a greater understanding of the socialization experience that occurs as students are inducted into the profession of medicine. The roots of many attitudinal and values dilemmas among physicians, such as whether to adopt a stance toward patients that is more slanted toward the technical or toward the humanistic, or how they position themselves in relation to suffering and death, are laid down during their four years of medical school. This makes it imperative that we understand in depth both the positive and negative effects of training on students, so that we can enhance the former and ameliorate the latter. We can learn much of importance by examining students' writing, as a type of origin myth – that is, "this is where I became a real doctor."[12] The attitudes of physicians originate in and are shaped by their medical school years. The physicians of tomorrow emerge from the medical students of today.

REFLECTIVE WRITING IN MEDICAL SCHOOL

Increasingly, medical students are being encouraged to engage in written reflection as a means of processing their experiences, to achieve additional personal and clinical insight, and even at times as a kind of healing from the pressures and strains of training. One of the few outlets that students have for honest self-probing and interrogation is reflective writing that gives them space, if they choose, to wrestle with and look deeply at their own ongoing experience. A literary sub-genre exists that documents the experiences of medical students.[13-15] However, these and similar books represent only the perspective of a single physician in training. The two anthologies of medical student writing of which I am aware are the collection entitled *Let Me Listen to Your Heart*,[16] which includes both original prose and poetry from a group of medical students doing rotations in Cooperstown, NY, and *Body Language: Poems of the Medical Training Experience*,[17] a broader range of poetry that also includes work by medical residents and prominent physician-poets. However, these books contain little or no textual analysis of the student writings.

Branch and colleagues[9,18–20] have spent almost two decades encouraging learners to interrogate their experiences through narrative accounts. Their analysis of critical incident reports has identified core themes in learners, such as balancing empathy and acculturation into medicine, the search for identity and values, disillusionment and despair, and hope and reconciliation. Other scholars have also examined medical students' original writing, in order to understand specific concerns related to medical education. Anderson[21] divided medical student stories into four categories:

1   those that encode the knowledge necessary to become a physician
2   those that create and maintain identity
3   those that problematize the normative world of medicine
4   those that heal the teller.

Other representative themes identified in the literature include role confusion, exploration of professional identity, consideration of medicine as a calling, physician privilege and power, the limits of medicine, and identification with the patient.[22] Reflective writing has also been used to help medical students to probe the perspective of patients,[23] as well as to understand their own physicality and personal experiences of illness.[24,25] Other medical educators have called attention to the value of journal writing by students in encouraging self-awareness and self-examination, as well as breaking down barriers between faculty and students.[26]

Reflective writing in any form is a useful vehicle for deepening understanding of medical students. Whereas scientific communication styles privilege objectivity, generalizability, categorization, and elimination of the particular, the subjective, the emotional, and the personal, all forms of reflective, creative writing give permission to reinstate these elements. Five aspects of this type of writing – voice, particularity, alternative perspective, emotion, and healing – have been identified that may facilitate catharsis and insight for students as well as provide improved understanding for scholars.[27]

Voice in this context refers to the expression of personal, subjective observations, feelings, and values.[5] Voice in student writing provides medical educators with the opportunity to focus on unique aspects of learners' personality, life experience, and perception, one student at a time. *Particularity* is the aspect of this writing that encourages focus on subjective details of importance to the teller, whether or not they signify on a broader scale or are pertinent in formulating a differential diagnosis.[28] Through the particularity of reflective writing, we can learn about the details that matter to students, the small things that mean a lot. *Alternative viewpoints*[29] – the capacity to recognize that multiple perspectives and stories exist in any given illness encounter – are useful because they enable us to appreciate the ways in which students apprehend patients and their families. Reflective writing also makes space for the expression of the whole gamut of subjective *emotions* that are evoked by the complex clinical situations to which students are exposed.[30,31] In the emotional tone of the writing, we can detect how students really feel about what they encounter during training, what distresses them and what brings them joy. Finally, because of the potential for writing to promote psychological and perhaps even physical *health and well-being*[32] through the restoration of a sense of control and the act of witnessing in response to difficult events,[33] we can begin to understand more deeply what helps to heal students' training-related traumas and wounds.

Many literary scholars have observed that stories are used to maintain power and control, especially by institutions. However, stories can also enable exploration and freedom,[34] and these are some of the motivations that lead medical students (and patients) to write about their experience. Their writing becomes a personal chronicle of their rite of passage, not as seen by the "elders" of the tribe who have imposed their narrative on this experience, but by the young men and women living it. Through writing (as well as reading), students develop the capacity to understand and be moved by the meanings of singular stories about individual human beings[23,35] – in other words, to develop narrative competence.

Broadly speaking, narrative competence is the ability to envision people's lives as coherent stories.[36] Narrative competence includes many knowledge- and skill-based dimensions. Some of the more important of these include sensitivity to voice, character, temporality, and plot, to the multiplicity of perspectives and therefore truths, and to the meaning assigned to events. The aspiring physician must learn to tolerate and bear witness to the pain, unfair circumstances, and suffering of patients, and to develop tenderness and courage, as well as the ability to comfort. Of great importance is the fact that narrative competence restores the writer's ability to think personally rather than abstractly, to focus on the individual and particularistic as a source of truth and meaning.[37] Writing seeks to maintain the personal aspect by re-embodying both writer and those written about in their particular lives. Narrative competence also includes what has been termed "perspectival vision,"[29] or the ability to cultivate empathy based on deeply experiencing the viewpoints of others. By stimulating narrative imagination, creative writing enhances the ability to appreciative perspectives other than one's own.[38] Writing helps to "lure" students into perspectives other than the biophysical, and helps them to see beneath the surface of things.[10] "Alternative" textual formats, such as poetry and fiction, allow medical students access to language from which they have become estranged, such as metaphors and symbolism, which are not used in medical-speak.[39]

NARRATIVE TYPOLOGIES

Patients and medical students write about perturbing and taxing experiences. Pathography – stories of illness – has been defined as a way to bind the narrator back to life and reality.[40] Frank[33] has categorized patients' stories as stories of chaos, restitution, quest, or witnessing. A chaos story is a kind of anti-narrative, in which a sense of despair and isolation paralyzes the patient's ability to formulate a coherent narrative. The patient is inarticulate, overwhelmed, and agonized. Restitution stories are quintessential modernist stories – the patient becomes temporarily "broken", is fixed by medical science, and returns to their pre-illness life. Quest or journey stories follow Joseph Campbell's hero's journey,[41] in which a reluctant hero (the patient) is summoned (by illness) to confront monsters and demons (both symptoms and medical treatment). Along the way, however, the hero also encounters wise guides and mentors. After surviving great trials, the hero returns to share their insight and knowledge with others. Stories of witnessing are the most post-modernist type of story in that they confront uncomfortable and ignored truths, they do not reach an easy resolution, and they provide testimony rather than answers to suffering and injustice. In addition to these Frankian categories, I also make use of a type of story that some scholars refer to as "transcendent,"[42] characterized by a transformational, epiphanic shift in consciousness.

Medicopedography – stories about medical education – may serve a similar function to pathography for its authors in that such stories are attempts to make sense of confusing and troubling experience, and to explore new identities and shape a meaningful place in the new order in which they find themselves. Such narratives serve many interrelated purposes. Student narratives are necessarily dynamic, constantly in flux with both the demands and the limitations of the cultural repertoire on which they draw[43] – in this case the culture of medicine. Students adopt, manipulate, resist, and expand upon those norms as they develop their own stories. They tell dominant narratives but at the same time they tell conflicting narratives characterized by less resolution, more confusion, ongoing loss, and suffering. These storylines compete and conflict.[44] Storytelling, whether through prose or poetry, represents students' efforts to make corrections, adjustments, and adaptations to their formal rite of medical passage, to fill in the gaps, and to prepare themselves more authentically for their future roles as physicians. I shall briefly discuss each of the narrative typologies noted above, remembering that most writing moves between several of these typologies within a given work. Furthermore, although each narrative typology emphasizes or enables the elements that I describe, some of these elements may also appear in other typologies, although to a less significant degree.

Chaos stories
Cry for help
A student's cry for help through writing[45] is similar to Frank's chaos story. It is inchoate and disorganized – a drowning person waving her hands above the encroaching waves. It struggles to find a narrative capable of containing its traumatic pain.[46] The student is aware that she is sinking, and is overwhelmed. However, writing carries her no further than this realization. Once achieved, the student feels panic and despair, and can only cry out, "Help me! Help me!" It is not an easy form for a student to articulate, but it may be somewhat easier to do this in written form than as a verbal appeal. Writing, however chaotic, provides a layer of insularity between student and audience, which grants the drowning student a little self-protection. Furthermore, there is usually an element of witnessing in a chaos story, in that the author is able to rise above chaos sufficiently to articulate it.

On Receiving the News That You Have Lost Your Nerve   By: Brian McMichael
UC Irvine. 2005

In that moment, when the horror of an accidental mutilation
Gets to you and you wish it not to be
And wish you could escape from the situation

You are transfixed into the smallest of vector quantities
You do not want to witness this; you are not fascinated
You gave up everything to become a doctor

In your shame and indecision, you stay and watch
You have no hope that the reattached body parts will survive
You are sickened at the pretense; what are you going to do now?

Students are sometimes caught between their desire to learn and their horror at what they are witness to, the largely unacknowledged reality that learning in medicine is filled with moments of revulsion, shame, doubt, and meaningless intervention. In the poem "On Receiving the News . . .," a student observing surgery to reattach a body part wants to turn his back on the gruesome pointlessness of the situation, but as a learner he is simultaneously transfixed. The student adopts the second-person voice, addressing himself with scathing condemnation. He yearns to escape, to flee, and not to stand as a witness to this procedure, futile at least from the patient's presumed priority of regaining function. Reluctantly, the narrator reminds himself that "You gave up everything to become a doctor," and he decides to stay and watch. The student knows that the reattached parts will not survive – the pretense of surgically going through the motions sickens him, but he has made his choice and is afraid to leave. As the poem's title suggests, the student concludes that both he and the patient have "lost [their] nerve."

Restitution stories
Self-reassurance
Students may also write to reassure themselves, a kind of self-soothing.[45] A restitution reaffirms the basic moral rightness and order of the world. Although things become broken, they can be fixed again. This type of narrative may accurately reflect certain situations (previously smart student is overwhelmed by all that she doesn't know – student receives training and studies hard – student becomes competent again), but it may also be an effort to too readily incorporate the prevailing dominant discourse: "My training is hard but worthwhile, my teachers are helpful, my patients are nice, and my life is good."

Piriformis By: Curtis Nordstrom
Originally appeared in The Yale Journal for Humanities in Medicine *2004, Yale University School of Medicine*

I pray for piriformis.
In my mind, the physician sizes me up, asks me
"Can you palpate this patient's piriformis?"
And I oblige her, dumbfounding the staff
With my deft and unhesitating actions.
Please, God, piriformis; I can find piriformis.
Piriformis is my only friend in this sterile
Jungle of mystical medical science.
In my mind, I sing your praises, piriformis
O taut, precious band of muscle. All hail piriformis!
But . . . no.
Alas, the patient presents with
    an upper respiratory infection.
I am so screwed.
She is so screwed.
"Listen," commands the physician.
    I listen. My stethoscope works.
"Feel," she directs.
    I feel. My fingers almost work.

"Observe," she smiles at me.
    I observe, and I am chastened in my ignorance.
"Learn," she does not say.
    I learn.
The physician is not angry with me.
She was me, once.
The patient is not angry with me.
She is grateful. She takes a slip of paper
From the physician, who knows far more than piriformis.
As she prepares to leave, I am relieved.
I am sad. She is my new best friend.
As she slides down from the treatment table
I quickly and silently, from the corner of my eye
Survey her posterior hip.
Piriformis.

This poem acknowledges chaos but ultimately tells a restitution tale. In this humorous rendition, a student calls the piriformis muscle his "only friend in this sterile / Jungle of mystical medical science", because it's the only part of the patient's anatomy he knows how to find. As a result, during rounds, the student prays that the attending physician will ask him to demonstrate palpation of a patient's piriformis. Instead, the patient presents with an upper respiratory infection, and the student laments, "I am so screwed / She [the patient] is so screwed." In this case, the student's ignorance resolves into a restitutive happy ending. The attending physician is a patient teacher who is not angered by the student's lack of knowledge, because she sees herself in him. The patient, who receives proper and useful treatment from the expert doctor, is also satisfied. However, as the patient departs, the student unobtrusively locates with his eyes her piriformis muscle, thus demonstrating his own limited, but documented, expertise. The student's ignorance and out-of-control feelings are balanced by a competent attending physician and an understanding patient. Stability and homeostasis are restored.

Sometimes this type of story is not thought through sufficiently or interrogated carefully enough. It is not that this is a false story, but it can be excessively simplistic, an anxiety-propelled papering over of more convoluted realities. It too casually borrows the dominant tropes of the medical education experience without questioning their veracity for the particular writer. I have labeled this related narrative type as an (anti)-restitution story. These stories can be recognized by an element of blame and judgment, usually directed toward a patient or family member. In these stories, restitution would be possible were it not for the noncompliance, uncooperativeness, demandingness, and even self-destructiveness of the ungrateful object of the doctor's attention.

It was my first day of preceptorship . . . By: Michael Shapiro
Originally appeared in Essentials of Patient Care II. 2005
University of Florida College of Medicine

It was my first day of preceptorship
And all through the clinic
Uncontrolled cholesterol
Was turning me cynic

The patients were friendly
But overwhelmingly ungrateful
As the hard-working doctor
Tried to prevent endings fateful

Running amok was diabetes
Obesity and high blood pressure
"Is everyone this irresponsible?" I asked
"Not everyone," he assured

It was nearing the end of the day
Ten hours of standing on my feet
And in rolled our last patient
One whom I really wanted to meet

Sarah was bright-eyed and all smiles
Ten or eleven years old
Her mother pushing her wheelchair
Which is why I say in she rolled

She was in for a checkup
And seemingly happy as can be
And what she had brought for the doctor
Was a miniature Christmas tree

"What a thoughtful gift," the doctor said
As she urged him to see it alight
He brought it to his office and plugged it in
And everyone seemed full of delight

In the exam room I introduced myself
She said hello and shook my hand
And as mother and doctor talked
I learned that Sarah had never been able to stand

"Developmental delay" he called it
I wondered what had delayed her such
Behind closed doors the doctor told me
Years ago the babysitter shook her too much

I became flooded with emotions
Sadness, pity, and disgust
I couldn't believe the damage done
Inflicted by someone you're supposed to trust

They discussed back surgery down the road
But they must wait until she was more grown
And it had still yet to be seen
If she'd be able to bear children of her own

I could see Sarah listening intently
As her mother and the doctor talked

And at the opportune time in the conversation
Young Sarah exclaimed, "I want to walk! I want to walk!"

It was all I could do to fight back the tears
If only what was done I could undo
But if mother and daughter could keep their spirits up
Then I guess I could, too

It seemed that of all the patients
Sarah and her mother had the most right to be downtrodden
So much had been tragically taken away
But it was what they still had that was not forgotten

They saw that in some ways they had something special
In some ways they were a fortunate pair
They had found a doctor who might not be able to cure
But one who was overflowing with care

I thought that of all his patients
She was the only one to bring a gift
I realized that it's those few special patients
Who have the power to uplift

I shook Sarah's hand as they left
Honored to meet such a special girl
Touched knowing that showing you care
Might make all the difference in the world

This example contains both anti-restitution and restitution elements. In this poem, the narrator initially records his cynicism about patients who are "irresponsible" and "overwhelmingly ungrateful." These patients are contrasted with a "good" patient, an innocent child who is a wheelchair-bound victim of physical abuse. Despite having many reasons to be resentful and bitter, this patient and her mother are happy, upbeat, and appreciative (they bring the doctor a gift). The doctor is also kind and caring, and helps both patient and mom to realize how "fortunate" they are. Although elements of anti-restitution are apparent in the opening stanzas, by the end of the poem order has been restored. The patient is kind and grateful to her doctor, the doctor is devoted, the student is honored, and he has made "all the difference in the world" by his caring attitude.

Journey stories
Self-discovery and identity formation
Another type of writing positions the student narrator as the (often unlikely) hero who undertakes a valiant quest, suffers hardships and obstacles, encounters enemies and demons, finds wise teachers and guides, learns and grows as a result, and intends to use their new-found knowledge to help others. The journey story, while peopled with many characters, places the self at the center of the drama, and the action is ultimately in service of the evolution of the self, although the fruition of this personal growth may be the societal good. Journey stories may take either a restitutive or a more somber, reflective turn. All journey narratives look backward and ask "What have I learned as a

result of my experiences?" The restitutive journey story at its most extreme can convey a sense that all of the anguish and loss experienced along the way – by self and others – is justified by the outcome of the hero's positive development. In these narratives, the emphasis seems to be on the "heroic" part of the journey. In the more reflective narratives, the stress is on the journey component, and the tone is more humble and introspective.

Regardless of the dominant mood of the journey narrative, this kind of retrospective reflection allows the writer to reconsider, reframe, and perhaps reinterpret the past as represented in the journey,[28,47,48] to place events in a larger context, and to revisit the meanings and implications of an experience.[49,50] Humanities scholars[5,51] have observed that writing is a way for students to "interrogate" their experiences during medical training, and to slow down "the whirlwind of medical education." Reflecting on the student's personal journey helps to reconcile the narrative expected according to the norms of the culture in which the writer is embedded with what actually transpired according to the writer's subjective, felt experience.[52] Usually, in recounting the tale of their journey, the student is in part engaging in a task of self-redefinition.

As Charon observes, this writing is not only reporting about the self, but also becomes a process of self-discovery and self-creation.[53] By engaging in self-examination, the student is able to question her own assumptions, biases, and preconceptions.[54] Writing "unmasks" the student, not least of all to herself.[55] Building on Montello's insights,[56] writing in the journey mode requires "departure, performance, and change." Once the student begins to tell the story of her journey, she has the opportunity to "depart" from the normative discourse that has up to this point defined the chronicled event. As she revisits the scene, she begins to embody and "perform" the events and characters in different ways, choosing which lessons offered are worthwhile and deserve to be incorporated in the self, and which should be rejected. Discovering how to reaffirm self and not be consumed by the master discourse of medical education that surrounds the learner[57,58] is an important potential function of the journey story.

Campo writes that poetry is forgiving because it can embrace and accept a more authentic, albeit altered, self.[30,59] A journey narrative may increase self-complexity by helping the narrator to see the self more flexibly and to expand the sense of what is allowable.[60] Anderson frames storytelling as a way in which medical students can move toward a more integrated professional and social self, an attempt to reconcile "original and new identities,"[21] while maintaining an authentic sense of personhood and humanity.[61] Contemplating the journey of the self is one way in which the pieces of the self that may perhaps have become fragmented during the course of medical education can be made whole once again.[62]

My Hand By: Dennis Chang
UC Irvine

"I've never been sick a day in my life."
I think, you have HIV.
"I don't know why this is happening to me."
I think, you have Hep C liver cirrhosis.
"I just threw up 5 cups of blood!"
I think, with surprise, that's no big deal.
The team's seen worse . . . and things are under control.

He says, "Tell me he's old enough to do this."
I tell him, "He's well-trained. He's good enough."
I think, my intern is only 27.
He says, "Tell me it won't hurt."
I tell him, "It's just a central line.
We need to give you blood and fluids."
I think, my intern must be sweating bullets.

He says, "I'm scared."
I tell him, "Don't move. You can squeeze my hand
but just don't move."
I think, He can't move. Not when my intern
does the stick, he can't move.
I read my intern's eyes. He's scared too.
But we know what we have to do.

He grabs my left hand. I smile.
Internally, I gasp. It's crushing.
"Anesthetic going in," R2 says. I say comforting words.
Inside, I grimace in pain. He's breaking my hand.
"Don't move," R2 says. "Putting in line."
The patient grits his teeth and moans.

I can no longer feel my hand.
But I smile and I tell the patient
"Good job."
Because he didn't move.
He didn't move.
He didn't move.

It's over and he thanks me.
I smile. I feel like a member of the team.
I think, maybe medical students are good for something
after all!
As I leave, I give him my hand with a smile.
My right hand.

The above example is a journey story in which intern, resident, and medical student work together to place a central line in a patient. The experience is essentially a rite of passage. The poem begins with the student's initial judgmental attitude toward a patient who seems to deny the severity of his medical condition (HIV positive and hepatitis C), as well as the student's blind faith that the medical team's competence will keep things "under control." However, when an inexperienced intern needs to place a central line (the demonic obstacle), the student (a reluctant hero) realizes that his help, in the form of reassurance, calmness, and hand-holding, is needed as well. As the student admits his own vulnerability and fear, the patient, previously a kind of monstrous "other," becomes more human to him. The student learns to literally suffer along with the patient, as the frightened patient squeezes his hand to a pulp. As a result, the experience for the student becomes a journey toward wisdom. By the end, the student writes, "I smile. I feel like a member of the team." The student moves from judgment and unquestioning confidence in medicine to facing his own vulnerability and fear. By suffering along with the patient, the student graduates to becoming a useful member of the medical team.

Witnessing stories
Examining suffering

Writing is not only or even primarily about the self, although it is inevitably filtered through the self. Writing may bear witness, albeit always imperfectly and partially, to the experiences and suffering of others. By writing the stories of suffering others (and given the distance that writing inevitably provides from one's self, this may at times include writing about the suffering of the self), one necessarily adopts a posture of speaking out on behalf of these others, and becomes a potential agent of change.[63] Writing that witnesses suffering and injustice is therefore not only about the individual sufferer, but also includes a critique (however implicit) of social values, and as a result involves efforts not only toward personal healing but also toward public healing.[47] In this form of writing, students can problematize and challenge their experiences, develop a critical position in relation to this experience, ask questions that have been ignored or marginalized within the larger system, and focus on occurrences that have been judged unimportant to everyone (clinicians, scientific researchers) except the student and/or the patient.[28] Stein[64,65] points out that writing can be used to help the writer to identify and reflect on not only personal, interior themes, but also organizational narratives, secrets, and conflicts that are usually considered forbidden and off-limits – what in medical education has often been called the informal curriculum that, as is discussed in Chapter 5, exerts such a powerful influence on students.[66]

Building on Cassell,[67] Verghese asserts that illness has two dimensions, namely physical deficit and spiritual violation.[68] The patient's suffering derives from the intersection of these dimensions, resulting in a feeling that what ought to be whole is now sundered, perhaps irrevocably. Suffering is by definition distressing. Suffering that is voiceless, impervious to expression, becomes something completely alien, unknowable, and unshareable,[69] an experience that overwhelms and isolates the sufferer.[70] When students step forward to help the patient to speak their suffering or even provide (an imagined) voice for the patient, in effect they are creating a container, a therapeutic holding space, for the patient's disheartening, demoralizing, or tragic life experience.[71] Whether a potential hurt is bearable or not depends in part on whether it can be articulated, whether useful metaphors and analogies can be found through which to filter it.[72] Constructing a narrative filter works not by sugar-coating trauma or reducing its immensity, but rather by expanding the self to include and absorb the trauma, to be able to be present with rather than turn away from it.[60] Expanding the self in this way to prioritize and bear witness to the patient's suffering may be a step toward reducing isolation for the patient and increasing moral maturity for the student.

ICU Rounds* By: Sheila Chan
UC Irvine, 2008

Beverly
Elizabeth
and Tim.

---

* After Frederico Garcia Lorca's "Fable of Three Friends to Be Sung in Rounds."

The three of them were hiding:
Beverly in a bog of edema
Elizabeth in a diaphanous sheath of skin
Tim in a thick grove of shattered bones.

Elizabeth
Tim
and Beverly.
The three of them were running:
Elizabeth from her four bloody bowel movements per day
Tim from a fourth-story window
Beverly from uber-gregarious coagulation factors congealing in her blood.

Tim
Beverly
and Elizabeth.
The three of them were bleeding:
Tim into his drunk, desperate head
Beverly into her gut of gagging arteries
Elizabeth into lungs weakened by her weary will to live.

Beverly
Elizabeth
and Tim.
In my hands the three of them were
three sacks of ether
three mounds of organs groaning despair
three ancient stars shedding light and heat, shedding time.

One
one
and one.
The three of them lasted each day
with the towering pyramids of medicines
with the EKG trails and IV streams
with expectations crumbled into an obstinate pile of debris.

Two
two
and two.
The three of them shut their eyes
rotten eggs lying limp
the fumes, the stench
dripping crusty moldy tears.

Three
two
and one.
I saw them lose themselves, panting and sighing
in the ancient stone

in the night that shed its stars
in my sorrow full of cracked eggshells and drenched petals
in my chest of mottled knowledge and desires
in my vortex of numbers spinning recklessly
in my fingers clenching the stink of rubber gloves discarded into a garbage can.

I had written their stories
On blue sheets of paper, between black boxes and thin lines
ink rushing through mountains
gurgling headstrong into a vast extreme.
Elizabeth
Tim
and Beverly.
Dying is hard
but sometimes its arms are cloaked with clouds
lavender songs and hushed eyebrows
where the fissures relax in tranquility.

When the curtains closed
and the words ceased
I knew they had gone away.
I searched for them in the monitors, the vent, the trickling IVs
I raked my hair, my heart, my brains, the crevices of my empty hands.
But I couldn't find them anymore.
I couldn't?
No, I couldn't find them.
They had joined the moths fluttering against the light
and then – singed!
powdered wings dispersed into the sky.

This poem is an example of witnessing the dying of three ICU patients. In form and content it is patterned on Lorca's mysterious poem which involves the deaths of three boys, whom at one point the narrator says he "holds in his hands." Paradoxically, in Lorca's poem, the narrator notes that the three friends have also "murdered" him. Lorca's poem itself is based on a children's counting game, made ominous by the context of death, corruption, contamination, and oppression.

In the student's writing, she, like Lorca, introduces her three patients, who then become a kind of Greek chorus throughout the poem. Although these patients are adults, referring to them by first name only makes them seem childlike and innocent. The poem quickly introduces the idea of "hiding," as in the child's game of hide-and-seek. However, what they are hiding from is not playfulness, but rather severe, uncompromising disease. In the next stanza, the three patients are running away, but again in this game they are not teasing each other. Instead, they futilely flee their frightful symptoms. As in Lorca's poem, there is an uncomfortable juxtaposition of childhood play and imminent death.

The student-narrator, like Lorca's narrator, holds her patients in her hand. In her own game of hide-and-seek she searches for metaphors to describe the experience of holding these lives. They are ephemeral like ether, inescapably tangible ("mounds of organs"), and memorably dying stars that will be extinguished even as their light still reaches us. Implacably, the narrator chronicles each devastating stage of the patients' decline until, at last, in this most awful hide-and-seek game, they "lose themselves" despite the student's sorrow, despite all her medical knowledge, her accumulation of numbers that are supposedly definitive but ultimately powerless, and above all despite her desire to save them. Literally, they slip through her fingers.

For a while the student continues her hopeless game of hide-and-seek, but with no success. Although she searches through all the tools and symbols of medicine, and even inspects her own body, especially the hands that once held these patients, they are nowhere to be found. Finally, although the student notes ironically that she has "written their stories" in their chart notes, as though this act has somehow bound them to life, she admits that she has lost them forever. Like moths circling a flame, they have been consumed, only the wings (of their souls?) suffused into the universe.

Manifesting resistance

Another version of witnessing is writing as an act of resistance.[42] In this case, the student rejects co-option by the prevailing cultural norms and expectations of medicine. In this writing, the student seems to assert that "I am *other*, and will remain so. I will not be coerced into fitting into the expected mold. I will stand against indifferent or unethical behavior. I refuse to be *you*." Here, the writer uses the creation of text to challenge the existing hegemonic discourse, and simultaneously to assert a countervailing alternative.[73] In this sense, resistance is a way of declaring agency and is therefore self-empowering at the same time that it seeks to empower the disenfranchised, demoralized other. It is counter-hegemonic in that it rejects the perceived oppression and control of the medicalized patient (and sometimes the medicalized student as well). This mode of writing contests who is normally allowed to tell a story and what can be told in it by defying conventional mechanisms for describing doctors and patients.

Complications By: Dina Seif
UC Irvine, 2003

So, Doctor, you're saying there's less than one percent chance of complications . . .
I hear you say, "pulmonary embolism, infarction, perforation,"
But what do those words mean?
"Death." I know that one.
No, I guess that's not too serious . . .
What would you do?
Of course. You would go ahead with it.
A fraction of one percent — what are the chances?
But what if I am that fraction?
What if I am the less-than-one in one hundred who dies of your "routine"
    procedure? Then I guess it's a hundred percent for me.
Do you still get paid if I die? Just wondering.
Oh, if I don't do it, I may drop dead next week.
Can you tell me the chances of that?
Didn't think so.
Fine, I'll do it. I'm feeling lucky.

Hey, maybe I'll buy myself a lotto ticket, too.
What are the chances of winning the jackpot AND dying on the same day?
Maybe it will be my un-lucky day.

Here the student adopts the voice of the patient to confront the standard complacencies about the risk of surgical complications. While the physician in this poem dances around the possibility of death, hiding behind medicalized language, the patient names this potential consequence baldly. When the patient asks what the doctor would do in her* shoes, she rejects the nonchalant answer that she receives. She sees through the doctor's superficial empathy, and realizes that she will be the only one gambling. Rather than accept the conventional medical perspective, which emphasizes the unlikelihood of serious complications, the student witnesses to the fear and helplessness of the patient confronting the possibility of death.

Building community

It has been pointed out that the creation of narratives involves connection, mutuality, and relatedness between teller and audience.[34] The dialogic aspect of narrative is of particular significance in witnessing. Writing that functions as witnessing cannot be viewed solely as an inner experience – it is also a public act.[45,74] Its goal is acknowledgment of injustice or wrongdoing and restoration of the connectedness between individuals that has been disrupted by both illness and its political ramifications[75] in a process that Coulehan[76] refers to as symbolic healing. By telling, hearing, and recognizing a story, a group of people is turned into a community.[73]

Transcendence stories

Healing

Occasionally in the telling of a story there is a moment of grace. It is not so much that the writer has "discovered" the essential core of an experience through careful excavation, or that the writer has meticulously "created" profound meaning through brilliant insight and the exercise of her craft. Rather, something beyond the student's intention has occurred, and the writing becomes simply an effort to represent that transformative event. Writing has the potential to offer, sometimes unexpectedly, alternative modes of being in the world. Anderson[47] suggests that by using writing to explore different responses to traumatic events, it is possible for transformation to occur – a kind of strengthening of the spirit.[77,78]

A story of transcendence is a story of (at least temporary) healing. Although the epiphanic moment of insight may be transitory, its effects are often long-lasting in the sense of providing a kind of paradigm shift. Once she has realized that her story is broken,[79,80] incomplete, or narrow, the student is open to the narrative revisioning of a transcendence story. The act of writing from this perspective literally explores, examines, and ultimately can recreate a preferred narrative, which the student is free to accept, reject, or continue to refine. In this sense, the reconstructed narrative becomes the student's origin myth, the foundation of that individual's life narrative as an adult person and professional. Such moments of grace allow for the possibility of the student becoming aware of a new way of being in the world.

---

* To avoid awkward linguistic construction, I have arbitrarily designated the patient as female in this poem.

More broadly, transcendent writing heals by helping the writer to reorganize the chaos of her inner world, by helping her to make sense of surrounding confusion and unclarity.[81] James Pennebaker[32,82] and others[83] have theorized that the therapeutic value of narrative lies in its ability to structure, organize, and create meaning out of complicated emotional and stressful events, such as trauma and loss. Anderson[47] argues that because writing allows both permanence and revision, it empowers the writer and provides an additional measure of control. The act of converting emotions and images into a narrative has the potential to dramatically change the way that the person organizes and thinks about stressful experiences.

Rekindling awe and mystery

Transcendence stories are a way of exploring what the poet Keats called "negative capability" – that is, the capacity to rest comfortably in uncertainties, mysteries, and doubts.[84] One of the great gifts of a transcendent narrative is that it brings the opportunity to understand old experience in a new light, and to perceive what is routine and familiar through fresh eyes. This sense of renewal and discovery can remind students of the awe and mystery that surround them both in their personal lives and in their profession.

Admittedly, it may be difficult at times to distinguish between a journey narrative and a transcendent narrative, and both share elements of healing and awe. Frank puts a rather modernist spin on "journey," and I have followed his lead. A journey narrative has several predictable elements – reluctant hero, good companions, wise guides, evil demons, trials and testing. Most importantly, it has a kind of contractual dimension. If the hero endures, he or she will be rewarded with wisdom and learning. Insight is hard-earned, and granted in reward for effort and hard work. By contrast, transcendence occurs as an unexpected, unpredictable act of grace.

Isolation: 5 South By Virginia Agnelli
UC Irvine, 2001

The flag waves freely
Mocking those stifled – away from the breeze.
Palms stand at attention
Faded and dusty in the warm sun.
Beyond, the bustle of 7th Avenue
The mottled greens of SoCal foliage
A cobalt dome stands
Timidly offering salvation among the chatter.
The ocean – just a hint –
At the hazy horizon
Dotted with oil platforms
Marring the deep blue.

Step back.

The view obscured by the vinyl mini blinds
Sealed within double panes –
A barrier, rigidly guarding, protecting
Imprisoning.

Step back.

The steel rail, locked in place
A cold reminder of frailty
Dependence . . .
Blocks the view to the cold glass
Separating you from the warmth outside.

Step back.

A sickly-looking man with
Eyes that twinkle above the tubing of the O_2 cannula.
A devilish grin as tales are spun
And memories fill the room.
Whispers discuss sedation
Sundowning as the sun
Shines brightly beyond.

Step back.

Beyond the solid door
Windowed yet blinded
A sign, blue like the dome
Announcing isolation —
Masks required.
Another of the myriad barriers
Past which many never stray.

Step in.

From the cold sterility of the corridor
Into the warmth of his spirit
I join in and my loneliness fades.

In this illustration of transformation, a student initially feels imprisoned on the ward, separated, barred from the outside world of breeze, palms, and ocean. The repetitive chorus "Step back," perhaps representing the detachment and separation of the medical profession, repeatedly urges the narrator to withdraw still further, to insulate herself behind double-paned windows and shuttered blinds. The "devilish grin" and interesting tales of the patient may tempt the lonely student. However, much still urges her toward distance, including the myriad tubes, the patient's sickly demeanor, and the professional whispers focusing on medication and diagnostic symptoms. In addition, the patient is in an isolation room, which requires all who enter to don protective gear. Yet, in a moment of grace, the chorus of "Step back" shifts to an invitation to "Step in." Daring to risk emotional connection with this seriously ill patient overcomes the student's own loneliness and fear: "From the cold sterility of the corridor/Into the warmth of his spirit/I join in and my loneliness fades." A transformative moment of connection between patient and student occurs.

LIMITATIONS OF WRITING
Accommodation to dominant discourse
Before proceeding to an examination of students' poetry, we must also acknowledge some of the limitations of writing and what we can learn from these. Writing has been criticized on many grounds. On the one hand, it can be too accommodating to dominant discourses, too ready to simply parrot public conventions, rather than finding the author's voice. When narrative becomes too quickly and easily smooth and coherent, it is only a story about a story. It lacks authenticity, and borrows too heavily from conventional dominant social discourse. Such a story becomes a culturally acceptable account, without being clearly authenticated by the author.

Indulgent, apolitical, and exploitative
On the one hand, some scholars assert that writing is too self-indulgent, too personally absorbed and not sufficiently aware of the social and political context of issues[73,85] – what has been referred to as the "weepy world of confessions and revelations that is a fundamentally egocentric sort of self-absorption." Others are more concerned to protect students, and worry that writing may become excessively confessional, thereby jeopardizing the student's privacy and placing the student in a position of additional vulnerability.[84] A somewhat different perspective[86] highlights the risk of expropriating the patient's voice and story, either in the service of student self-exploration and discovery or, even more prosaically, to complete an educational assignment. As Arras[87] has noted, such issues raise critical questions about who gets to tell the story and what they are allowed to say.

Truthfulness revisited
Finally, it is important to remember that writing is not "the truth" – it is always about self-presentation. It may contain lies, omissions, or distortions, either advertent or inadvertent.[88] Any writing is inevitably based on a conscious selection and organizing of information for various purposes, such as creating an effect, reframing an experience, etc. However, precisely because writing is not the unmediated outpourings of an originating self, bur rather the performance of a constructed self, it can make change and healing possible.[73] At the same time, it is important not to simplify the effects of writing. In Henderson's words, writing is not a benign, risk-free experience. It is not always obviously healing. It may equally be transgressive and outrageous.[5]

REFERENCES
1 Aull F, Lewis B. Medical intellectuals: resisting medical orientalism. *Journal of Medical Humanities* 2004; **25**: 87–108.
2 DasGupta S. Reading bodies, writing bodies: self-reflection and cultural criticism in a narrative medicine curriculum. *Literature and Medicine* 2003; **22**: 241–56.
3 Kaiser R. Fixing identity by denying uniqueness: an analysis of professional identity in medicine. *Journal of Medical Humanities* 2002; **23**: 95–105.
4 Poirier S. Voice in the medical narrative. In: Charon R, Montello M (eds). *Stories Matter: The role of narrative in medical ethics.* New York: Routledge; 2002. pp. 48–58.
5 Henderson SW. Medical student elegies: the poetics of caring. *Journal of Medical Humanities* 2002; **23**: 119–32.
6 Suchman AL, Williamson PR, Litzelman DK, *et al.* for the Relationship-Centered Care

Initiative Discovery Team. Toward an informal curriculum that teaches professionalism: transforming the social environment of a medical school. *Journal of General Internal Medicine* 2004; **19**: 501–4.

7 Branch WT Jr. Deconstructing the white coat. *Annals of Internal Medicine* 1998; **129**: 740–42.

8 Good BJ, Good MJD. "Fiction" and "Historicity" in doctors' stories: social and narrative dimensions of learning medicine. In: Mattingly C, Garro LC (eds). *Narrative and the Cultural Construction of Illness and Healing.* Berkeley, CA: University of California Press; 2000. pp. 50–69.

9 Branch WT Jr. Supporting the moral development of medical students. *Journal of General Internal Medicine* 2000; **15**: 503–8.

10 Spatz LS, Welsh K. Literature and medicine as a writing course. In: Hawkins AH, McEntyre MC (eds). *Teaching Literature and Medicine.* New York: Modern Language Association; 2000. pp. 141–50.

11 Shapiro J. Listening to the voices of medical students in poetry: self, patients, role-models and beyond. *Journal of Poetry Therapy* 2006; **19**: 17–30.

12 Stein HF. The coming again of age of clinical narrative in (family) medicine. *Families, Systems, and Health* 2001; **19**: 135–45.

13 Shem S. *The House of God.* New York: Dell Publishing; 1979.

14 Klass P. *A Not Entirely Benign Procedure: Four years as a medical student.* New York: Penguin Books; 1987.

15 Ofri D. *Singular Intimacies: Becoming a doctor at Bellevue.* New York: Beacon Press; 2003.

16 Svahn D, Kozak A. *Let Me Listen to Your Heart: Writings of medical students.* New York: Basset Healthcare; 2002.

17 Jain N, Coppock D, Brown Clark S (eds). *Body Language: Poems of the medical training experience.* New York: Boa Editions; 2006.

18 Branch WT Jr, Pels RJ, Lawrence RS, Arky R. Becoming a doctor – critical-incident reports from third-year medical students. *NEJM* 1993; **329**: 1130–32.

19 Hupert N, Pels RJ, Branch WT Jr. Learning the art of doctoring: use of critical incident reports. *Harvard Student British Medical Journal* 1995; **3**: 99–100.

20 Brady DW, Corbie-Smith G, Branch WT Jr. "What's important to you?" The use of narratives to promote self-reflection and to understand the experiences of medical residents. *Annals of Internal Medicine* 2002; **137**: 220–3.

21 Anderson CM. "Forty acres of cotton waiting to be picked": medical students, storytelling, and the rhetoric of healing. *Literature and Medicine* 1998; **17**: 280–97.

22 Hatem D, Ferrara E. Becoming a doctor: fostering humane caregivers through creative writing. *Patient Education and Counselling* 2001; **45**: 13–22.

23 Charon R. The patient–physician relationship. Narrative medicine: a model for empathy, reflection, profession, and trust. *JAMA* 2001; **286**: 1897–902.

24 Goldstein M. Medicine and poetry: pathway of communication. *The Pharos* 1997; **60**: 12–14.

25 DasGupta S, Charon R. Personal illness narratives: using reflective writing to teach empathy. *Academic Medicine* 2004; **79**: 351–6.

26 Ashbury JE, Fletcher BM, Birtwhistle RV. Personal journal writing in a communication skills course for first-year medical students. *Medical Education* 1993; **27**: 196–204.

27 Shapiro J, Stein HF. Poetic license: writing poetry as a way medical students examine their professional relationship systems. *Families, Systems, and Health* 2005; **23**: 278–92.

28 Downie G. Telling: detail and diagnosis in medical poetry. *Medical Humanities Review* 2002; **16**: 9–17.

29 Charon R. Reading, writing, and doctoring: literature and medicine. *American Journal of the Medical Sciences* 2000; **319**: 285–91.

30 Campo R. *The Healing Art: A doctor's black bag of poetry.* New York: WW Norton & Co.; 2003.

31 Stein HF. *Prairie Voices: Process anthropology in family medicine.* Westport, CT: Bergin & Garvey; 1996.

32 Pennebaker JW, Seagal JD. Forming a story: the health benefits of narrative. *Journal of Clinical Psychology* 1999; **55**: 1243–54.

33 Frank AW. *The Wounded Storyteller: Body, illness, and ethics.* Chicago: University of Chicago Press; 1995.

34 Spiegel M, Charon R. Narrative, empathy, proximity. *Literature and Medicine* 2004; **23**: vii–x.

35 Silenzio VMB, Irvine CA, Sember RE, Bregman BE. Film and narrative medicine: cinemeducation and the development of narrative competence. In: Alexander M, Lenahan P, Pavlov A (eds). *Cinemeducation: A comprehensive guide to using film in medical education.* Oxford: Radcliffe Publishing; 2005. pp. 9–18.

36 Griffin FL. The fortunate physician: learning from our patients. *Literature and Medicine* 2004; **23**: 280–303.

37 Shattuck R. A brief history of stories. *Literature and Medicine* 2001; **20**: 7–12.

38 Frank AW. Asking the right question about pain: narrative and phronesis. *Literature and Medicine* 2004; **23**: 209–25.

39 Smith P. Inquiry cantos: poetics of developmental disability. *Mental Retardation* 2001; **39**: 379–90.

40 Hawkins AH. Pathography and the enabling myths: the process of healing. In: Anderson CM, MacCurdy MM (eds). *Writing and Healing: Toward an informed practice.* Urbana, IL: National Council of Teachers of English; 2000.

41 Cousineau P (ed.). *The Hero's Journey: Joseph Campbell on his life and work.* New York: Harper and Row; 1990.

42 Gray DR. Accommodation, resistance and transcendence: three narratives of autism. *Social Science and Medicine* 2001; **53**: 1247–57.

43 Gale DD. Negotiating values in stories of illness and caring on St. Kitts. *Storytelling, Self, Society* 2005; **1**: 38–52.

44 Drew S. The Delta factor: storying survival and the disjuncture between public narratives and personal stories of life after cancer. *Storytelling, Self, Society* 2005; **1**: 76–102.

45 Borkan J, Reis S, Medalie J. Narratives in family medicine: tales of transformation, points of breakthrough for family physicians. *Families, Systems, and Health* 2001; **19**: 121–34.

46 Holmes L. Narrative in psychotherapy. In: Greenhalgh T, Hurwitz B (eds). *Narrative-Based Medicine: Dialogue and discourse in clinical practice.* London: BMJ Books; 1998. pp. 176–84.

47 Anderson CM. Writing and healing. *Literature and Medicine* 2000; **19**: ix–xv.

48 Rennie DL. Storytelling in psychotherapy: the client's subjective experience. *Psychotherapy* 1994; **31**: 234–43.

49 Mishara AL. Narrative and psychotherapy – the phenomenology of healing. *American Journal of Psychotherapy* 1995; **49**: 180–95.

50 Branch WT Jr, Paranjape A. Feedback and reflection: teaching methods for clinical settings. *Academic Medicine* 2002; **77**: 1185–8.

51 Reifler DR. "Poor Yorick": reflections on gross anatomy. In: Hawkins AH, McEntyre MC (eds). *Teaching Literature and Medicine.* New York: Modern Language Association; 2000. pp. 327–32.

52 Garro LC, Mattingly C. Narrative as construct and construction. In: Mattingly C, Garro LC (eds). *Narrative and the Cultural Construction of Illness and Healing.* Berkeley, CA: University of California Press; 2000. pp. 1–49.

53 Charon R. The body and the self: the seamless experience of being. *Medical Humanities Review* 2002; **16**: 40–50.

54 Hawkins AH, McEntyre MC. Teaching literature and medicine: a retrospective and a rationale. In: Hawkins AH, McEntyre MC (eds). *Teaching Literature and Medicine.* New York: Modern Language Association; 2000. pp. 1–25.

55 Cady J. In brief: a literature seminar in clinical medical education. In: Hawkins AH, McEntyre MC (eds). *Teaching Literature and Medicine.* New York: Modern Language Association; 2000. pp. 333–7.

56 Montello M. Narrative competence. In: Nelson HL (ed). *Stories and Their Limits: Narrative approaches to bioethics.* New York: Routledge; 1997. pp. 185–97.

57 Anderson CM, Holt K, McGrady P. Suture, stigma, and the pages that heal. In: Anderson CM, MacCurdy MM (eds). *Writing and Healing: Toward an informed practice.* Urbana, IL: National Council of Teachers of English; 2000. pp. 58–82.

58 Johnson TR. Writing as healing and the rhetorical tradition: sorting out Plato, postmodernism, writing pedagogy, and post-traumatic stress disorder. In: Anderson CM, MacCurdy MM (eds). *Writing and Healing: Toward an informed practice.* Urbana, IL: National Council of Teachers of English; 2000. pp. 85–114.

59 Campo R. Healing and poetry: representations of illness in contemporary American poetry. In: Donley C, Kohn M (eds). *Recognitions: Doctors and their stories.* Kent, OH: Kent State University Press; 2002. pp. 25–38.

60 Honos-Webb L, Sunwolf, Shapiro JL. Towards the re-enchantment of psychotherapy: the container model of storying in treatment. *Humanistic Psychologist* 2001; **29**: 70–97.

61 Carson RC. The hyphenated space: liminality in the doctor–patient relationship. In: Charon R, Montello M (eds). *Stories Matter: The role of narrative in medical ethics.* New York: Routledge; 2002. pp. 171–82.

62 Saliba M. Story language: a sacred healing space. *Literature and Medicine* 2000; **19**: 61–83.

63 Charon R. *Narrative Medicine: Honoring the stories of illness.* Oxford: Oxford University Press; 2006.

64 Stein HF. The inner world of workplaces: accessing this world through poetry, narrative literature, music, and visual art. *Consulting Psychology Journal: Practice and Research* 2003; **55**: 84–93.

65 Stein HF. Organizational totalitarianism and the voices of dissent. *Journal of Organizational Dynamics* 2007; **1**: 1–25.

66 Haidet P, Stein HF. The role of the student–teacher relationship in the formation of physicians: the hidden curriculum as process. *Journal of General Internal Medicine* 2006; **21**(Suppl. 1): S16–20.

67 Cassell E. *The Nature of Suffering and the Goals of Medicine*, 2nd edition. Oxford: Oxford University Press; 1991.

68 Verghese A. The physician as storyteller. *Annals of Internal Medicine* 2001; **135**: 1012–17.

69 Morris DB. *Illness and Culture in the Postmodern Age.* Berkeley, CA: University of California Press; 1998.

70 Clark MM. Holocaust video testimony, oral history, and narrative medicine: the struggle against indifference. *Literature and Medicine* 2005; **24**: 266–82.

71 Allen G. Language, power, and consciousness: a writing experiment at the University of Toronto. In: Anderson CM, MacCurdy MM (eds). *Writing and Healing: Toward an informed practice.* Urbana, IL: National Council of Teachers of English; 2000. pp. 249–90.

72 Scarry E. *The Body in Pain.* New York: Oxford University Press; 1985.

73 Ryden W. Stories of illness and bereavement: audience and subjectivity in the therapeutic narrative. *Storytelling, Self, Society* 2005; **1**: 53–75.

74 Shapiro J, Kasman D, Shafer A. Words and wards: a model of reflective writing and its uses in medical education. *Journal of Medical Humanities* 2006; **27**: 231–44.

75 Smyth J, Gould O, Slobin K. The role of narrative in medicine: a multitheoretical perspective. *Advances in Mind-Body Medicine* 2000; **16**: 186–93.

76 Coulehan JL. The word is an instrument of healing. *Literature and Medicine* 1991; **10**: 111–29.

77 Orban C. Writing, time and AIDS in the works of Herve Guibert. *Literature and Medicine* 1999; **18**: 132–50.

78 Scheurich N. Reading, listening, and other beleaguered practices in general psychiatry. *Literature and Medicine* 2004; **23**: 304–17.

79 Taylor D. *Tell Me A Story: The life-shaping power of our stories.* St Paul, MN: Bog Walk Press; 2001.

80 Brody H. "'My story is broken: can you help me fix it?" Medical ethics and the joint construction of narrative. *Literature and Medicine* 1994; **13**: 79–92.

81 Gerkin CV. *The Living Human Document*. Nashville, TN: Abingdon Press; 1984.

82 Pennebaker JW. Telling stories: the health benefits of narrative. *Literature and Medicine* 2000; **19**: 3–18.

83 Hastings SO, Hoover JD, Musambira GW. "In my heart for eternity": normalizing messages to the deceased. *Storytelling, Self, Society* 2005; **1**: 11–25.

84 Holt TE. Narrative medicine and negative capability. *Literature and Medicine* 2004; **23**: 318–33.

85 Payne M. A strange unaccountable something: historicizing sexual abuse essays. In: Anderson CM, MacCurdy MM (eds). *Writing and Healing: Toward an informed practice*. Urbana, IL: National Council of Teachers of English; 2000. pp. 115–57.

86 De Moor K. The doctor's role of witness and companion: medical and literary ethics of care in AIDS physicians' memoirs. *Literature and Medicine* 2003; **22**: 208–29.

87 Arras JD. Nice story, but so what? Narrative and justification in ethics. In: Nelson HL (ed.). *Narrative Approaches to Bioethics*. New York: Routledge; 1997. pp. 65–88.

88 Hardwig J. Autobiography, biography, and narrative ethics. In: Nelson HL (ed.). *Narrative Approaches to Bioethics*. New York: Routledge; 1997. pp. 50–64.

3 *Why Study Medical Student Poetry?*

Where I Left Off By: Meghann Kaiser
UC Irvine, 2002

Inspiration is
Taking up where I left off.

Rosarito is a place for new mornings.
Or at least new to me.
At sixteen, I can't remember the last time I was up before sunrise.
And had time to see it.
Or cared to.
But here, the cool is almost acidic, the dew dense
The ocean water skitters audibly, incessantly, insensibly
Over a dimpled shore two blocks past
And I am lying on the rooftop of an old shoe factory
Negotiating the unmatched tooth of my sleeping bag's zipper
Exposed
Enthralled
Awakened
At last.

Don't worry, I'll teach you how to write.
(High school English projects still induce anxiety)
Close your eyes.
Turn, turn, turn.
Stop when you feel dizzy and don't know where you are.
Stop.
What do you see?
The ocean, a cinder block wall on the beach, pumpkins growing behind it.
The waves moving over the sand
Rusted with red tide, and shining.
Good.
What rhymes with shining?
Three more lines, you can set it all to music.
You can sing anything to the tune of
Amazing Grace.
Or Jingle Bell Rock
And Peaceful Easy Feeling
By The Eagles.

That's easy, I'm going to be a poet.
I'm going to workshops
Learning to express my precise persona

In haikus about white lilies.
I'm majoring in literature, I'm mastering the subtle finesse of
Aggressively applied alliteration
Ominous onomatopoeia
Aesthetically aligned couplets, and
Well-wired metaphors.
Words strung on fish line – puppets to the poet
Tip-toe, quiver along the circumference of
Just outside of
Won't intrude on
The unconscious
The unexpected.

Don't worry, I'll teach you how to write.
Forty students, the next generation of intuition
Gather at the tidepool
And scoop out running slivers of enlightenment
Hauled home within their backpacks.
False fluorescent lighting finds them
Methodically outlining the groundbreaking point
Slosh dilapidated Dixie cups of acrid saline
Send dribbles of poetic drool down their fronts
Watch the granules sift within an artificial motion
Listen for rhythm
The water resists
Inertia declines
The poet imposed.
And wait for waves.

That's harder. I'm going to be a doctor.
I'm living in Irvine.
And spending time with specimens of humanity
    strewn schematically on stainless steel.
Trivia, textbooks, and ultimately
Science, with which we label wonder repeating.
Here, the climate is pre-programmed on my thermostat
The hour I rise determined by insomniac panic
Of the impending exam.
The ocean is five miles away, I have not once visited it.
And sunrise is a swelling Venetian slat of clarity across my slurring notes
Tells me I'll be late for class.
I will recreate my art form in the image of myself.
The inner tide I carry with me still
Too scarlet for seas.
The sound I can't escape
In Rosarito
Not in Irvine
It is me, but not mine made.

> Take up your scalpel
> And write.

This poem reflects on the nature of writing itself, and gives us insight into what we can learn about the relationship between writing and doctoring. The poem commences with an intriguing definition of inspiration as "taking up where I left off." This beginning is an indication that the poem will be a reflection on "inspiration" as it relates to the integration of the self. The narrator then jumps back through time, to re-encounter and reclaim the moment when she became "awakened" – her 16-year-old self on a school trip to Rosarito Beach in Mexico, where she learns to write.

What follows is a deconstruction of the process of writing, which seems to share many similarities with the medical student experience. First, one must be willing to enter into a state of disorientation and uncertainty, spinning until one is lightheaded and no longer sees life through a conventional lens. Feeling dizzy "until you don't know where you are" is also a phrase that well describes the medical student's initial experience of medical school.

Next one learns to see anew – observational skills, but not just any old observation, rather observation that is particular, detailed, penetrating, and prepared for unusual associations and connections. Observation, too, of course is a critically important part of learning to make medical diagnoses. Ideally, the student learns to pay attention to the information obtained from all of their senses, and even to listen to what is not said.

After observation comes description – the way in which words, language, metaphors, images, specificity, and clarity are used to represent that which is perceived, whether it is the rusty red sea or a suffering patient. Like the language of medicine, the language of literature is governed by certain rules and techniques – metaphor, alliteration, onomato-poeia, rhythm, and rhyme. However, the narrator knows that writing is not only about the expert shaping of an external product, but also about the expression, sometimes unexpected, and often emerging from the unconscious, of the self. Writing is not only about technique, but also about "intuition." Similarly, although strict conventions guide the construction of the patient's chart, the physician in training perceives that there are many other stories about the patient which are waiting to be told.

The decision to become a doctor is harder for this student than her early yearnings toward writing. The poem contrasts the natural rhythms and beauty of her past experience in Mexico with the regimented life of a medical student. Medicine is all about studying and "science." Apparently, no two things could be more different than poetry and medicine. Yet the student avers that she "will recreate [her] art form in the image of [herself]." What links the past with the present, and intuition with science, is the continuity of the person who is both writer and doctor (to be). The "inner tide" discovered so many years ago still resides within her because it *is* her. In the concluding couplet, the narrator unites art and science, as well as the various dimensions of herself. Suddenly she addresses herself in the second person, and issues herself a command: "Take up your scalpel/And write." Dissection becomes an act of creation. She is writing herself on the body of her cadaver.

WHY STUDY MEDICAL STUDENT POETRY?

The above analysis of writing still does not explain why we should focus analytic attention on medical student poetry in particular. Why examine poetry in preference to prose? The literature is replete with medical students' prose writing – for example, first-person narratives, critical incident reports. Why not study these as well? Of course, such writing should be (and has been) studied. And there is no definitive reason at the moment for restricting a study of student writing to poetry alone. Partly, I admit, it is a matter of personal preference. I *like* reading the poetry of medical students. However, it is also true that poetry can provide a unique window into medical students' subjective perceptions and concerns as they proceed through training. Poetry offers a singular and distinctive source of information and insight through which to search out the minds and hearts of medical students. This is because it is so different from standard forms of medical communication, including its reliance on metaphor, image, and rhythm to address issues of meaning. Poetry is uniquely suited to deepen our understanding of complex issues without simple answers. I elaborate below on certain key aspects of poetry, and why they are particularly suited to developing insights into medical students' experience.

UNIQUE FEATURES OF POETRY
Limits of the language of science
Medical students work very hard to master the scientific language of medicine. According to some estimates, students must learn at least 13 000 new words in their first year of medical school alone.[1] Clearly, becoming fluent in this language helps medical students to conceptualize disease processes and to communicate efficiently with supervisors and peers. Yet Stein has pointed out that, at some point, professional language "fails" its possessor, in that it no longer illuminates or brings understanding of what is happening. Poetry, by contrast, speaks from the interior of experience, eliminating the safe distance that is created by the language of science. Stein goes on to say that literature in general can be a "bridge back" when individuals have become alienated from their world through fear or pain.[2]

Understanding incoherent narrative
Poetry has been criticized because it does not always present a coherent narrative arc (although sometimes it does). However, it is possible to argue that poetry in all its allusiveness, brevity, ellipticism, and indirection is more like actual unruly human narrative than the smoothed and polished narratives that we construct when writing prose. Everyday stories that real people tell are often undeveloped, fragile, incomplete, inconsistent,[3] and characterized by fragments of speech, abrupt figurations, and unexpected shifts.[4] In fact, these stories sound much more like poetry than we'd like to admit. The fact that poetry is often unruly, ambiguous, and unresolved makes it closer to the way that life actually unfolds than a well-structured, well-organized narrative. Poetry is especially good, in Keats' famous phrase, at creating a space of negative capability, where uncertainty, mystery, and doubt can flourish. As one author puts it, poetry is "keener" in terms of exploring human ambiguity.[5]

Boundary crossing
I would argue that, overall, poetry has greater potential than prose to be transgressive and boundary-crossing, at least when wielded in the hands of medical students.[6] Although poetry has its own potentially restrictive rules and regulations, perhaps fortunately these are by and large unfamiliar to medical students (with the somewhat common

exception of the use of rhyme schemes). Thus poetry avoids the formalized codification of storytelling and offers students an opportunity to shake up their ways of thinking and expressing themselves.[7-9] Straightforward narratives (for example, critical incident reports) run the risk of becoming formulaic, closing off choices and opportunities, and trapping the teller.[10] Such stories become accommodations to the dominant discourse.[11] It is tempting to create "functional narratives" that rely on cliché, and which devolve into merely a "story about a story."[12] In this case, the experience has not been excavated, much less described, but only labeled. When narrative too quickly prioritizes coherence and resolution, it also becomes distant from actual experience.[3] Poetry is less governed by the conventions, rules, and social codes of conversational language / communication than other forms of writing. Thus it is more likely to be authentic and revealing than a carefully crafted story that slips into traditional linguistic and discourse practices.

New ways of seeing things

It has been claimed that poetry in particular can create "rotation"[13] – that is, the experiencing of events in new, fresh ways that challenge the habitual thinking to which one tends to revert in moments of stress and crisis. This claim raises the interesting possibility that one of the best ways of processing problematic and challenging situations is to write a poem! Poetry "defamiliarizes the familiar" and is a way of "consenting to see with close and compassionate attention."[14] Its reliance on metaphor and imagery can take both writer and reader to new and unexpected places.[7] By linking two things that are not normally considered synonymous or similar, by making unexpected connections,[15] a poem can create new understandings that are different from ordinary experience. These unexpected relationships in turn are more likely to lead to a kind of counter-existence or counter-reality consisting of different, unpredictable, and unanticipated possibilities.[16] Because poetry combines patterns, knowledge, and emotion in new ways, it allows the writer to overcome habitual forms of thinking.[17] In all these ways, poetry allows access to language, images, and associations that are not normally used by physicians and physicians in training – forms from which they have become separated and alienated.

Epiphanic insight

Along similar lines, others have asserted that poetry is especially useful in describing ineffable, epiphanic moments that other media cannot entirely capture.[18-21] Precisely because it operates outside ordinary individual and institutional boundaries, it can provide rapid insight.[22] It is possible that poetry better conveys the richness of certain experiences that cannot be totally understood in narrative form. In the words of medical anthropologist Howard Stein, "[Poetry] transforms the experience of an It, a thing, into a relationship with a Thou."[22] Poetry addresses things that cannot always be said directly, and that perhaps are only sensed intuitively rather than logically apprehended. As James Joyce expressed it, poetry can provide a moment of "radiance" that leads to a sudden profound understanding. Because it does not rely entirely on ordinary logic, poetry has greater potential than prose for tapping into depth meanings[23] that transcend the limits of what can be known through conventional analytic modes of thinking.

Truthfulness

Finally, there is the question of the "truthfulness" of poetry. Poetry is fiction, not fact. Poetry is imagined, not real. If we want to understand medical students, why not just ask them what their experience is like? Of course, this is a valuable method of approaching the medical student perspective. However, as I hope to have established in the above discussion, I believe that the poems of medical students illuminate aspects of their experience that they have trouble putting into other, more conventional words – aspects of their experience of which they may not even be fully consciously aware. In this regard, I choose not to make an absolute distinction between fact and the "fiction" that is poetry. As Chambers and Montgomery have noted,[24] there are no unplotted stories. All narrators, even "factual" ones, shape the story to tell the tale. Truth is always to some degree particular and incomplete. There is always a gap between narrative discourse and the actual life lived. Every text distorts and selects.[25]

Subjective particulars

Writing poetry legitimates the subjectivity of students' observations and imagination,[26,27] regardless of idiosyncrasy or variance from more prevalent social norms. The poems of students often focus on mundane details that clinical experience and scientific research might regard as inconsequential. In doing so, they become a way of supplementing standard "medical telling",[28] allowing students to concentrate on those elements of an encounter that might have mattered to them or to patients and families, if not to their attending physician. Because in poetry students are not required to state events "correctly" or to distinguish in the approved manner between what is relevant and what is tangential, particulars of the events students experience that are normally discarded as irrelevant may be retrieved, contemplated, and savored in verse. In particular, using metaphor appears to allow students to enter their clinical (or life) experiences from unexpected vantage points, gaining new insights and understanding in the process.

Emotional experience

Furthermore, poetry locates the author directly within emotional experience by removing the safety net of scientific discourse.[29] Rather than attempting to ignore or set aside emotional reactions as unprofessional,[30] writing a poem gives students an opportunity to examine emotion fully, to experiment with different ways of expressing it, and to explore its varied potential meanings and implications. For example, many student poems address issues that generated considerable personal confusion and suffering for them, such as how to break bad news to patients or how to deal with their anger and frustration at the limitations of medicine.[31] In an insightful article, Henderson[32] analyzed students' poetry in order to explore their evolving views of death and dying, and noted their struggles to avoid dehumanization and emotional detachment. One medical student anecdotally reported turning to poetry to explore her personal experience with illness as well as to develop more emotionally authentic communication with her physician.[33]

METHODOLOGY

In terms of the methodology employed, I read 576 poems written by 386 medical students who ranged from the first to the fourth year of their training. The distribution of number of poems written by a single student was as follows: 1 poem, $n = 302$; 2 poems, $n = 54$; 3 poems, $n = 11$; 4 poems, $n = 9$; 5 poems, $n = 8$; 6 poems, $n = 3$; 7 poems, $n = 3$; 8 poems, $n = 1$; 10 poems, $n = 1$. Using several Internet list servers, I solicited examples of medical student poetry from schools of medicine faculty working in the area of medical humanities. In response, I received literary journals from 15 institutions, containing the original creative work of students (and sometimes of faculty and staff as well). These journals represented medical schools located on the East Coast and West Coast, and in Southern and Midwestern states, as well as a medical school in Qatar. I restricted my project to the poetry of medical students. About 55% of the poems reviewed came from students at my home institution, which provides opportunities for students to use a range of creative media to reflect on their medical school experiences on average once a year as part of required or elective coursework. All poems quoted in their entirety in the text are reprinted with the permission of the author.

Content analysis

I performed a content analysis and interpretation of each poem, and then organized my insights into the thematic categories that emerged from a grounded theory analysis[34] of all of the raw data. The themes that emerged inductively from my review were as follows: the anatomy experience; becoming a doctor; becoming a patient; doctor–patient relationships; student–patient relationships; two subsets of the student–patient relationship; language and culture differences and death and dying; the nexus of societal issues and medicine; and students' reflections on life and love. By systematically categorizing and then interpreting a large body of medical student poetry, I was able to reach conclusions about what topics are of importance to students who write poetry, how they use poetry to address these topics, and what conclusions we are able to draw from their poems.

The themes identified through this process were subsequently organized to represent a developmental approach to medical education, starting with students' first introduction to medicine in the gross anatomy lab, and progressing through their initial superficial contacts with patients to deeper connections and commitments over the course of training. Of particular importance was the emergence of problematic relational issues in medicine, including observing and interpreting difficult physician–patient encounters, dealing with negative professional role models, reflecting on their own relationships with patients, coming face to face with the limitations of medicine, confronting death and dying, and balancing their personal and professional lives. Although others will certainly identify additional themes to the ones discussed in the text, no one can disagree with the importance of the topics selected for focus.

Narrative typologies

In addition to a content analysis, I also focused on the narrative types that could be identified in student poetry. Narrative scholars have expressed concern that the dissection of text, while offering much of value, can also result in overlooking or ignoring the overall sense of the story.[35] In an attempt to capture this larger perspective, a global narrative coding for each poem was also developed. Narrative typologies, such as tragedy, comedy, romance, and satire, have long been identified in the literature.[36] Other common prototypes are stable, progressive, and regressive narratives.[37] There is considerable controversy as to whether these are archetypal, universal story lines. Hogan, for example, asserts that certain narrative types, such as heroic tragi-comedy and romance, occur with remarkable consistency across cultures.[38] Post-modernists, however, dispute the existence of any universalizing narratives.[39] In either case, narrative typologies have been successfully applied to the analysis of storytelling.[40] Adame[41] developed a typology of narratives of mental illness that she concluded was quite different from that of narratives told about physical illness. Ezzy[42] explored the role that broader social forces play in how people tell stories about job loss, describing the heroic job loss narrative, which emphasizes personal agency, and the tragic job loss narrative, which emphasizes victimization at the hands of larger social forces.

For this work, the narrative framework that I judged to be most relevant was based on the work of medical sociologist Arthur Frank.[43] As was discussed in Chapter 1, Frank identified four major types of illness narratives – chaos, restitution, journey, and witnessing. However, these narrative types refer to stories told by patients. Frank's theoretical work has recently been supplemented in the literature by articles examining how such stories actually appear in patient accounts.[44,45] After reading many student poems, I was struck by the similarity in overall form of the poems to the Frank typologies originally identified through studying patient stories. To increase their relevance to the student poems, I refined and modified Frank's original categories somewhat. For example, the chaos category was primarily conceptualized as a cry for help. The restitution story took form as a kind of self-reassurance and rapid repair of uncertainty and ambiguity (or anti-restitution, when patient intransigence interfered with the re-establishment of order and normalcy). The journey story included self-discovery and identity formation through personal growth and learning. Witnessing narratives could bear witness to the issue of patient suffering, but could also take the form of an act of resistance, and were focused on the creation of community, whether between student and patient or as a bridge between the patient and the larger, indifferent society. In addition to the original four categories, I included an extra category, namely transcendence – stories characterized by epiphanic transformation and healing.

Most of the poems that I reviewed made sense within these Frankian-influenced narrative typologies. However, this does not mean that the fit was always comfortable or simple. As can be seen in the numerous examples that have been included, many of the poems not only addressed multiple content themes but also incorporated more than one narrative type. For example, many poems started in chaos, only to embark on a journey, achieve restitution, or end up witnessing. These categories slip and slide, merge and collide with each other in ways that make them not so much rigid "either/or" choices as conceptual "beginnings" or triggers that I hope will stimulate further thinking and discussion. Therefore the narrative typologies are not offered as one-dimensional categories, and the object is not so much rigid classification of student poetry as a framework for interpretation – a framework that is recognized as provisional and imperfect.

Conceptual metaphors

Two overarching metaphors dominated my conclusions. One of them is alluded to in the work of the social philosopher Susan Sontag, who referred to illness as "a foreign land."[46] Other scholars, such as anthropologist Robert Murphy,[47] sociologist Arthur Frank,[43] and neurologist Oliver Sacks,[48] have also usefully worked within this metaphor. This text incorporates the same conceit, and through these poems explores in what sense illness is unfamiliar territory not only for the patient but also for the student-physician, examines some of the vulnerabilities and pitfalls in exploring this terrain from the learner perspective, and finally considers ways in which writing poetry helps learners to begin to apprehend this world from the inside out.

The second metaphor is that of the heroic journey, as articulated in the writings of Joseph Campbell.[49] Medical students in some respects are similar to the often ordinary, reluctant and struggling heroes of myth and fairytale. Like physicians in training, these heroes leave familiar environments, confront dangers, battle demons, discover new companions and wise guides, acquire self-knowledge, develop unsuspected depths of courage and compassion, and finally return home to serve their kingdoms. It is important to note that both of these metaphors are employed in a post-modernist context, so that the medical sojourner is less expert than confused and lonely castaway, while the medical hero is less god-like presence than wounded healer. The two metaphors of stranger in a strange land and Everyman's journey combine nicely to help us to understand how students use poetry to make sense of important aspects of their own and their patients' experiences.

QUALITATIVE DATA ANALYSIS OF POETIC TEXTS

This book is predicated on the argument that poetry can be understood as a form of qualitative data, and that techniques of analysis developed for other sources of qualitative data (such as interviews, focus groups, and textual narratives) can be applied to an understanding of poetry. Many might argue that the terms "poetry" and "data" do not belong in the same sentence, except in an oppositional way. The *Oxford English Dictionary* defines "a datum" as "something known or assumed as fact, and made the basis of reasoning or calculation." Few would claim that poems are primarily facts, although they may certainly contain facts and even numbers (one of the most moving poems I ever read is composed entirely of the "numbers" of a patient admitted to an intensive-care unit, who eventually expires[50]). The relative absence of factual, objective, universally verifiable evidence in poems may initially appear to be a disadvantage in exploiting the possibilities of poetry as data. However, as the British physician and researcher Denis Burkitt observed, "Not everything that counts can be counted." In the post-modern era, it makes sense to consider the extent to which we might be able to expand the sources of knowledge that we admit as legitimate data to our scholarly canons.[51] How can we approach the concept of "poetry as data" in a way that retains both literary and scientific integrity and somehow enhances each of these?

Theoretical foundation

The theoretical basis for approaching poetry as data is found in conceptual models of ways of knowing, as pioneered by Jerome Bruner,[52] who distinguished between logico-scientific and narrative modes. Howard Stein[22] points out that knowing in medicine, as in other areas of life, is not singular but rather various. What we "know" in medicine is surely derived in part from empirical research and scientific data, but it is also derived from multiple other sources, including possibly poetry. In fact, we ignore multiple ways of knowing at our peril. For many purposes related to healing, scientific terminology is deficient in comparison with poetic expression.[2,29] Poetry speaks from the interior of human experience in a unique way that science can never do, and indeed does not wish to do.

POETRY AS QUALITATIVE DATA

The idea of using poetry as data is unusual but not unprecedented. The basic assumption underlying this approach is that poetry can be subjected to hermeneutic analysis as well as content analysis, just as can be done with any other text. From this perspective, poems may be considered as specific pieces of information or evidence. Other scholars have approached medically related poetry in this manner,[29,31,32,53,54] scrutinizing poems by medical students, nurses, physicians, and patients, as well as formally trained poets, in order to explore and understand aspects of professional development, the illness experience, and the doctor–patient relationship. Poetry does not represent the sort of data that conform to tenets of reproducibility, generalizability, and objectivity, which are found in quantitative research. Rather, although it is quite different from empirical research, it contains its own veracity consistent with the reality that it describes through insight, personal vision, and interpretation.[55]

Some assumptions of qualitative research appear to be amenable to considering poetry as a source of data. For example, qualitative approaches are interested in questions of meaning. Poetry also may be understood as an inquiry into meanings.[29] Qualitative research further favors the view that its task is not to verify or predict a single, enduring "truth", but to discover and better understand multiple, socially constructed realities.[51,56] Such research is interested in relationships and circumstances in which the explanation of action is not straightforwardly causal, linear, or unidirectional, but rather due to multiple interacting factors, events, and processes. Similarly, poetry is not concerned with prediction. Rather it provides a kind of deep understanding of subjective experience that is difficult to access in other ways, and is capable of presenting diverse, often contradictory, narratives and images simultaneously.[2] Because of its belief in coexisting various, inconstant realities, qualitative research approaches knowledge as local and specific. Poetry, too, is particularistic and concrete.[28] As Campo[29] writes, it is one of the few ways available to us of preserving "the fragile details of the human experience of sickness" (p. 98).

Qualitative research generally identifies two interrelated aspects of dealing with data:

1 analysis, or the process of bringing order to the data by organizing it into patterns, categories, and basic descriptive units

2 interpretation, which involves attaching meaning and significance to the analyses, explaining descriptive patterns, and looking for relationships and linkages among descriptive dimensions.[57]

Qualitative approaches are very much concerned with the informant's frame of reference,[58] and in poetry we find what has often been called a unique entry into the subjective experience and point of view of others, especially others unlike ourselves. In some respects, poetry is like instant anthropology. The power and immediacy of its language take us in short order to places we never thought we would be, and into lives that perhaps we did not initially wish to know. Qualitative research takes as a given that inquirers cannot maintain objective distance from the phenomena which are being studied – at best, they can only acknowledge and reflect on their own subjectivity. Poetry likewise requires reflexivity about self, others, and the world. In terms of assessing the validity of conclusions, qualitative guidelines of trustworthiness and credibility[59] are relevant to poetry. Poetry continues to survive as a mode of expression because of its capacity to create useful, credible, and trustworthy truths that are hard to discover in other ways.

POETIC EXCEPTIONALISM?

Should poetry be treated like any other text? Clearly, poetry is not the same as prose, but especially when written by untrained medical students, nurses, physicians, or patients, it is sometimes difficult to specify precisely why. One author[32] has speculated that, because of their requirement for reflection, analysis, and organization of ideas, as well as their inquiry into meaning, poems provide a uniquely critical position from which to "interrogate" salient life experiences. Poetry may offer students certain unique possibilities for reflection that are less evident in more analytic, logical forms of writing or in verbal communication.[60] The indirection of poetry may allow learners to more easily examine intangible aspects of their experiences in medical school. Issues that seem straightforward when organized through the well-defined and prescribed formulas of the case presentation yield other interpretations when explored in verse. The often ambiguous, complex, and imprecise nature of the quandaries that students encounter makes exclusive reliance on logico-scientific reasoning inadequate in expressing and addressing their concerns.[61] Thus, methods of narrative analysis[62] and textual analysis used by social scientists[63] are relevant to the concept of poetry as data. However, they may also do violence to the aesthetics of poetry. As Henderson goes on to point out, "A simple mapping of . . . techniques that apply to poetry in one cultural domain onto poetry in another domain is problematic."[32]

Because of its predilection for imagery and metaphor, meanings may emerge in poetry of which the author herself is not always completely aware, and which may not be entirely intentional, yet which have their own inherent validity and signification.[64] This characteristic of poetry raises fascinating questions about how, or even whether, consensual interpretations can be reached in treating poetry as data. It even suggests the possibility that outliers or negative cases might be found within a single poem that simultaneously contains their contradiction. One way to mitigate this problem of differing meanings within a single poem is to encourage the full inclusion of poetic text in the reporting of findings. This allows readers to act as triangulated investigators in their own right. In addition, we need to understand more about how the artistic signification of this form of self-expression influences the poetic data that we are analyzing and interpreting.

Poetic data analysis should strive to achieve qualitative guidelines of trustworthiness, credibility, dependability, and utility by following practices such as establishing an audit trail, theoretical saturation of the data, triangulation of data sources, and involvement of more than one researcher. In attempting to draw any conclusions from these student poems, we must not forget that poetry bears only an imperfect relationship to actions and events in real time. We cannot assume that these poems were entirely authentic. There is always a gap between the poem and the actual experience.[25] Nevertheless, on balance it is reasonable to apply qualitative methods of investigation to an examination of poetic text.

The literary value of medical student poetry

Although my purpose here is not to address the literary and aesthetic attributes and value of the poems that I reviewed, I would like to make a personal observation in this regard. It is true that much of this writing is imperfect, unpolished, lacking in formal craftsmanship, and does not appear to pay attention to the formal structural or rhythmic conventions of poetry. However, Berman, a professor of English literature, has argued[65] that when students write about what is important to them, they write very well, often better than when they are writing to complete graded assignments. Matarasso[66] notes that although there are varying degrees of integrity, ability, technique, and originality, "the poetry of a mental health service user and the poet laureate use the same method." Similarly, Bolton[7] writes that "poetry does not have to be great so long as it is useful to the writer and to an appropriate audience." In my view, when students write authentically about their own experience, the results are uniformly moving, compelling, and impossible to ignore. While these qualities are not identical to literary merit, they provide strong arguments for the inherent "value" of such work.

REFERENCES

1 Blackwell B. Drug therapy: patient compliance. *NEJM* 1973; **289**: 249–52.
2 Stein HF. *Prairie Voices: Process anthropology in family medicine.* Westport, CT: Bergin & Garvey; 1996.
3 Kirmayer LJ. Broken narratives: clinical encounters and the poetics of illness experience. In: Mattingly C, Garro LC (eds). *Narrative and the Cultural Construction of Illness and Healing.* Berkeley, CA: University of California Press; 2000. pp. 153–80.
4 Hartman G. Narrative and beyond. *Literature and Medicine* 2004; **23**: 334–45.
5 Stripling MY. *Bioethical and Medical Issues in Literature.* Westport, CT: Greenwood Press; 2005.
6 Verghese A. The physician as storyteller. *Annals of Internal Medicine* 2001; **135**: 1012–17.
7 Bolton, G. *Reflective Practice: Writing for professional development.* London: Sage; 2001.
8 Heath I. Following the story: continuity of care in general practice. In: Greenhalgh T, Hurwitz B. (eds). *Narrative-Based Medicine: Dialogue and discourse in clinical practice.* London: BMJ Books; 1998. pp. 83–92.
9 Munson P. Criminal language and poetic jailbreak: writing chronic fatigue immune dysfunction syndrome. *Literature and Medicine* 2000; **19**: 19–24.
10 Garro L. Narrative representations of chronic illness experience: cultural models of illness, mind, and body in stories concerning the temporomandibular joint (TMJ). *Social Science and Medicine* 1994; **38**: 775–88.
11 Sunwolf. Rx Storysharing, prn: stories as medicine. *Storytelling, Self, Society* 2005; **1**: 1–10.
12 MacCurdy MM. From trauma to writing. In: Anderson CM, MacCurdy MM (eds). *Writing and Healing: Toward an informed practice.* Urbana, IL: National Council of Teachers of English; 2000. pp. 158–200.
13 Lantos J. Why doctors make good protagonists. In: Elliott C, Lantos J (eds). *The Last Physician: Walker Percy and the moral life of medicine.* Durham, NC: Duke University Press; 1999. pp. 38–45.
14 McEntyre MC. Getting from how to why: a pause for reflection on professional life. *Academic Medicine* 1997; **72**: 1051–5.
15 Little M. Does reading poetry make you a better clinician? *Internal Medicine Journal* 2001; **31**: 60–1.
16 Pearce SS. *Flash of Insight: Metaphor and narrative in therapy.* Boston, MA: Allyn & Bacon; 1996.
17 White MT. Fire-fighting at the bedside. *Medical Humanities Review* 2003; **17**: 41–5.
18 Coulehan JL. A suitable measure of redemption. *Journal of Medical Humanities* 2000; **21**: 189–98.
19 Hawkins AH. Medical ethics and the epiphanic dimension of narrative. In: Nelson HL (ed.). *Stories and Their Limits: Narrative approaches to bioethics.* New York: Routledge; 1997.
20 Charon R. Time and ethics. In: Charon R, Montello M (eds). *Stories Matter: The role of narrative in medical ethics.* New York: Routledge; 2002. pp. 59–68.
21 Hawkins AH, McEntyre MC. Teaching literature and medicine: a retrospective and a rationale. In: Hawkins AH, McEntyre (eds). *Teaching Literature and Medicine.* New York: Modern Language Association; 2000. pp. 1–25.
22 Stein HF. The inner world of workplaces: accessing this world through poetry, narrative

literature, music, and visual art. *Consulting Psychology Journal: Practice and Research* 2003; **55:** 84–93.

23 Hawkins AH. Pathography and the enabling myths: the process of healing. In: Anderson CM, MacCurdy MM (eds). *Writing and Healing: Toward an informed practice.* Urbana, IL: National Council of Teachers of English; 2000. pp. 222–46.

24 Chambers T, Montgomery K. Plot: framing contingency and choice in bioethics. In: Charon R, Montello M (eds). *Stories Matter: The role of narrative in medical ethics.* New York: Routledge; 2002. pp. 77–84.

25 Garro LC, Mattingly C. Narrative as construct and construction. In: Mattingly C, Garro LC (eds). *Narrative and the Cultural Construction of Illness and Healing.* Berkeley, CA: University of California Press; 2000. pp. 1–49.

26 McLellan MF. Literature and medicine: the patient, the physician, and the poem. *Lancet* 1996; **348:** 1640–1.

27 Spatz LS, Welsh K. Literature and medicine as a writing course. In: Hawkins AH, McEntyre MC (eds). *Teaching Literature and Medicine.* New York: Modern Language Association; 2000. pp. 141–50.

28 Downie G. Telling: detail and diagnosis in medical poetry. *Medical Humanities Review* 2002; **16:** 9–17.

29 Campo R. *The Healing Art: A doctor's black bag of poetry.* New York: WW Norton & Co.; 2003.

30 Smith RC, Stein HF. A topographical model of clinical decision making and interviewing. *Family Medicine* 1987; **19:** 361–3.

31 Poirier S, Ahrens WR, Brauner DJ. Songs of innocence and experience: students' poems about their medical education. *Academic Medicine* 1998; **73:** 473–8.

32 Henderson SW. Medical student elegies: the poetics of caring. *Journal of Medical Humanities* 2002; **23:** 119–32.

33 Goldstein M. Medicine and poetry: pathway of communication. *The Pharos* 1997; **60:** 12–14.

34 Charmaz KC. *Grounded Theory: Methods for the twenty-first century.* London: Sage Publications; 2005.

35 Kuper A. Literature and medicine: a problem of assessment. *Academic Medicine* 2006; **81:** S128–37.

36 Frye N. *The Anatomy of Criticism.* Princeton, NJ: Princeton University Press; 1957.

37 Gergen M, Gergen, K. The social construction of narrative accounts. In: Gergen M, Gergen K (eds). *Historical Social Psychology.* Englewood Cliffs, NJ: Lawrence Erlbaum; 1984.

38 Hogan PC. *The Mind and its Stories: Narrative universals and human emotions.* Cambridge: Cambridge University Press; 2003.

39 Freedman J, Combs G. *Narrative Therapy: The social construction of preferred realities.* New York: WW Norton; 1996.

40 Riley T, Hawe P. Researching practice: the methodological case for narrative inquiry. *Health Education Research* 2005; **20:** 226–36.

41 Adame AL. Representing madness: how are subjective experiences of emotional distress presented in first-person accounts? *Humanistic Psychologist* 2006; **34:** 135–58.

42 Ezzy D. Fate and agency in job loss narratives. *Qualitative Sociology* 2000; **23:** 121–34.

43 Frank AW. *The Wounded Storyteller: Body, illness, and ethics.* Chicago: University of Chicago Press; 1995.

44 Auxiliadora C, De Benedetto M, Blasco PG, *et al.* "Once Upon a Time . . ." at the Tenth SOBRAMFA International and Academic Meeting, São Paulo, Brazil. *Journal for Learning Through the Arts: A Research Journal on Arts Integration in Schools and Communities,* 2006; **2:** Article7; http://repositories.cdlib.org/clta/lta/vol2/iss1/art7.

45 Whitehead LC. Quest, chaos and restitution: living with chronic fatigue syndrome/myalgic encephalomyelitis. *Social Science and Medicine* 2006; **62:** 2236–45.

46 Sontag S. *AIDS and its Metaphors.* New York: Picador; 1989.

47 Murphy RF. *The Body Silent.* New York: WW Norton; 1990.

48 Sacks O. *An Anthropologist on Mars: Seven paradoxical tales.* New York: Vintage; 1995.

49 Cousineau P (ed.). *The Hero's Journey: Joseph Campbell on his life and work.* New York: Harper and Row; 1990.

50 Cramer SC. ICU. In: Kaiser M (ed.). *Plexus: UCI College of Medicine Journal of Arts and Humanities.* Irvine, CA: UCI College of Medicine; 2004.

51 Frank AW. Asking the right question about pain: narrative and phronesis. *Literature and Medicine* 2004; **23**: 209–25.

52 Bruner J. The narrative construction of reality. *Critical Inquiry* 1991; **18**: 1–21.

53 Oiler C. Nursing reality as reflected in nurses' poetry. *Perspectives in Psychiatric Care* 1983; **21**: 81–9.

54 Rucker L, Shapiro J. Can poetry make better doctors? Teaching the humanities and arts to medical students and residents at the University of California, Irvine, College of Medicine. *Academic Medicine* 2003; **78**: 953–7.

55 Saunders L. "Something made in language": the poet's gift? *Management Decision* 2006; **44**: 504–11.

56 Greenhalgh T, Taylor R. Papers that go beyond numbers (qualitative research). *BMJ* 1997; **315**: 740–3.

57 Patton MQ. *Qualitative Research and Evaluation Methods,* 3rd edition. Thousand Oaks, CA: Sage Publications; 2001.

58 Ventres WB, Frankel RM. Ethnography: a stepwise approach for primary care researchers. *Family Medicine* 1996; **28**: 52–6.

59 Lincoln YS, Guba EG. But is it rigorous? Trustworthiness and authenticity in naturalistic evaluation. In: Lincoln YS, Guba EG (eds). *Naturalistic Inquiry.* Beverly Hills, CA: Sage; 1986. pp. 73–84.

60 Shapiro J. Can poetry be data? Potential relationships between poetry and research. *Families, Systems, and Health* 2004; **22**: 171–7.

61 Shapiro J, Stein HF. Poetic license: writing poetry as a way medical students examine their professional relationship systems. *Families, Systems, and Health* 2005; **23**: 278–92.

62 Charon R. Literature and medicine: origins and destinies. *Academic Medicine* 2000; **75**: 23–7.

63 Elwyn G, Gwyn R. Stories we hear and stories we tell: analyzing talk in clinical practice. *BMJ* 1999; **318**: 186–8.

64 Kociatkiewicz J, Kostera M. The anthropology of empty spaces. *Qualitative Sociology* 1999; **22**: 37–50.

65 Berman J. *Diaries of an English Professor: Pain and growth in the classroom.* Amherst, MA: University of Massachusetts Press; 1994.

66 Matarasso F. "No appealing solution": evaluating the outcomes of arts and health initiatives. In: Evans M, Finlay G (eds). *Medical Humanities.* London: BMJ Books; 2001. pp. 36–49.

4 Living Anatomy: The Experience of Cadaver Dissection

Although the necessity and utility of anatomy laboratory dissection experiences have been questioned, with some schools substituting virtual training for actual cadavers,[1] the course has also been defended as the first, and crucial, training ground for aspects of professionalism, such as respect for patients, accountability for one's actions, teamwork, and social responsibility,[2] as well as various humanistic attitudes.[3,4] In this sense, dissection has a key role in a student's journey towards becoming a physician.[5] Anatomy is sometimes regarded as the student's first clinical experience, with the cadaver viewed as the student's first patient.[6] Rizzolo[7] observed that anatomy introduces students to the idea of the donor and, by extension, of the patient as a person.

Despite its great potential in both professionalism and academic domains, anatomy can be a challenge for medical students. The research is equivocal about the extent to which students are bothered physically or emotionally by anatomy. Several older studies[8–10] report serious psychological distress in anatomy students. However, more recent studies indicate that anatomy is only moderately or not very stressful,[11] and in fact generates considerable enthusiasm and excitement among the large majority of students.[12] A similar study[13] indicated that students generally do not find cadaver dissection aversive, but rather see it as "a positive and challenging life event." Whether or not anatomy is stressful for students, there is evidence that learning how to manage emotions that arise during anatomy may improve test performance.[14]

The anatomy lab can be the beginning of a physician's training in how to isolate and restrict affect, or how to deal appropriately with affective responses.[15] Unfortunately, an unintended consequence of human dissection is that it may create in medical students an inappropriate and callous "property of easiness" in dealing with death and the human body.[16] To combat this tendency, some anatomy programs have used self-reflection,[17] art,[15] journaling,[18] and group discussion[19] to encourage students to explore their emotional responses to dissection. Other curricula combine anatomy with material on death and dying.[20]

The gross anatomy course is frequently regarded as the first rite of passage for medical students. Anatomy is the students' first formal opportunity to bear witness to another's suffering (in this case, the "suffering" of the cadaver), as well as to their own suffering as a result of participation in the anatomy lab and the dissection process. Most commonly, students express identification with the cadaver, and readily recognize the way in which they are connected to each other through shared vulnerability. The poems are variously cries for help (chaos stories), processes of self-interrogation and identity formation, and expressions of solidarity and resistance.

Primum di, primum nocer
[First day, First harm] By: Alex Cuenca
Originally appeared in Panacea *Summer 2005, p. 25*
University of Florida College of Medicine

The room is meant to be cold
Like the metal stands that
Prop up the last stage of 21 lives
Ghosts sealed up tight in their skin suits
Drunk and toxic with preservative
God's fixed image . . . for us.

We learn in this discreet
Polysyllabic apathy because we need to . . .
Do I need to?
How is it to disassemble and not dissolve?
To violate and still respect?

I mean, I see these poor marionettes
Of tendon and sinew
Wonder how that last caress of their grandchild's cheek
Must've coursed so deep through that long web of nerves

I know.

The intent here is to fill
But I feel a little bit more hollow today.
I am etching lines into me with the shards of my innocence
Tempted to wedge it tightly
between my curiosity and my humanity.
Everyday that passes
We unravel the twine our biology
And I see the chaotic but
delicate stitches that nature has woven us into . . .

What is it you want me to see?

I'm trying to not wear through this purpose
   Lose it in the lines and volumes of text
      Drown it in the hours of lecture
         And menial aspects of my own immature consumptions . . .

I'm trying.

This work provides an appropriate poetic introduction to medical students' experience of the gross anatomy course. The title is the first warning that the student is writing in some confusion, if not distress. "First day, first harm" puns on one of the most revered strictures in medicine, primum non nocere (first, do no harm). It also hints at the troubling realization that the practice of medicine inevitably involves harm, sometimes in the service of a greater good, sometimes unintentional and accidental.

Like many poems written about anatomy, "First day, first harm" is written in the first-person-singular voice of the medical student. First, the narrator sets the scene – an intentionally cold, metallic room. However, it is the description of the cadavers that grips us. They are represented not by names but only by a number, 21, that now "sums" them up. They are no longer living but toxic ghosts, "drunk" on formalin. Both the numerical designation and the non-human, threatening apparitions who dwell in another plane encourage a sense of distancing and danger.

Then, in an abrupt U-turn from this somewhat repellent and threatening metaphor, the poet reverses himself. The cadavers are not a dangerous and contaminating "other." In fact they are, like all of us, made in God's image (although in their case the image is "fixed" – punning on the way that the preservative acts on the corpse, as well as suggesting a profound difference between students and cadavers, the quick and the dead). Nevertheless, the use of this religious reference unmistakably suggests the sacred nature of the human form. This reminder is quickly and ironically followed by the phrase "for us," intimating that even the image of God is not safe from the depredations of first-year medical students.

The narrator proceeds in a series of questions that speak to some of the deeper dilemmas of anatomy. Is dissection really necessary? As noted above, some medical schools, especially in the UK, have answered this question in the negative, using prosections and digital technologies to simulate cadaver dissection. The poem also asks whether it is possible to disassemble another human being (albeit one no longer living) without in some respect doing violence to the humanity of the self. And finally, how can one simultaneously engage in a practice so inherently disrespectful from any ordinary perspective and retain an attitude of respect, even reverence (as suggested in the first stanza) for the cadaver?

The poem then turns to a brief reflection on the cadaver's past life, contrasting the woodenness and deadness of a marionette (which evokes comparisons to Pinocchio, a wooden boy who magically came to life) with a poignant picture of a grandparent's last caress. Many student poems try to imagine the life of the cadaver as a way to connect with, humanize, and reconcile the present reality of the lifeless body with the living spirit that once inhabited it.

Perhaps the primary focus of this poem is the relationship between the student and the cadaver. The narrator expresses concern for the cadaver, and is worried about violation and disrespect. He is also concerned about whom he is becoming as a result of the dissection process. While he acknowledges that the goal of dissection is to "fill" him (presumably with knowledge), he admits to becoming empty – in his words, "hollow" (evoking TS Eliot's "hollow men"). The poet identifies a parallel process between self and cadaver that appears in many other student poems, with reference both to cadavers and to patients. Although he is dissecting the cadaver, he is also cutting into himself. In the process, his innocence is shattering, a theme that is also replicated in other poems. Here he answers the question that he posed in stanza two – there is something in the brutal nature of dissection (which at various points requires a fair amount of pulling apart) that does inflict violence on the perpetrator as well as on the "victim." The narrator also recognizes that the proper "place" in which to hold the "shards of my innocence" is "between my curiosity and my humanity." This insight pays tribute to the balance that students must strike between enthusiasm, excitement, the "joy of discovery" at the wonders that dissection reveals, and a basic human attitude of compassion and respect.

The next line, emphasized by its singular status, sounds in our ears like a cry for help. It represents a dramatic change in the voice of the poem, moving from discussing the 21 cadavers generally in the third person to appealing to one specific cadaver directly in the second person: "What is it *you* [italics added] want me to see?" The answers, which we can only infer but which are suggested by all that has gone before, are likely to be multiple. Yes, appreciate the intricacy, complexity, and marvel of the human body. Learn from me so that you can help others. But perhaps most importantly, see my humanity, see my wholeness as well as my brokenness. The final stanza confirms this deeper interpretation when the student concedes the ease with which he may succumb to the superficial – the endless studying and lectures, even his "own immature consumptions," the latter word referring literally to the student's "consumption" of the cadaver as well as referring metaphorically to an attitude of grasping and taking, and reminding us of the earlier reference to being filled. The student runs the risk of becoming so focused on "consuming" the cadaver that he may miss the essence of the cadaver – its humanity. In the final line of the poem, the narrator continues the intimacy that he has now established with his cadaver. "I'm trying" is a promise to the cadaver that he will do his best not to lose sight of what this process is really all about.

ANATOMY AS A RITE OF PASSAGE
Restitution stories

Anatomy is the mini-rite of which medical school itself represents the larger rite. In most of these poems, anatomy marks the transition from normal life to medical life – it is, in the words of a poem quoted in its entirety in Chapter 2, "The End of Innocence." What this student means is that anatomy is an impermeable barrier between the world of medicine and a "normal life" that is now irretrievably in the past. In another poem, the student acknowledges anatomy as their first real entry into the profession's mysteries. A more humorous take on this dramatic change in one's life is captured in a poem that refers to spending "quality time with our cadavers, our newest best friends." In another poem, the student experiences total immersion in anatomy, but despite the smells and long hours, desires it: "I never get enough." The narrator feels an "inseparable bond" with the cadavers. Just as dissection "consumes" the cadaver, the student is consumed by anatomy. It becomes her life, but in a way that enlivens her.

Living Anatomy By: Yassi Omidvar
UC Irvine, 2007

The fumes seep through my pores
burning my glands
rupturing every remaining cell that is left in my body.
Long hours . . .
The smell, taste, and feel of everything distorted as I leave the building
in my dirty, worn-out scrubs.
And yet again I go back the next day
forming an inseparable bond with the bodies of
someone's mother, father, brother, or sister.
I don't understand why I feel that I never get enough
of anatomy – tensor veli palatine, superior thyroid artery
bicepts brachii, levator ani – all the body parts floating

in my memory — so close yet so far
fading, reforming, and fading again . . .
The cycle is never ending
I am consumed by it all
And it is consumed by me.
This is the process of learning, feeling, breathing, and living
A-N-A-T-O-M-Y . . .

Rite-of-passage poems tend to be part of a restitution metaphor because of their strong implication of forward progress. Students endure the trial by fire that is anatomy, but the reward is a new and privileged way of life.

THE CADAVER AS A GUIDE AND TEACHER
Restitution stories
It was common for students to assume the first-person voice as the cadaver – in other words, speaking from the cadaver's point of view, addressing the medical student. Poems written in this voice are often restitution stories, adopting a reassuring, even protective tone towards the medical student. The restitution that is occurring takes the form of restoring "normalcy" to an initially brutalizing, non-normative, and disturbing act (dissection). Through the cadavers' voices, the students extend reassurance, protection, and validation to themselves. Students often imagine that their cadavers want to take care of them. One cadaver repeats the refrain, "It will be fine" – a comforting voice imagined by a student possibly filled with trepidation. In this poem, the soul of the cadaver kindly lingers until "the first cut" is successfully completed, getting the student off to a benevolently supervised start, so to speak. A similar poem written from the perspective of the medical student imagines the cadaver watching over her in a concerned, guiding role as she performs the dissection. In another poem, the cadaver gives students permission to proceed by telling them bluntly to "sharpen [their] knives."

Since the cadavers are generally much older than the students, it is natural that students should project on to them nurturing parental and even grandparental roles. For example, one poem conceptualizes the cadaver as a selfless father, a generous man who continues to give of himself even after death. In a poem that expresses a similarly nurturing stance on the part of the cadaver, the students are envisioned to "sail" on the "ocean" of the cadaver, who caresses them with a soothing "lullaby." Here the disconcerting sensation of unsteadiness is combined simultaneously with one of parental safety and comfort. Another student ("For OG", quoted later in this chapter) refers to the cadaver as "My first, my best teacher," and as a good parent: "You reared me / My medical father."

In a typical restitution story, dissection becomes an act of liberation / completion for the cadaver. The poem insightfully plays with near double entendres, mirroring the differing perspectives of student and cadaver. The student's anatomical terms remind the cadaver not of body parts but of aspects of living – its brevity, its suffering, and the vitality inherent in living. Nevertheless, the cadaver is reassuring ("You're going to help so many like me") and comforting. She liked sharing with the student, hopes the experience made the student a better person, overcomes the student's own doubts and confirms her worth ("I believe in you even if you don't"), and gives the student permission to carry on, to save lives. Mourning the cadaver is unnecessary ("Don't cry for me when I go"), because the cadaver has been "set free."

Untitled By: Natalie Hoffman
UC Irvine, 2007

What do I look like inside?
Now you know the parts I hide.
What do you think about the real me?
I feel like I've been set free

So many words you speak
Have double meaning to me.
Femoral! You shout
I hear Ephemeral, and think about
How short life is.
Brachial! You shout
I just think about my Breakdown.
Liver! You shout
And I just want to Live.

I know I'm a person you'll never forget.
Don't feel like you're in my debt
I'm glad I could share this with you
Now it's time to move on to something new.
So let me live on in your memories
Be part of your stories
And make you better than you were.

You're going to help so many like me
You followed your calling on what to be.
I believe in you even if you don't
As for failing, you won't.

So I guess it's time to say farewell
But I'm already in heaven or hell.
Don't cry for me when I go.
As for my fate, I already know.

Another restitution story, also told from the point of view of the cadaver, observes that the student seems more freaked out, panicked, and anxious than the cadaver. The cadaver points out the parallels between them ("I gave up my body for your sake / You give up your life for that of others") and recognizes that "I am no longer myself / Neither are you." But then the cadaver adds a reassuring restitutional note: "But my life was worthwhile / As will be yours." The sacrifices that the student is making will all prove to be worthwhile.

Under the knife By: Steven Le
UC Irvine, 2007

The bandage wrapped tightly around my head
    and yet, you feel lightheaded.

With eight snips my heart was loose
> but it is yours that jumps out of your chest with eight seconds left
> on question number eight

My lungs were lying on my legs so that you could see my sympathetic chain
> yet you are the one with the nerve to say that you cannot breathe.

You accidentally severed my median nerve
> but it is your hand that fumbles helplessly.

My brain was carelessly pried from my skull
> but it is your mind in disarray.

I gave up my body for your sake.
> You give up your life for that of others.

I am lifeless, I am underappreciated, I am no longer myself:
> Neither are you.

But my life was worthwhile.
> As will be yours.

In another representative poem, a student writes of standing "at the window to her [cadaver's] soul . . . / As I stood there, I saw him teaching." She imagines the cadaver smiling in "joyous wonder" at the good he has done and the knowledge he has conveyed, finally realizing that "he left behind a perfect gift." This student uses the cadaver's smile throughout the course to guide and reassure her.

Students also imagine the cadavers hoping that the students will be appreciative and respectful towards them in their work. This too represents a kind of restitution, in that the students feel that they can fulfill these hopes, thereby bringing a sense of civility and normalcy to the "interaction" between cadaver and student. In one poem written from the cadaver's point of view, the cadaver begs the student not to "fail" her, not to become "too familiar", or too judgmental about the cadaver's physical flaws and imperfections. After all, as the cadaver somewhat cattily reminds the student, *she* (the cadaver) is not making any judgments about *her* (the student). In another poem, the cadaver gratefully reports that the student "even held my hand at times / as if feeling sorry for having to cut through me." The students in many of these poems make promises to their cadaver that they will treat them with care and dignity. One student writes that although she knows her cadaver can't feel anything, she still tries to make her "comfortable" before each dissection.

THE STUDENT AS A CONDUIT OF KNOWLEDGE
Restitution stories

A related theme that emerges portrays the student as a conduit of knowledge flowing from cadaver through students to patients. The gift of one's body carries with it a responsibility, a "call to action" to make good use of what has been given. This responsibility sometimes elicits vows to "never forget" the anatomy experience. Students promise that they will learn as much as possible from the cadavers, that they will utilize this knowledge to improve the care of future patients, and that they will not betray the cadaver's trust established through the act of donation. One student called this an unending "chain of giving." In a poem written from the cadaver's point of view, the cadaver anticipates that students will "go on with knowledge to serve others," and recognizes that, in dissection, they have already begun this process of service. The cadaver has given "vast" knowledge and "shared selflessly." With effort and luck this gift might some day "turn back or deflect the advance of death." Such poems also represent restitution narratives – normalcy and balance are restored through the promise of respect and learning. In some of these poems, the student appears to make a bargain with the "devil" – the student can convert horror to good if she agrees to put what she learns from the cadaver to a beneficial and virtuous end.

Another student uses metaphors of "teacher" and "parent" to honor the selfless giving of the cadaver. This poem also links the cadaver to future patients. When the student finally sees a child with an earache or a grandmother with an arthritic knee, he will remember the first ear, the first knee that he saw, which belonged to the cadaver. Although the cadaver will never know any of the student's future patients, "Yet you gave even to them / Through me." The chain of giving is established and confirms and justifies the cadaver's dissection.

For OG By: Dipti Barot
Originally appeared in Body Electric *Anniversary Issue, 2005, pp. 18–19*
first published in Body Electric *Vol. XX, 2004*

You did not know me
Yet
You gave of yourself
Nay, you gave yourself
To me.
You did not know me
My first, my best teacher
You reared me
My medical father
Oh the sheer honor
I beheld your lungs
Held your heart
Cupped between trembling palms
You did not know me
My first, my best teacher
Yet you gave yourself
To me.
And years from now
You will not even know
the runny-nosed eight-year-old
Who comes in with an earache
My eyes will peer through light
While the imprint of your ear
That first ear to teach me
Will still remain
Etched in my brain.
You will not know

the seventy-five-year-old grandmother
Who presents with arthritis in her knee
Yet your knee
That first joint I study
Will still remain
Etched in my brain.
No, you will not know any of my patients
Yet you gave even to them
Through me.
No, you did not know me
And yet
Yet
I feel I know you
Sweet Soul
Who gives from the hereafter
You did not know me
Yet I feel I know you
Sweet Soul
Who gives the greatest gift
For ones
You do not know.

In another poem, the student promises to do his best to find all the connections that link what was learned in anatomy to patient care and to life. Yet another student vows to extract all that he can, to cherish the secrets and truths he gains from dissection, and to give them to others. One student writes a haiku visualizing, somewhat humorously, the gratefulness of future patients for whom students were forced to cram their brains so full of anatomy. This poem, too, implies a great chain of knowledge stretching from cadaver to student to patient. A poem in the voice of the cadaver builds on this image by lauding students, with perhaps a touch of grandiosity, as the future "healers of the world." The students' future greatness – the endpoint of the chain – is offered up as justification for the grim tasks associated with dissection. A similar restitutive theme views the cadaver as the student's first patient. One student writes about getting to know this "patient" through frequent "visits," and ironically notes that, from this patient at least, she has had "Not a single complaint to date." This is a conclusion that provides easy reassurance to the student in the face of natural anxieties about the complexities of actual patient interactions.

DONATION
Restitution stories

Other poems represent attempts to sublimate anxieties about the act of donation itself. There is an element of chaos in some of the poems that focus on donation, because students have difficulty believing that people would really donate their bodies if they knew in detail what awaited them. However, in the majority of cases, these poems usually take a restitution turn, imagining that the cadaver is happy to give, and often does so as a final teaching, or to give their life one last bit of meaning. Donation is viewed variously as a gift, a sacrifice, a sacred trust, a final defiance of death, and a final great accomplishment.

One author hopefully imagines that, from the cadaver's perspective, the anatomy lab is not the cold and sterile environment he experiences it to be, but rather a companionable, sociable place where cadavers chat animatedly about the day's dissections: "We laugh and dance in the anatomy lab at nights." In this rendering, the cadavers do not regret their decision to donate their bodies, but rather are glad that they could make this contribution to student learning: "Yes, you said, with pride or resignation or foresight/Yes, you may." In this poem, the donation is conceptualized as "one final mockery of death," and the cadaver smiles, "knowing that [he has] pulled one over on the old bastard." In another poem, the student imagines a dying patient consenting willingly to donation.

Still another poem, based on Hamlet's famous soliloquy, has the cadaver speculating: "To give – or not to give, that is the question." This ambivalent cadaver ultimately concludes that donors' motives are altruistic, and decides to proceed. A somewhat different approach, expressed in a poem entitled "Redemption, the hard way," uses the voice of a cadaver, a veteran suffering from post-traumatic stress disorder, to speculate that perhaps he agreed to have students "cut me to pieces" because "I need some good to come out of all this/You gotta make this count." In this interpretation, donation is conceptualized as a final act to make life meaningful.

Another poem, based on Robert Frost's famous poem, speculates about the cadaver's choice to donate, wondering whether the donor felt afraid, was religious, or experienced pain. The narrator concludes by considering making the same decision at the end of life, but is ultimately noncommittal: "One day I may make the same leap/But I have promises to keep/And so much living left to reap/And miles to go before I sleep." This poem, too, recognizes not only the living ahead for this student, but also the "promises" that she must fulfill, including presumably one to put to good use the gift of the cadaver.

Stopping by Lab on a Lonely Evening By: Janessa Law
UC Irvine, 2007

What life you lived I'll never know.
Your body lies in this lab room though
You'll never see me standing near
With thanks for the knowledge I'll sow.

But how were you not filled with fear
Knowing that you'd be laying here
Unable to utter a sound
Even if pain should start to sear?

Had you no want of hallowed ground
Having never felt Him around?
Or, even if my cut went deep
To your flesh were you never bound?

One day I may make the same leap.
But I have promises to keep
And so much living left to reap
And miles to go before I sleep.

THE CADAVER AS A PERSON
Witnessing

Students often speculate about the person of the cadaver. Who *was* this body, now so lifeless, preserved in formalin, before them? In these poems, the tone is quite different from the restitution narratives discussed previously. These poems are a kind of witnessing, because there is less possibility of resolution. Rather they are an act of imagined testimony to the life of the patient. Since students are often not provided with identifying information about their cadavers, they frequently give free rein to their imaginations, and envision whole lives for their cadavers – wives, husbands, children, military service, jobs, losses, dreams, and hopes. They contrast these imagined passions, worries, and inspirations with the empty corpse that is being dissected. Several of the poems contain questions directed towards the cadaver: Why did you donate? How did your family feel? Who were you? Where are you now? How do you feel about what the students are doing?

A representative poem imagines the life of the cadaver through touching various organs, muscles, and veins, and fantasizing what these body parts might have meant. Ultimately, however, for the student, this exercise falls short. Although he studies the body with careful attention, and honors the trust bestowed on him, he regrets that he never knew the cadaver's smile, the aliveness of the cadaver. The poem is a witnessing to the "gaping" emptiness left in the wake of a vanished life.

I'll never know By: Sumudu Dissanayake
UC Irvine, 2007

I cradled your heart in my palms
Imagined the pulsations breathing warmth into your day
I strung the muscles of your hand
Enchanted by the notes resonating from your violin
I peeled away the thinnest of skin
Soothed the grimaces of papercuts long forgotten
I followed the narrowest of vessels
Wondered if my own were equally tortuous
I stared at the dark nodules around your lung
Felt my stomach drop as you first grasped the news
I studied the tracts followed by your children
Saw them still waking every day with you in their thoughts
I honored your trust in sharing with me your everything
Filled in a few gaps left by nature's variation
But all the rest
Remained forever gaping
I will always regret
Never knowing
Your smile

Another author recognizes that the fundamental question "Who are you?" can only be answered to a very limited extent by dissection. In the following poem, the student uses the simultaneously beautiful and horrifying simile of creating origami out of human flesh. He knows that the body tells certain stories – of disease and of repair – but not the stories he most wants to hear, nothing of the cadaver's dreams. Without seeing the "hidden" face, there can be no full "knowing." Although the student's efforts are all directed towards stripping away the layers of the cadaver, ultimately he remains undiscoverable. The poem is suffused with the longing of the narrator to experience his cadaver as a person.

Confession By: Michael Doo

Originally appeared in Plexus *2002, p. 3. UC Irvine School of Medicine*

That finally-first cut, not deep enough
Folding of skin to the side, like some twisted
origami played with human flesh
Picking, picking, picking, picking, picking

Once gleaming instruments of steady
deconstruction
Now encrusted with biological remains
Work to fill bright red bags costumed in their
proclamations of danger and avoidance

You are at once
A careful explosion of autumn-greens and yellows
reds and browns
But at times too recognizable all the same

Your scars and staples and solid masses
What stories your body tells me
A history of surgeries, and diseases
But nothing of your dreams

The smell is like hickory smoke
Sickly sweet and oh-so sticky
I wash myself religiously

Some choose to tie you with string
impale you with nails
Tag you with labels
The paper windowed by grease

My stomach rumbles during almost every lab
I eat meat
But I think of you and hesitate

Your shaved head, shrouded
I have sliced through your skin, fingered your
organs, broken through your bones
Still I do not know your face

Why did you choose this?
Did your family object?
Would you care what I do now?

Such thoughts to be cast aside
As part of the recipe:
Heaping layers upon myself while stripping yours away

I stand in the twilight
That first step toward isolation?
I will grow into this responsibility.

Students yearn to "know" the cadaver more fully, and try to achieve this through the only path they have available – the body itself. This effort to attain personal knowledge of the cadaver is best understood as a kind of witnessing that affirms the vanished humanity of the cadaver. Often students try to imagine this person through the few details they are able to discover from the body itself – tattoos, nail polish, the scars left from surgeries, implants, physical anomalies. In the following poem, the student contemplates a tattoo on the arm of her cadaver, and fantasizes a life for him – sexual, exciting . . . and memorable. The outline of a mermaid becomes infinitely more intriguing to the student than the deltoid muscle on which it rests. It is the narrow doorway through which she might slip to encounter his life, part by imagined part, much as she dissects the actual parts of his body.

Untitled By: Diana Katsman
Originally appeared in Plexus *2003, p. 29, UC Irvine School of Medicine*

One afternoon of his life
Was spent on a mermaid
Tattooed onto his left deltoid
So I could study her in more detail
Than the deltoid she is tattooed on.

Once, perhaps more, he was worried
Rushed, exalted, thrilled, inspired . . .
Wishing it to go on forever
To skip the thrust
That will collapse his tomorrow into dust.

Now he rests motionless on a steel table
While a group of studious medical students
Myself included
Are picking apart his every part

Detail by scrupulous detail
Like perhaps once a jealous girlfriend
Picked his character apart
Part by scrutinized part.

That is one way to prolong your stay here
Impressing yourself onto the memories of those
Whose time has not yet come
Mermaid by mermaid.

Students often write about the hands of the cadaver, and their face, which seem to evoke emotions of connectedness and awareness of humanity. The face is particularly mysterious and haunting, because it is often shrouded until the final days of dissection. As one student observes, without seeing the face, there is never the possibility of full "knowing." Another student uses the experience of holding the cadaver's heart in her hands to speculate about the cadaver's feelings and life. She wonders about the dreams, fears, joys, and sorrows that this heart experienced, and employs the metaphor of the heart as a flower to better understand the man that was: "Was his heart a shy bud, peering out suspiciously to the world before him / Or a bold blossom, sharing its beauty without inhibition?" She realizes that while some of the heart's secrets can be discovered by scalpel and probe, others can only be understood through the imagination.

PHYSICAL INTIMACY
Witnessing (resistance) stories

Some students tackle the delicate issue of the necessary physical intimacy between student and cadaver. After all, it is a relationship in which one person spends a great deal of time with his or her hands inside the body cavity of the other (former) person. Exploring this topic is another example of witnessing, with a specific emphasis on resistance. Even acknowledging that such intimacy exists resists the dominant narrative of dichotomous separation between living and dead, and dares to cross a seemingly impervious boundary by suggesting a physical intimacy between cadaver and student. In one such poem, as the student develops "the confidence of a surgeon" and her skills increase, the cadaver wonders, in a subjugated, implicitly sexualized question, "Have you mastered me?" Another poem also uses sexualized language in addressing the cadaver: "You did not know me / Yet / You gave of yourself / Nay, you gave yourself / To me."

Another poem is more callous. It starts out with the student telling his cadaver, "I can't get bogged down in anything / Beyond a purely physical relationship" because, as he asserts, he doesn't have "the time." Yet in the middle of the poem, he interrupts his distancing and self-protective statements to marvel at the beauty of the cadaver's body. He notices, almost against his will, that he "treasures" the cadaver, and wonders how he can dissect this precious body. However, by the end of the poem the student has retreated again emotionally: "I am under a great deal of stress / And I just don't have time for anything more / Than a physical relationship." His thoughts turn involuntarily towards themes of belonging and violation, but he fears such thinking because it may lead him towards a more intimate connection with the cadaver. The language of this poem is reminiscent of negotiating a sexual relationship that the speaker wants to be contained within strictly physical, non-emotional bounds.

A different student recognizes that she is "exposed" to her cadaver, just as the cadaver is exposed to her. She acknowledges the cadaver as a former sexual being: "A man once despaired / To hold you so close." She compares this enforced familiarity to the intimacy of love and sexuality, and in fact, the addressing of the poem in the second person to the cadaver rather than the lover intimates that she may feel closer to the former than to the latter. This author finds multiple parallels between her lover's actions and her own actions towards the cadaver. She realizes that both the body of the cadaver and her own emotional vulnerability are exposed.

Exposed By: Sarah Mourra
Originally appeared in Plexus *2005, p. 10, UC Irvine School of Medicine*

Thick lenses
Thinly veil
Burning eyes that watch
His hand brushing your hand
As his had brushed mine
Tracing figure eights
On a flowered and fluttering tablecloth
Blown by warm wind
On an empty hilltop street.
Hands that hold your heart
As his had held mine
Refreshing its tattered caverns gently
In a warm bath
Extracting dark blood
That had stopped cold
For so long.
Stinging eyes watch him cover
Your mottled veined skin with a thin cheesecloth
And remember
Him pulling the sticky linens of this morning
Over my nakedness.

In another interesting poem, the student longs for a lover to help to mitigate the stresses and strains of anatomy – a sweet smell to balance out the fetidness, someone to share a meal with, someone to drive home to, to have sex with. He would practice his anatomy on her sweet, supple, and alive body: "You see, this is a case of need/A case of academic necessity." If he had a real body that he loved to pay attention to, he thinks all the anatomy would really sink in, and that he would return again and again to everything he had learned. And if pure memorization of anatomy was too boring, he would invent stories that he would tell his lover to amuse and fascinate her. Listening to her heart would not merely be a matter of lub-dub, lub-dub, but of listening "to the poetry/ your heart writes every day." If this were a moral universe, "the only just reward/for a cadaver's cold body/would be a warm one/waiting for me at home." This poem of yearning is a form of chaos narrative, a cry for help in confronting the loneliness of the world.

IDENTIFICATION WITH THE CADAVER
Witnessing (resistance) stories
The sense of a bond between cadaver and student, and even identification, comes through in many poems. Identification with the cadaver is most often a form of resistance because the proper identification should be, according to the dominant medical discourse, with the physician, not the patient, and particularly not with the cadaver – a contaminated and unclean body. Defying this convention, one student writes that the essence of the cadaver has become part of the student, and continues by

asserting that student and cadaver have a depth of relationship that even lovers lack. This view stresses the mutuality of the connection between cadaver and student. While the student "owns" the cadaver for the period of the anatomy class, the cadaver also owns "a piece of" the student, because the cadaver is now part of the student's life. They share a special intimacy. Another student marvels at the togetherness of student and cadaver: "My spirit can still hold you in rapture," the cadaver tells the student.

In the following poem, a student describes a late night visit to the anatomy lab. She is searching "for that one structure" that will make both the cadaver and herself complete. The poem expresses identification with the cadaver's body – it is her own, "as complex and torn up" as she is. Paradoxically, the student seeks completion of self through dissection of the cadaver. Although she is exhausted and desperate, she will continue the exploration. Instinctively, she understands that she must discover something in this process of taking apart that will result in wholeness.

Picture This By: Katherine Freeman
Originally published in Body Language: Poems of the Medical Training Experience *edited by Neeta Jain, Dagan Coppock and Stephanie Brown Clark, 2006, p. 23 Reprinted with the permission of BOA Editions, Ltd. www.boaeditions.org*

Picture this:

Two a.m., Thursday night. I'm trying to find myself
amidst a brachial plexus of fibers; my nerves
shredded from picking at a torn-up stylopharyngeus, muscles
aching from overarching my secondary curvature, back
stiff as the epiglottis pierced with my blunt scalpel.

Yet I keep standing, searching, for that one structure
that will make this body complete, that will make my self
feel found in this body that I now feel is my own
as complex and torn up.

JOURNEY OF CADAVER AND STUDENT
Journey stories

Anatomy is also conceptualized as a meeting of two people who will journey together and experience adventure, risks, and the unveiling of secrets. This is obviously a paradigmatic journey narrative. In these poems the cadaver is most similar to the classic wise guide in journey narratives – "a teacher of truth" who helps the hero to grow and mature, as well as teaching esoteric knowledge that is unavailable to most people. A different poem notes that the cadavers will "mold us into healers." They teach not only anatomy and pathology, but deeper wisdom as well. As one student writes ironically to his cadaver, "You opened yourself up to us . . ." to teach unselfishness and altruism, putting others above self.

In this model, the cadaver is one among many along the path that the student has begun to travel. Student and cadaver adventure together for a time and collaborate on specific tasks. Then, however, the student moves forward, to further training, and the cadaver is left behind. One student affirms for the cadaver that this portion of the journey "we take together." Another notes that for a period cadaver and student must work together to pursue knowledge. However, in this poem the student also realizes that their shared path will come to an end. Cadaver and student will eventually part to follow very different futures. In this case there is the clear recognition that the relationship between student and cadaver is temporary.

Transcendence stories

Occasionally, there is a moment of transcendence, an undeserved experience of grace. In one such poem, the narrator's consciousness shifts as he realizes that he must accept dissection as "Macabre and beautiful at the same time." The poem concludes that the experience has added immeasurable meaning to the way that the student understands life. In a similar poem that moves from journey to transcendence, the student first appears mercilessly dissecting the cadaver. The author introduces the metaphor of a valet bringing in the suitcases (the cadavers in their vinyl bags); unpacking the bag parallels the dissecting of the cadaver. However, although a valet can be conceptualized as a low-level servant, objectified as a means to an end (not unlike the way that students can think of the cadaver), the metaphor also introduces the idea of service in a deeper sense, and suggests ways in which the student may serve both the cadaver and perhaps future patients. In "gazing" at the cadaver, the student experiences a moment of transformational awareness. The cadaver is "exalted," and the student is "exonerated." As a result of this occurrence, the student is healed.

EMOTIONAL RESPONSES TO DISSECTION

Students catalogue a range of emotions that they experience during the anatomy course, including sadness, shock, gratefulness, happiness, enjoyment, amazement, concern, curiosity, disgust, guilt, and shame. Expression of emotions tends to be a cry for help that either stays the same, resolves into a restitution story, describes a journey, or occasionally achieves a kind of transcendence (awe and wonder). A handful of students are persistently fearful and troubled. A typical poem expresses fear, powerlessness, and a sense of being overwhelmed. For another, the emotional journey commences with the student feeling frustrated and disheartened, but later she begins to enjoy and appreciate the experience of dissection. Another student expresses a similar trajectory of worry and trepidation resolving into curiosity and amazement.

Transcendence stories

The most common emotion expressed by students towards the cadaver is gratitude. Students often marvel that people are willing to donate their bodies for dissection purposes, and are filled with appreciation and thankfulness for this opportunity for hands-on learning. These poems convey an elevated emotional experience that often seems closer to transcendence than restitution. It is as though the student has moved beyond guilt, beyond rationalization. The student experiences dissection as a great gift, and stands in awe of the almost unimaginable sacrifice that the donor has made. One student refers to dissection as an "honor." Another cadaver is eulogized as a "Sweet Soul/Who gives from the hereafter . . . /Sweet Soul/Who gives the greatest gift/For ones/You do not know."

Other common emotions are awe and wonder, both being examples of a transcendent narrative. During the anatomy experience, several students are struck by the sacredness of the human body, or at least filled with awe at its complexity. One student experiences this when she holds a human heart in her hands. Another student realizes that what he used to think of merely as bones have become "the map of a bright and sudden life/ the soft powder a butterfly sheds from its wings/before it arcs above the trees." The bones are transformed into an awe-inspiring map that guides this student in an amazing exploration. Students describe the knowledge that they gain about specific nerves and organs as "intimate and special." In one less usual counter-example, the student laments that, through dissection, the body has lost its mystery for her. She addresses the cadaver directly, complaining that she can no longer see "you as simply you" because the mask guarding the secrets of the internal body has been peeled away.

VIOLATION REQUIRING FORGIVENESS
Chaos stories

Although most students view anatomy as a generous gift for learning, a few students find the experience unremittingly appalling, even sacrilegious. The sense of violation is predominantly a cry for help, a reflection of the chaos that the student is experiencing. Anatomy has left these students feeling part of something ugly and inhumane. There is no sense of resolution or absolution. One student, for example, perceives dissection as killing and a violation: "A hundred times I killed you, more." He reports that he "thought nothing" of splitting the cadaver in half, and laughed when the heart slipped to the floor. He didn't worry when he misplaced a lung. He writes callously, "You were nothing to me", but then caught a glimpse of the cadaver's eyes and realized that the cadaver had been watching his disrespectful, heartless behavior. Now the student confesses to having committed a crime, and seeks pardon. A similar poem is structured so that the words "Please Forgive Me Father For I Have Sinned" are both integrated into the poem and can be read vertically down its margin. Here dissection is conceptualized as a hubristic, self-gratifying quest seeking knowledge, secrets, and gifts, but troublingly, it is also a sin, for which the writer beseeches forgiveness. This poem concludes with the powerful and disturbing image of the student realizing that, beneath the shroud that covers the cadaver's face, the cadaver may be grinning at the transgression the student is about to commit.

Other poems also express concern about the "wrongness" of dissection. In one poem, the author argues that the cadavers should be in heaven instead of in the anatomy lab. He is wracked with guilt at having participated in their mutilation, at having lost sight of the "real worth" of the cadavers, their humanity, and at having lost his guilt. For this student, although he has experienced death before, there remains a vast gulf between what happens to beloved dead and what happens to cadavers. Yet it is not for the dissection itself so much as for this moral lapse that he pleads for forgiveness, moving from the distance (which he speculates may have been necessary to learn the requisite anatomical lessons) of the third-person voice to a direct and intimate second-person address.

Forgive Me By: Daniel Chun
UC Irvine, 2003

Death surrounds me
Sixteen entities within a room
Clothed in blue and white garments

It is not heaven that they experience
but instead the cold steel of the blade
I feel guilt, guilt having been lost over time.
A question arises, Will they forgive me?

Yes, I have experienced death.
Grandfather, great grandmother
Fellow high school student
Victims of something inescapable.
Lives lost to the wind
Returning to the earth
To decay into nothingness.
Life is precious I know
I claim to have experience.

Yet these bodies fallen to blackness
They lay before us still and mutilated.
Looking upon them, cold and pale
We rank the bodies according to
their color and smell.
The ease of isolating and identifying
has become their worth.
How sad that I have forgotten
What these men and women have endured.

I have lost sight of your real worth.
I ask for your forgiveness.

Perhaps it is a necessity that
We distance ourselves from their plight
To fully learn the intricacies
Of their physical domain.
I am thankful for their sacrifice
To be torn apart and sliced to pieces
So that we could perhaps one day
Save someone from the darkness.

I will not again forget your value and worth.
Forgive me.

One powerful poem addresses the cadaver as "our lady of the tank," evoking intimations of divinity and holiness, and notes her "graveless state." She makes him think of the "trivial time" we have on earth going from birth to grave. The student wonders whether the cadaver "submits to the ingracious exploration of fools," or rather despises "our semester of eternity." After the final exam, there is literally nothing left – the "blanks" (of the exam) have been filled in, but the cadaver's skull is empty, as is the student's thanks. The cadaver is described as "gross," "petty," "decayed," "displayed," "plucked," "pickled," "shredded" and a "mess."

SUPPRESSION OF AND DETACHMENT FROM EMOTIONS
Chaos stories

Several students try to cope with the troubling aspects of anatomy by detaching from their emotions. Detachment represents an effort to create a restitution narrative, acquiescence to the dominant discourse that draws a clear distinction between doctor and patient, student and cadaver. Occasionally, the cadaver is dehumanized in an effort to cultivate this emotional distance. Instead of being a patient, teacher, or friend, the cadaver is turned into a lesson, an instrument, a device to train students, a kind of formerly alive but now very much inanimate Harvey (mechanical life-size model used to teach students about heart and lung function). This kind of objectification is a defense mechanism to protect against chaos, and supports the restitution story of maintaining firm boundaries as the method of tolerating the disturbing aspects of dissection.

Most poems about emotional detachment ultimately take the form of a chaos narrative, because their attempts to disconnect fail or make them disillusioned with medicine and disappointed in themselves. One poem written from this perspective is primarily characterized by the emotion of dread, and the student can think only of "dissected parts and vanishing faces." She dreams of cadavers and dreads these dreams. This student briefly wonders about the person of the cadaver, but acknowledges that she prefers this question to remain unanswered. Another student's poem reflects her embarrassment that on her first exposure to the anatomy lab, she runs out and bursts into tears. She subsequently deals with her agitation by suppressing all feelings and tricking herself into thinking that "the bodies weren't real / And I wasn't supposed to feel." At the end of the class she expresses the wish that she had done things differently. In particular, she writes, "I wish I could have felt / But there was no time for feeling." This poem conveys the impression that emotions are inappropriate in medicine.

In the previously quoted poem, "Forgive Me," the student admits that, although he has experienced death before through the loss of family members and friends, when he looks at the cadavers, he quickly forgets their humanity and suffering. He and his peers catalogue them remorselessly by color and smell. This same student ponders whether it is "a necessity that / We distance ourselves from their plight" in order to learn the requisite anatomy. Like many of her fellow students, another student reports flagging compassion for her cadaver in the face of curiosity about the cadaver's implants. Yet another student defiantly boasts of her intestinal fortitude, and insists that the sights and smells of anatomy have not in the least affected her ability to eat meals (a common student complaint). In the last line of her poem she agonises as to whether this vaunted imperturbability has not turned her "heart to stone."

Dinner By: Vinita Jain
UC Irvine, 2001

Somehow things aren't as gross as they used to be,
Since I started anatomy.

I can talk about dissecting scrotums at dinner,
And how penile implants don't make one a sinner.

Maybe retching versus vomiting is not appropriate,
But it doesn't seem to bother me one bit.

Cracking ribs or vertebrae is no problem,
As long as bone marrow doesn't ooze out of 'em.

Isn't it funny how this steak looks like pectoralis major?
But it sure does have some great flavor!

I know diarrhea is not a popular subject over dessert,
But I'm trying to tell you what makes your stomach hurt.

I hope my heart has not turned to stone
because I always end up eating alone.

Yet another poem of this type warns the cadaver not to reveal his name or who he was to the student. Even more directly, the student admonishes the cadaver: "Do not try to move me." He arrogantly asserts that all he needs are his "damned" utensils, and professes not to care about any other aspect of the cadaver. Later he admits that he does not dare to risk thinking of the cadaver as a person, because it would make it impossible to continue his grisly task.

Witnessing stories

At times, students are able to step back and question the benefits of emotional detachment. For example, one student challenges the boundary implicit in emotional detachment – that is, the creation of a clear distinction between student and cadaver, and between life and death. This poem points out that really very little separates the cadaver from the student: "All it takes is one little tear / a pinprick in your glove / and we are / one." The "barriers" erected to keep the student distinct from the cadaver, such as masks and gloves, are woefully insufficient. When the student tries to reduce the cadaver to a dismembered body, the cadaver intervenes, chiding the student for not taking the time to really look at her, really recognize her, one person to another.

Still another poem reflects on the narrator's increasing callousness, and notes a devolution in his thinking about the cadavers from "dead people" to "bodies." As the bodies were deconstructed, their "remnants of self" disappeared. The student perceives that he is participating in a process of "debauchery," and employs a Darwinian metaphor of lions devouring a zebra. He recognizes that both lions and students feel "utter satiation" upon completion of their "respective butcheries." This student witnesses the brutality of dissection, while also recognizing it as a necessary means to a valuable end.

Untitled By: Nikhraj Brar
UC Irvine, 2007

When I first entered the anatomy lab 5 months ago, I saw dead people.
Now all I see are bodies.
Any remnant of their self that ties them
to their former worldly existence
has nearly disappeared in my eyes.
Limbs severed, bones broken, ribs cracked
organs removed, skin cut –
no, it's not a pride of lions who have devoured a zebra
on the open plains of Africa.

This debauchery was done by med students.
Med students? Debauchery?
Surely the med students did not rip these bodies to shreds
like the savage beasts of the wild.
They made fine cuts. Deep incisions.
They used every precaution possible
to preserve some semblance of normal bodies.
And of course the no brainer . . .
the med students did not kill the people
who once inhabited these bodies.
Yet who can blame the hungry lion?
Ah! But these med students are not so different
from the beastly lions after all.
Both feel utter satiation
after they have done their respective butcheries –
the lions fill their starving stomachs with a full meal
not knowing when they will next have this feeling again.
The med students fill their minds with knowledge
that will serve them a lifetime.
And oh so much knowledge has been gained!
As anatomy comes to a close
I realize that although I see bodies
I am always mindful that they belonged to people.
As the lions finish their meal
and leave the carcass for the vultures
and wait for their next kill;
the med students will always be grateful
and mindful of the individuals
who once so kindly donated their earthly remains
to the pursuit of knowledge.

PHILOSOPHICAL REFLECTIONS ON LIFE, DEATH, AND LOVE
Transcendence stories

Some students are moved by their experience in gross anatomy to reflect on ultimate questions. Most of these poems are best conceptualized as transcendent narratives, because the students move beyond their daily concerns to awareness of what makes life truly meaningful. In a typical poem, the student is struck by the preserved body as a lumpish "mass," in contrast with the meaningful loved and loving person who must once have existed. She concludes that the difference between a cadaver and a human is simply love – human and divine – that creates bridges across souls and between life and death. If we do not acknowledge the mysterious breadth and depth of our existence, we will be limited within the finite borders of flesh and bone.

Life, death and the in-between By: Roya Saisan
Originally appeared in Plexus, *2004, p. 29, UC Irvine School of Medicine*

A body which lies upon the table
A mass of tissue, bone, cartilage

Caught in a tug-of-war between
its preservation by our chemicals and putrid decay

It is caught between what it was in this life
On the surface of the Earth
And what it was once before
Absolutely
Nothing

Although it is this mass we study
Learn meticulously hover over and inhale
It is not
The dad who adores us
The mom who loves us
The man who holds us

It is a mass.

What keeps us afloat in this state, life, is beyond
any border of vertebra
any border of pleura
Beyond all the earth
and the moon and the sky
Beyond all comprehension
by our inadequate imaginations

What keeps us afloat in the space of air
is just what we cannot see
lying still in a puddle of phenol on a steel table

Love
Between the souls of this existence
The breath of life, death and the unknown
Beauty
Within every soul that blooms

Desire
To know the creator of that soul

God
For if we do not acknowledge
the depth of our own existence
it only reaches that distance
dictated between the borders of our skin.

Similar thoughts are expressed by a student who finds "a glimpse of immortality" in his cadaver. Even in a poem that begins by expressing only an intellectual commitment to the acquisition of knowledge, towards its conclusion its author begins to wonder what it is he is really looking for in the act of dissection: "And can I be sure / The Answers are buried / At the center of you?" Another poem reflects on the cycle of death and renewal, and sees anatomy as part of this recurring process. This poem uses the metaphor of a phoenix to symbolize both cadaver and medical student, each rising from their own imperfect ashes. This image soothes the student's anguished mind because in it he finds healing and an affirmation of life. Another meditation on the cycle of life and death frames death as liberation. It sets us free from the karmic cycle: "round and round and round . . . / Until suddenly . . . / No longer they no longer we no longer you no longer me . . . / but Free."

One student starts by "reflecting" on "passing" anatomy, then turns this reflection into an opportunity to explore various implications of reflection – as careful thought, as anatomical technique ("reflect the fascia"), as (expected but undiscoverable) mirror image between student and cadaver, and in the sense that everything that ensues eventually will "reflect on" the narrator well or poorly, in terms of how she treats, talks to, and touches her patients. In a similar manner, she also explores the various implications of passing, as in passing the class, the anatomy knowledge so painfully gained passing away through the erosion of memory, the class itself coming to an end and passing away, and the passing on of the cadaver, who has died. The narrator speculates about what will be left in the reflection of others when the class, the cadaver, and her life itself are gone.

Reflections on Passing By: Meghann Kaiser
UC Irvine, 2003

If anatomy is a rite of passage
(Assuming I pass)
Where will I end up? And what will I take away
In passing?

"Reflect the fascia"
The second line of any given protocol
As if it might take you, oh, thirty seconds or so
These three words account for three hours.
And then you're finished
And the finished product
Looks remarkably little like the atlas ideal.
Nights of neck-numbing frustration over bodies and books
Yet I know that in six months
Immersed in the panic of
Pharmacology, pathology, and microbiology
I will be lucky if I can still find my own knee.
Even now, I cannot help but wonder
If it is not already
Before my own eyes
Passing away.

I cannot see my own reflection.
And I suppose I must have expected to.
But the dead woman's face, when I finally dared look
Was already peeled, chipped, and defrocked to its
Intimate, muscular origins
And very little else.
I suppose this is the inevitable exchange

That at the expense of discovering a tendon of mastication
I can no longer tell how old she is.
She has no wrinkles
No evidence of ever having experienced life
Or sheer time, if nothing else. Or reality.
And yet, I know at some point all this was there.
So where did it go
When she finally
Passed away?

It will all reflect on me.
For the time being, anyway.
How I treat, talk to, and touch my patients
How it is I live when I have left here, and her.
This existence, evaporated off a frozen face
Now reinvented in my own.
But how could I expect to have any more than she had?
Or why should I think I will hoard it
When she has more than taught me
All this time spent
In lab and in life
Remains only in the flicker of reflection
Not knowledge, but knowledge gently taught
Not life, but life lived for renewal of my friend
Continues to live
When all of this
Passes away.

SUMMARY

These poems confirm that the anatomy course is indeed an important training ground for various aspects of professionalism, including relationship with the cadaver, how to balance enthusiasm for learning with respect and compassion, and how to preserve a humane sense of self. The writings of these students also suggest that anatomy is emotionally demanding – not simply "stressful," but requiring them to ask and attempt large questions of who they are and what the practice of medicine is all about.

Students sometimes conceptualize the anatomy course as a rite of passage – their first initiation into their chosen profession. These are generally restitution stories that try to create a happy, fulfilled outcome. When speaking in the voice of the cadaver, poems are usually encouraging, reassuring, permission-giving, nurturing, guiding, and sometimes even admiring and respectful in relation to the students. Students often view their cadaver as their first guide and teacher, who most often tells them reassuring stories of restitution. Often students seem to engage in a process of restitutive bargaining. They make promises of respect and learning to their cadavers and rationalize dissection because of what it will contribute to their future ability to help the living through the knowledge they have gained. When students speculate about the cadaver as a person, they are more likely to tell stories of witnessing. Often they look for clues in the physical body to help them to imagine a life they will never know. They are less focused on their own anxieties and more committed to paying tribute to the life that was. Donation is an anxiety-ridden subject, because students are not sure whether donors really understand what happens to their bodies during dissection. These poems vacillate between chaos and restitution.

There can be an intimate connection between cadaver and student, an awareness of being involved in a journey that they take together, a sense of bondedness and possibly identification, and there are even issues of physical intimacy that arise when students contemplate their relationships with their cadavers. Such poems witness honestly to the complexity of their connection with the cadaver. Students experience a variety of emotions in response to dissection. The most common of these is gratitude, but they also register awe and wonder. Some students are overcome with feelings of horror and guilt. Expressing their revulsion in chaos poems, these students perceive dissection as a sacrilegious violation that requires forgiveness. Sometimes students try to cope with the anxiety engendered by dissection through suppression of and detachment from emotions. In the service of this goal, the cadaver is at times dehumanized and regarded simply as a vehicle for learning. However, poems of detachment and dehumanization usually end in chaos because the students do not find these emotional strategies morally satisfactory. Occasionally the anatomy experience gives rise to philosophical reflections on the purpose and meaning of life.

REFERENCES

1 Lempp HK. Perceptions of dissection by students in one medical school: beyond learning about anatomy. A qualitative study. *Medical Education* 2005; **39**: 318–25.

2 Swartz WJ. Using gross anatomy to teach and assess professionalism in the first year of medical school. *Clinical Anatomy* 2006; **19**: 437–41.

3 Rizzolo LJ, Stewart WB. Should we continue teaching anatomy by dissection when . . .? *Anatomical Record Part B: The New Anatomist* 2006; **289**: 215–18.

4 Kostas TR, Jones DB, Schiefer TK, *et al.* The use of a video interview to enhance gross anatomy students' understanding of professionalism. *Medical Teacher* 2007; **29**: 264–6.

5 Bender J. From theater to laboratory. *MSJAMA* 2002; **287**: 1179.

6 Wenger DCK. It's not your parents' anatomy course. *Academic Physician and Scientist* 2006; March issue: 1–3.

7 Rizzolo LJ. Human dissection: an approach to interweaving the traditional and humanistic goals of medical education. *Anatomical Record* 2002; **269**: 242–8.

8 Finkelstein P, Mathers L. Post-traumatic stress among medical students in the anatomy dissection laboratory. *Clinical Anatomy* 1990; **3**: 219–26.

9 Horne DJ de L, Tiller JWG, Eizenberg N, *et al.* Reactions of first-year medical students to their initial encounter with a cadaver in the dissecting room. *Academic Medicine* 1990; **65**: 645–6.

10 Dickinson GE, Lancaster CJ, Winfield IC, *et al.* Detached concern and death anxiety of first-year medical students: before and after gross anatomy course. *Clinical Anatomy* 1997; **10**: 201–7.

11 McGarvey MA, Farrell T, Conroy RM, *et al.* Dissection: a positive experience. *Clinical Anatomy* 2001; **14**: 227–30.

12 Dinsmore CE, Daugherty S, Zeitz HJ. Student responses to the gross anatomy laboratory in a medical curriculum. *Clinical Anatomy* 2001; **14**: 231–6.

13 O'Carroll RE, Whiten S, Jackson D, *et al.* Assessing the emotional impact of cadaver dissection on medical students. *Medical Education* 2002; **36**: 550–4.

14 Saylam C, Coskunol H. Orientation lesson in anatomy education. *Surgical and Radiologic Anatomy* 2005; **27**: 74–7.

15 Stewart S, Charon R. Art, anatomy, learning, and living. *JAMA* 2002; **287**: 1182.

16 Francis NR, Lewis W. What price dissection? Dissection literally dissected. *Journal of Medical Ethics: Medical Humanities* 2001; **27**: 2–9.

17 Lachman N, Pawlina W. Integrating professionalism in early medical education: the theory and application of reflective practice in the anatomy curriculum. *Clinical Anatomy* 2006; **19**: 456–60.

18 Coulehan JL, Williams PC, Landis D. The first patient: reflections and stories about the anatomy cadaver. *Teaching and Learning in Medicine* 1995; **7**: 61–6.

19 Tschernig T, Schlaud M, Pabst R. Emotional reactions of medical students to dissecting human bodies: a conceptual approach and its evaluation. *Anatomical Record* 2000; **261**: 11–13.

20 Leung KK, Lue BH, Lu KS. Students' evaluation on a two-stage anatomy curriculum. *Medical Teacher* 2006; **28**: 59–63.

5 Am I a Doctor Yet? Becoming a Physician – Part 1

As I discussed in Chapter 1, entering the profession of medicine involves undergoing a lengthy process of acculturation that begins with students' matriculation and extends through medical school to residency and beyond. Students are both fascinated by and confused about what it means to be a doctor, and how to accomplish this goal. The meta-question on the minds of many of them is "How do I become a physician?" They may not ask it directly, but they are paying close attention to all possible sources of information to guide them in their socialization. They are sometimes persuaded by the formal curriculum of the medical school, which states explicitly that upon successful completion of its requirements, graduates will be qualified as physicians, represented through the granting of the M.D. degree. For example, one study found that its sample of medical students defined becoming a doctor primarily in terms of gaining biomedical knowledge and resultant curative powers.[1] Although these students recognized the humanistic and psychosocial aspects of doctoring, they did not expect these to be a central part of their curriculum. However, other reports indicate that students recognize the importance of discovering and metabolizing a core essence of doctoring distinct from specific content expertise.[2]

Students may initially view medical school as an idealized adventure, a culminating reward for hard work. These early expectations are quickly tempered by experience.[3] Although students express enthusiasm and positive attitudes towards their professional indoctrination,[4] and indicate enjoyment of opportunities to assume the roles and tasks of doctoring,[5] they can also wrestle more deeply with what it means to become a physician. For example, in a study that used creative projects to help students to reflect on their training experiences,[6] many of the students concentrated on the socialization process directly, exploring the expectations and role requirements of the medical student within the hierarchy of medicine, the stresses and, at times, harshness of medical school, and the balance between personal and professional worlds. Some students focused on the challenges of newly introduced clinical responsibilities, their limitations and sense of inadequacy, feelings of being overwhelmed by too much information and knowledge to master, and the humiliating experience of being questioned by superiors about their knowledge base in a condescending or hostile manner.

As their training proceeds, medical students begin to realize, subliminally if not always overtly, that being a doctor involves not only knowledge mastery and technical competence, but also joining a very specific culture, with its own preferred language, style of writing, modes of dress, symbols, rituals, and, most importantly, commonly held understandings, ways of thinking and behaving, and taken-for-granted aspects of interaction, both with patients and with superiors such as residents and attending physicians.[7] The culture of medicine has a profound influence on the attitudes and behaviors of aspiring physicians, because it shapes basic assumptions about what are "acceptable" and what are "unacceptable" medical practices.[8]

For the past decade or more, scholars in medical education have been writing about coexisting but not always aligned formal, informal, and hidden curricula in medical school.[9] According to the originator of these concepts, the formal curriculum is the stated, intended, and formally offered and endorsed curriculum, the informal curriculum is what is transmitted to medical students about becoming a doctor through the unscripted interactions, and the hidden curriculum refers to institutional and organizational influences. The non-formal aspects of the curriculum have also been described as the unofficial expectations, implicit messages, and unintended learning outcomes that are conveyed to students.[10]

Medical educators have argued convincingly that both the informal and hidden curricula exert a powerful influence on the types of doctors that medical students in fact become. This influence is probably much more powerful than that of the formal curriculum. Medical students interpret the informal curriculum as how things are "really" done, in contrast to how things are supposed to be done, and what really matters, as opposed to what is said to matter. Although the hidden or informal curriculum may be used to align with formally espoused actions, attitudes, and values,[11–13] in its present method of operation it often contradicts explicit curricular messages about embracing humanistic values and relationship-centered care.[14]

Students perceive that the informal curriculum prioritizes the acquisition of testable knowledge over less tangible attitudinal and values-driven actions in clinical settings.[2] They also believe that medical educators are more likely to evaluate external attributes of appearance, formality, and conformity in assessing student professionalism than virtues of honor, altruism, and responsibility, and to prioritize adherence to hospital etiquette, respect for academic hierarchy, and subservience to authority above patient-centered virtues.[15] As a result, students may conclude that doctoring is not so much a moral and principled way of being as the manifesting of certain attitudes and behaviors during evaluative and examination situations, without necessarily developing ownership of underlying virtues and principles.[16]

Some of the premises of the culture of medicine that are conveyed through the hidden and informal curricula are avoidance of uncertainty, belief in the perfectability of physicians, valuing outcome over process, the prioritizing of medicine over all other aspects of life, and the supremacy of hierarchy.[8] These pervasive, but usually unacknowledged, beliefs obviously exert an influence on physicians' relationships with patients, but they also have a substantial effect on acceptable ways in which students are indoctrinated into the medical culture. Specifically, in the informal curriculum, these foundational assumptions justify unquestioning deference to experts (physicians, especially subspecialists) and discounting of non-experts (patients, students), emphasis on top-down, passive transmission of information as opposed to wrestling with ambiguity and multiple truths, rationalization of chronic stress, distress, and imbalance as a necessary part of training, and the use of intimidation, public shaming, and humiliation of learners as an acceptable teaching approach. Other research has documented that shaming and blaming are not unusual pedagogical practices in medical school.[17–19]

In the past decade or so, greater attention has been paid to the emotional distress experienced by medical students. This is a welcome development in a system that historically, while privileging patient suffering, has generally ignored physician suffering.[20] Since institutions often serve their own purposes by blocking out the voices of members who are distressed or dissatisfied,[21] there are few mechanisms for acknowledging suffering within the medical school experience. Nevertheless, a body of evidence has accumulated which indicates that a significant number of medical students are stressed, anxious, and depressed.[22-4] Fatigue, sleep problems, and irritability are widespread.[25] Over the course of training, students' mental health worsens,[26] attention to their feelings and their ability to "repair" negative mood decreases, and they report significant increases in personal distress.[27] It is not uncommon for students to have doubts about or question the rightness of their career choice.[23] One study estimated that as many as 45% of American medical students experience burnout,[28] which is associated with impaired humanistic attitudes, decreased effectiveness, and lowered professionalism.[19] Sources of distress include workload, lack of feedback, anxiety about their physical endurance and intellectual competence, pedagogical shortcomings, and a non-supportive training environment.[29] Student distress can contribute to substance abuse, broken relationships, suicide, and attrition from the profession. It also leads to cynicism and may subsequently affect students' care of patients.[26] In one troubling study, behaviors that both preclinical and clinical students previously considered unprofessional became increasingly acceptable to them, while unprofessional behavior increased in clinical students after they had participated in clerkships.[30]

Investigations of the causes of medical students' emotional distress have often focused on internal psychological attributes of students (e.g. perfectionism and neuroticism[31,32]) or on traumatic personal life events (e.g. death of a family member). Although intrapsychic difficulties and personal variability in resilience no doubt contribute to stress-related outcomes, this line of research may suggest a primary explanatory model rooted in individual vulnerability or weakness. Students' interaction with a demanding and punitive educational system has not received sufficient attention in terms of understanding student stress and dysfunction.[24] Yet, by and large, students feel unwilling and unable to protest about these aspects of their education, motivated by a compelling desire to be accepted as part of the medical enterprise. Of course, as mentioned earlier, the overriding desire to become a member of this elite and somewhat mysterious profession can propel students towards greater altruism, caring, and humanism when they perceive these qualities to be highly valued and central to the physician enterprise. However, absorbing less desirable aspects of the culture of medicine as part of their socialization can have profoundly deleterious effects on these future physicians, both in terms of their own distress and in terms of their attitudes towards and interactions with patients.

Is being a doctor about something more than information and knowledge? When have you absorbed enough punishment to become a doctor? How do you know when you have mastered the important rules? What if you disagree with these rules? These are particularly elusive questions, which perhaps are best answered, or at least explored, through poetry rather than through didactic lectures. And in any case there are few lectures and little formal curricular time devoted to this topic, although it is the reason for everything. It is as though trying to determine how one becomes a doctor is too vast, too amorphous a question to consider, whereas there is a lot of certainty in learning the Kreb's cycle or how to place a central line. Medical education often seems to assume that all the pieces will fit together in the end, but until then, students must look around for themselves, trying to extract the right lessons.

I stare out By: David Kopacz

Originally appeared in Body Electric *Anniversary Issue 2005, pp. 6–7*
first published in Body Electric *Vol. IX 1993, University of Illinois – Chicago*

I stare out across the frozen lake
the water blends into the sky
the ice stretches out
the cars go by on Lake Shore Drive
the belly of the pregnant woman
stretches up toward the sky
the mustache of the resident
hides his upper lip
as he watches the screen while the ultrasound
slides over the belly of the pregnant woman
the dimensions of new life flash on that screen
as he reads them aloud
I memorize
I see the lake and the sky
there is no difference to me
I see a truck pulling a house on the road
and the lake and the sky and the ice
stretch on around
until I feel sad and imprisoned
because my life is not my own
because I am not sure what is left of me
as I think this
I boil with hate
at the forces shackling me
at myself
at the mustachioed resident
a personal hate for the mustachioed resident
who blew his top
when I didn't know on my first call
who threw the book at me
I look at the clock, 4:30 AM
"Then read the chapter on it," he says
I look at the clock, 4:40 AM
"You must really be dazed out
you're still on the first page," he says
I personally hate the mustachioed resident
particularly his mustache
it hides his upper lip
and I boil with hate
and I'm just tired, man
and I feel deflated with pain
for everything that binds every being
for the constrictions and dissatisfactions of life
I look out across the sleeping city

I am mostly awake
I can more than imagine the pain of life
the woman with the belly breathes and cries
new life born with a pungent mess
the baby breathes and cries
I breathe and remain silent.

This poem encompasses many of the issues that students strive to resolve during the four-year process of becoming physicians. The narrator presents a stultifying, bleak, and cold environment. The tone is detached and deadened. Everything that is described – whether the frozen lake, the cars going by, the mustache of the resident, or the belly of the pregnant woman – receives equal weight, and all seem equally unimportant and meaningless. Even the new life that is about to appear is reduced to an image on the ultrasound machine. The student at first only feels "sad and imprisoned." He is distraught because he feels trapped, out of control of himself, and no longer even sure who he really is. This loss of self – of self-sacrifice to the point of breaking – is a common theme in many student poems.

As soon as the student recognizes his grim mood, he becomes filled with hate. The target of his rage is the supervising resident, who apparently earlier threw a book at the student when he didn't know the answer to a question. This aspect of the poem speaks both to the inappropriate abuse that students sometimes experience at the hands of their superiors, and to the potentially oppressive effect of constantly being expected to know all the answers. This helpless fury towards teachers who humiliate rather than instruct is not an uncommon theme among other student poems, although students also write about positive role models. Here, the resident's mustache becomes a particular target, because of its capacity to hide presumably not only the resident's "upper lip", but also his humanity.

We also have a glimpse into how the oppressive environment, the long hours, and the constant pressure to acquire more knowledge burden and stifle the student. The poem effectively conveys the student's fatigue, lack of sleep, and pain. In the lines, "I feel deflated with pain/for everything that binds every being/for the constrictions and dissatisfactions of life," we begin to understand how even the student's empathy has overwhelmed and depressed him. Compassion has turned to despair. While the baby "breathes and cries", the student "breathes and remains silent," unable to share in the appreciation of life, probably wanting to cry himself. The student has lost the ability to express his emotions. Like the frozen lake, the cars, and the ultrasound machine, he is without sensation. At this point, he can only "stare out."

THE MEDICAL SCHOOL APPLICANT INTERVIEW
Chaos stories
This topic rarely occurred in the poetry that I reviewed. When it did, the poems often had elements of chaos narratives. One of the poems written by a student from Qatar reflects back on his interview for medical school. Preparing for the encounter, he struggles with self-presentation: "What do I tell them if they ask/Who I am and who I'm not." The student is afraid of revealing something that will make him appear vulnerable and imperfect. When he arrives at the interview location, it seems bizarre, alien, and almost unidentifiable in ordinary perception. The student employs the metaphors of lie

detectors and even torture to describe the interview process. Afterwards, although he cherishes every detail of the experience, it seems unreal, like a "nebulous dream." The narrator tries to identify with the reassuring objectivity and predictability of science that can guarantee him a coveted spot in the entering class, based on quantifiable, measurable performance ("curious scientist"), but he is "lost in space." It is difficult to convince himself of the reality of this enormous step in a bewildering new universe.

Interview Day By: Anas Abou-Ismail
Originally appeared in Paint the Walls, *2005, p. 8, Weill Cornell School of Medicine*

I looked at a crowd of stars
    Waiting for the sun to rise
The streets were empty of people and cars
    And slumber had escaped my eyes

What do I tell them if they ask
    Who I am and who I'm not
It might sound like a simple task
    But trust me, you have to plan and plot

Awaken by the spirit of New Year's Eve
    Wondering which tie to wear
I crossed my fingers ready to leave
    And in less than a century, I was there

The promised land looked bizarre
    A polyhedron? A pumpkin? Who can tell!
A Martian Spaceship parked in Qatar
    Or simply a building called Cornell

I closed my eyes and went inside
    A room that tortures me and you!
Near a detector that beeps if you lied
    A process called the "Interview"

But once it's over, you drift away . . .
    And like a curious scientist lost in space
You cherish every detail of that day
    Then it turns to a nebulous dream
        And you doubt if it ever took place . . ..

TRANSITION TO MEDICAL SCHOOL
Chaos stories
In contrast to the euphoria of a successful interview, the transition to medical school is often a shock. These poems sound like cries for help, the actual chaotic encounter with this new life. In the words of one student, college was mostly about play and sleep, whereas medical school is mostly about studying. Medical school exams are "like college finals on steroids." First-year students end up spending "quality time with our cadavers, our newest best friends." All in all, medical school is "a hostile takeover of my life." A similarly themed poem summarizes the life of a medical student as having a primary

relationship with his stethoscope. In a poem quoted in its entirety later in this chapter ("Along for the ride"), another student writes that, in medical school, he feels as though he is living in a dream, which every day seems more like a nightmare. He yearns to return to his previous world, which was "carefree, promising, easy."

The transition from "normal" to medical life is sometimes portrayed as "the end of innocence." One student, writing about the gross anatomy lab, reminisces about the life he once had, and the person he once was – an ordinary person leading an ordinary life. The narrator longs to escape to a place of quiet solitude, but deep down he knows that he must say "goodbye" to all that was. Still, he hopes that "somewhere down there in that mess / There's the same soft heart in each of us." In this poem, the "mess" refers both to the literal mess on the dissection table, and to the mess that medical school has made of their lives. This poem contains both a cry for help and the hope that things will be put back together the way they used to be.

End of the Innocence By: Andrew Sledd
UC Irvine
Adapted from "This is the End of the Innocence" by Jon Henley and Bruce Hornsby

Remember when from dusk to dawn
We'd live our lives like everyone
Didn't have a care in the world
With our hopes and dreams starting to unfurl
But happily ever after failed
And we've been tainted by these scary tales.
Teachers dwell on small details
When memory will suffice.

> Pre-chorus:
> Ha, but I know a place where we can go
> Still unseen by man.
> We'll sit and watch the hours roll
> And white stones in the wind.

> Chorus:
> You can lay your hands down on their chest
> And let your senses do the rest
> Offer up your best defense
> This is the end, this is the end
> Of the innocence.

Verse 2:
O beautiful unblinking eyes
Now those eyes are calling me
They're turning pencils into probes
For this tired old man with the bifocal gaze
Model warriors often fail
And we've been haunted by those fairy tales
Netter fills in all details
When others fall behind.

Pre-chorus Chorus

Verse 3:
Who knows how long this will last
Now we've come so far so fast
Somewhere down there in that mess
There's the same soft heart in each of us.
I need to remember this
So give me just one last list
Let me take a long last look
Before we say goodbye.

Restitution stories

Other poems recognize the transition dimension, but adopt a more restitutive tone. In one such example, a student struggles with identity issues. As the title of the poem suggests, he is questioning whether he is a scientist, a doctor, or both. The narrator starts out as a confident scientist, garbed to protect himself from "contamination" by the cadaver. His impressive status is established by possession of expert knowledge (access codes). The consummate scientist, the narrator is already identified not with the "specimen" on the laboratory table, but with his colleagues, and he wields his professional tool (the scalpel) with élan.

At this point the narrator experiences a moment of doubt. He stops and hesitates. Gazing at the cadaver, he becomes aware of her humanity. He notices her nail polish, her "peaceful" quality. Suddenly, the specimen table is a bed, and the cadaver is "resting calmly" with her head on a pillow. The "specimen" becomes "a mother, a wife, a daughter, a friend," a willing teacher ready to share herself, body and soul. She provides the bridge that unites science and humanity.

Scientist and Doctor By: Neal K. Kaushal
Originally appeared in Plexus *2007, UC Irvine School of Medicine*

I gather my instruments. I snap on my gloves.
I apply my personal protective gear, first my coat and then my safety goggles.
I enter my identification code.
Access to the facility is granted.

I file into the laboratory with my colleagues.
I take note of the chemicals, reagents, and wash basins that line the walls.
The smell of formaldehyde and phenol fills my nostrils.
The specimen has been prepared on the laboratory table.

I obtain a fresh blade for my scalpel.
I position myself for the primary incision along the thorax.
A wave of excitement swells over me.
A true scientist I am, ready for the day's work in the lab.

But then —
I stop.
I hesitate.

She lies peacefully on her pillow
blanketed by the royal blue canvas ensheathing her.
Her arms neatly tucked at her side, her nails polished with a glossy pink.
Her legs are outstretched, her feet facing towards the east.
She rests calmly in her bed.

She invites anyone to explore her soul and know who she was.
A mother, a wife, a daughter, a friend.
She lies ready to pass on knowledge about science and about life.
She lies at the bridge between science and humanity.

I adjust the grasp on my scalpel and wield it with poise.
I no longer hesitate. I feel at ease.
Silently, I express my gratitude toward her.
I thank her for allowing me to take part in her life.

No longer just a scientist am I
But now becoming a true doctor.

STULTIFYING ENVIRONMENT OF MEDICAL SCHOOL
Chaos stories

Students often reflect on their external environment – the world of the classroom, clinic, and wards that they have exchanged for a more natural setting. These narratives are most typically chaos stories and cries for help. Constantly spending time shut inside lecture halls strikes many students as depressing. They long for contact with the natural world. Walking alone through a rough neighborhood in the very early morning, a student contrasts the beauty of the rising sun and sinking moon with the confines of the lecture hall that awaits her. She longs to put the beauty of this moment in the pocket of her white coat ("with my reflex hammer and stethoscope") and carry them with her on "this long road" that lies ahead. The poem implies that the tools which the medical student usually carries with her will not be enough to sustain her in the long term. In a more poignant poem, a student does not see daylight for days at a time while on her surgery clerkship. When the sunlight pours in through a window, the entire surgical team is irresistibly drawn towards it, pressing their faces to the glass as if trying to absorb the warmth and light. Their souls are polluted, jaded "and mute to that which we are."

Another chaos poem discusses the narrator's belly, which is protesting against too much coffee and "venom." It wants to be set free, and is "begging to set out to farms and clouds and corn / to drink dark earth there as it was intended." Here it would be "soothed by the music of crickets and coyotes." Here the narrator could "snore in Morse / the tuneless song of the content." The poem expresses longing for leisure, idle space, and natural surroundings. In a sadder poem, an exhausted, unfocused young man studies at his desk in a sterile environment. Outside, nature is vibrant and alive. The young man laughs (or is it a sob?) and wishes that he could cry, "But truly / He did not know how." Nature is portrayed as soaring, vast yet relaxed, lazy, and idle. The student is portrayed as small, alone, and despairing. This poem contrasts the enormity and mellowness of nature with the sadness, isolation, and sterility of the student.

In a similar poem, the student sees life slipping away, and wants to experience it before it disappears altogether. The poem uses the metaphor of skating on black ice to describe his life as a medical student. Black ice, of course, poses special hazards to pedestrians and drivers because it is hard to recognize. The poem implies that what is happening to the student may be equally difficult to detect, and equally dangerous. In contrast to the cold, frozen quality of life as a medical student, the narrator's previous life was symbolically filled with warmth, sunlight, adventure, and sensuality. As the nurturing natural world recedes, so does the student's life, leaving only pain in its place.

Falling Through By: Michael Jacobs
Originally published in Body Language: Poems of the Medical Training Experience
edited by Neeta Jain, Dagan Coppock and Stephanie Brown Clark, 2006, p. 49
Reprinted with the permission of BOA Editions, Ltd, www.boaeditions.org

It feels as though my life has slipped away
Or I from it
So suddenly and slowly.
I've been skating on black ice, out on a frozen ocean.
I have broken through, each drop piercing
Each a single memory.
I don't want to see my life
Flash before my eyes.
I want to spread my soul out against the sun
So that my pain will melt away.
Leaving me my life to live.

I want to stay on the beach
And play in warm and shallow waters.
I want to dance the harmony of Mambo
Under the sun on Havana's Malecon.
I want to stand on the Great Wall of China
And wave to outer space
I want to explore the big white Alps
The way my tongue swirls about
This ice cream cone.

I want to taste my life
Before it melts away.

Witnessing stories
Occasionally, these poems adopt a position of resistance. In one such poem, the author intimates that she is wearing a mask of social conformity. When she is able to break free, she discovers a life that is fresh, intimate, clean, comforting, and carefree. She realizes that she has lost touch with the joys of nature. Now that she is able to re-appreciate the natural world, she is connected once again to "life's pulse." This is a poem of connection through resistance (witnessing) that results in a sense of community with nature, thus leading to an experience of liberation and transcendence.

SACRIFICE OF PERSONAL LIVES
Chaos stories
A sense of self-sacrifice is a common theme found in many poems, especially in terms of the cost that students pay relationally. These poems are also primarily cries for help,

sometimes tempered by a sense of journey with lessons learned. In one characteristic poem, the student reflects on all that she has lost in terms of time, sleep, friends, and family events to prove that she belonged to this exclusive fraternity. She asserts that she has paid the price and will keep on paying. Another student laments the death of her grandmother, who died before she became a doctor and could help her. Being a medical student meant that she was always too busy for her grandmother, although the grandma loved and supported her. The poem is filled with feelings of sadness and guilt while acknowledging the pride that the grandmother took in the student's medical career. The poem ends with a moral – prioritize your life, because "Time waits for no one."

In an angrier chaos poem, a student laments missing a series of significant family events in order to study. She feels more and more disconnected from her family and more and more lonely. Her grandmother has a stroke, but still the narrator cannot visit her for months. Being a "good medical student" is opposed to being a good member of her family. When the grandmother's condition suddenly deteriorates, the narrator ironically and bitterly comments, "How fortunate she declined at my convenience." Finally, she asks in despair, "What am I doing here?/Like ------- battle,/I fight to console myself each day." The poem conveys that the student has sacrificed what is most important in her life.

446 Miles Away By: Julie Tarn Ching Wu
UC Irvine, 2000

446 miles away
My cousin Roxanne gets married
My brother tells me there were many satirical moments
I picture them in my mind and laugh with him.

Come Christmas, 446 miles away
No one erects the artificial tree
The one we've had for over twenty years
I am at Hoag Memorial
Andy waits for me to get him.

446 miles away
My sister visits from Taiwan
I have not seen her for nearly three years
Her son is rapidly approaching five
Maybe I will see her in the next three years.

446 miles away
It's February, my grandma's birthday
The single event that brings the entire family together
I wonder who held her arm and guided her steps
Watched for hazards wherever she walked
Assisted her to the restroom
Selected soft foods for her to eat.

446 miles away
My cousin Johnny gets engaged
Who is his fiancée?

446 miles away
My grandma has a multi-infarct stroke
She cannot swallow and requires a G-tube
Her speech is at best barely comprehensible
She will never walk again
I do my best to resist rushing home and to finish
psychiatry, like a good medical student.

446 miles away
three weeks later
My grandma has a questionable number of strokes
Her condition rapidly declines
I take the next flight home
How fortunate she declined at my convenience
The boards can wait.

446 miles away
Mother's Day
I am on call at the VA
I called my mommy yesterday, just in case.

446 miles away
For two months now, my grandma lies in bed
At Death's door
After seven weeks and three days, I get to see her again
I did not catch her on a "good" day
I hope she heard my words
Remembered my plastic smile
Will there be another chance?

What am I doing here?
Like ------- battle
I fight to console myself each day.
Repeating these words over and over and over again:
But my heart is there
Four hundred and forty-six miles away.

One chaos poem focuses on the way that the student shies away from asking difficult questions not only of patients, but also of himself, his wife and his children. He has lost his ability to engage deeply with life, and instead must just skim the surface of things. The poem suggests that the narrator is afraid to take a long hard look at himself and his personal relationships, and is just trying to survive. Other chaos poems reflect the stress of multi-tasking. In one of these poems, the student complains that he is always accountable, whether to attending clinicians, patients, or family. He can't escape from trying to please others and keep them happy. The result is that he burns the candle at both ends and lets everyone down.

A funny, bitter poem describes the compromises and sacrifices that one must make relationally during medical school. The narrator likens having a relationship while in medical school to trying to build a doghouse for your dog (the presumably uncomplaining and devoted significant other). The student knows that the dog "needs a doghouse," but a million things (most of which have to do with medicine) interfere. Eventually, motivated by guilt, the student commences to construct the canine domicile. However, being made out of makeshift, haphazard materials, it is fragile, uncertain, and perpetually subject to the vagaries of wind, rain, and possum's breath. It barely functions, and serves almost none of the purposes for which it was intended. It is true that, every once in a while, love and companionship can be found "in the shade of the doghouse", but it is a far from satisfactory arrangement.

The Doghouse By: Meghann Kaiser

Originally published in Body Language: Poems of the Medical Training Experience *edited by Neeta Jain, Dagan Coppock and Stephanie Brown Clark, 2006, p. 84 Reprinted with the permission of BOA Editions, Ltd, www.boaeditions.org*

I'll tell you what having a relationship in med school is like.

It's like having a dog and thinking to yourself
He needs a doghouse but
Somehow there are always about a million other things to do
Papers, tests, rounds, residency applications . . .

Until one day you get to feeling so guilty
You decide you're going to build that doghouse
Come hell or high water, out of anything you can find
Rulers, masking tape, newspapers, toilet paper tubes . . .

And then you have a doghouse.

Only every time your dog actually goes inside that house
Or it rains, or the wind blows just a little too hard
Or a possum breathes on it wrong, your little doghouse has to be
Propped up, picked up, retaped, repaired . . .

So that in time you start to wonder, why you have one at all.
It's not like any other doghouse. It does
Hardly any of the things you hoped it would. All your neighbors
Point, laugh, roll their eyes, shake their heads . . .

But every now and then

I get home at 7 o'clock in the morning after a night on call
Lie down in the dew grass on the lawn beside my dog
In the shade of a makeshift doghouse.

Other poems emphasize the student's aloneness and isolation. One poet confesses that he was not prepared for the loneliness of medical school – the separation from the normal world, from friends and loved ones, and from life as he knew it. He asserts that he was drawn to medicine out of love, but now feels that he has sacrificed and delayed too much.

Lonely Life By: Stefan Samuelson
Originally appeared in Reflexions, *Vol. XII, Spring 2005, p. 26*
Columbia University College of Physicians and Surgeons

No one ever told me
That following my dreams
Of caring for the lives of others
Would leave me so alone

Never in my lifetime
Have I sat like this and watched the world slip out of reach
While I, amid exams and deadlines
Duties and unexpected pressures
Am withheld from life as a human

I find myself oftentimes at night
Sitting alone at my desk, gazing over the river
Wondering what happened to the warm interchanges
That once were the undercurrent of my day
The people I knew have lives – they live them ceaselessly

And I, the delayed gratifier
Lose more and more in sacrifice to the gods of my future.
I came to medicine out of love
No one ever told me I would feel alone.

Another student laments the loss of her old life. She no longer remembers the phone numbers of friends, or her mother's childhood lullabies. Instead of parents, she now has "white-coated lecturers bringing/simultaneous information/five forms of data." The student-author compares medical education to moving to a new town, but one that is filled with "radioactive ash" and that is "without telephones." In the same way that some people forget why they moved, she "may forget why she came" to medical school. Living in a radioactive town symbolizes all that this student has lost, including the reasons that inspired her to move in the first place.

At times, students strike a note of despair. In one desperate appeal, the narrator in another poem stands outside on a cold night, gazing at the stars. He is unable to be touched by love, happiness, warmth, or light. He feels as though his soul is dying. His emotions are "an overflowing ocean." He pleads for someone to "take my hand" and "understand my fragility." Togetherness would relieve his misery, but he is alone. In a disturbing cry for help, another student-poet appeals to the ocean for guidance to lead her to a simpler place and a happier time. She longs to find a home in the sea, and seeks to assuage her woundedness and pain in the comfort of its depths. Like the ocean, she is "blue, infinite, deep, and true," ever-changing, but now completely alone and forlorn. Another student writer uses the analogy of a "hapless moth" drawn to a flame to explain her relationship with medical school. Self-immolation cannot be avoided once the process has been set in motion.

FEAR, EXHAUSTION, AND BEING OVERWHELMED
Chaos stories

Other students focus on their sense of being overwhelmed and exhausted by their training. These are also typically chaos narratives. One student describes her first month on
the wards. She has a huge workload – constant fires to be put out, large patient volume,
blood draws gone wrong, diagnoses missed. She wonders disconsolately, "There had to
be a way out / I already wanted to retire." Another student finds her experience so crushing that she sees herself as more of a patient than the actual patient, and even wishes
that she could change places with her patient. This student is struck by the irony that
she is supposed to counsel and advise patients on healthy living and reducing stress, but
she cannot begin to achieve these things in her own life.

I find medical school hard By: Sheela Reddy
UC Irvine

I find medical school hard
overwhelming, there is always too much
to do. Sometimes I wonder
who is the patient.
Me
or the old woman in front of me?
I am supposed to counsel her –
exercise, meditate
eat healthy, maintain low stress
laugh, spend time with
loved ones, don't take life too seriously.
Sometimes I wish I were the patient
not she.

Another similarly exhausted student wants to change places with a hospitalized patient
because at least the patient has people who take care of her, and she is allowed to sleep.
Another student also admits to sleeping anytime, anywhere he can, but worries that he
will be judged negatively for "indulging in that simple pleasure."

In a final example, one student describes himself in a passive role, carried along by the
wild ride of medical school, in which he cannot slow down, cannot understand what is
happening, and cannot even fathom how he is changing. He knows that he is not who he
was, but he has no idea who he will become. Somewhere out there is a "carefree, young,
promising, easy" world, but it is no longer his. Instead, the narrator is carrying burdens
that are not even his (perhaps his patients), but which he has assumed nonetheless. He is
going faster and faster, out of control, and can only wait to see what the future brings.

Along for the ride By: Gabriel Herscu
UC Irvine

I am not who I was before I gave up
I am moving much faster this time
My obsession is like sour candy, unbearable, addictive
I am living a dream

Will I awake to find myself
before?
A world carefree, young, promising, easy
I am carrying too much
It's not mine
Am I carrying anything?
I can't slow down
I'm not steering
I'm out of control
I don't understand
all these things
And I am not who I will be
When they are clear

Some students focus on the all-consuming nature of the physician's role, even as train-ees. These poems are consistently cries for help. In one poignant poem, the student is leaving the hospital, anticipating a glorious weekend of freedom. As he leaves, he sees a very sick gowned and masked patient with an oxygen tank in a wheelchair accompanied by his wife, both also outside the hospital. The student crosses the street, leaving them behind. He glances back once, and then quickens his pace, "afraid to look back again." The poem contrasts the student's almost desperate urge toward freedom (shedding his white coat and "stethoscope necklace," loosening his tie, crossing against the "Don't Walk" sign) with the couple who are still tethered to the hospital. Why is the student afraid to look back? Perhaps he is afraid that he, too, is tied with invisible but equally strong chains. Another exhausted student also describes driving away from "my patients and their pain." She sees a tree covered with birds instead of leaves and wonders whether they are "mourning doves." The tree appears to be outside the normal course of things, just like the hospital. The tree is filled with mourning, again like the hospital. This poem intimates that no matter how hard the student tries to escape, she cannot get away from the suffering of her patients.

Restitution stories

Sometimes students attempt to resolve their distress through restitution – tasks and work paradoxically become the "solution" to stress. These poems have a sense that the immediate sacrifice and suffering will be redeemed because the student is doing a good job. A typical poem portrays the life of the medical student as one of sleeplessness and constant studying for exams. The only satisfaction in this hard life comes from the sense of "a job well done." In another example, the narrator ponders the problem of sleeplessness through a series of metaphors and similes. She hopes for "A reprieve from consciousness / not much to ask . . . / No? Okay, I have other tasks." Again, suffering is rationalized as necessary, and more effort is seen as the answer to stress.

One student describes the night before an exam, and the visceral feelings of stress that, as a medical student, seem to beset him constantly. Stress is like a flame that burns and "marks the skin." His poem is filled with images of his chest being torn open, bones and flesh exposed, twitching muscles, burnt skin, and difficulty in breathing and moving. However, he concludes somewhat abruptly that, as a medical student, one must learn to deal with stress. In another poem that also explores medical student stress, while driving home late at night the poet recognizes that stress can make one dissociate from the world around one, but then quickly reframes this process as a period of refuge and decompression. In both poems there is a kind of quickly appended, instant resolution. Stress is devastating, but one has to deal with it. Stress makes one dissociate and become isolated, but this is really a kind of regrouping.

Sometimes students actively embrace the pressures and challenges. In one such example, which is filled with military metaphors, medical students are described as young "soldiers." Attending clinicians and residents bark orders at them, and they work impossibly hard (the poem contains a repeating chorus of "hurry!"), but as patients get better, the students gladly work harder, always "ready for more." This is a restitution story because the students' exhaustion is justified by the patients' improvement ("a smile of content on our weary faces"). In a similar restitution-themed poem, a student describes participating in a surgery. The student endures for several hours. "On the 368th" minute, they start to feel resentment as a result of physical and mental exhaustion. However, in the 369th minute, the student is asked to close the incision, with the implication that this privilege compensates for the previous stress. Here, the student is reassured to realize that the "privilege" of closing the incision makes the hard training worthwhile. Everything now makes sense.

Transcendence stories

Occasionally, a poem about the stresses of medical school adopts a transcendent narrative. In a poem that illustrates this viewpoint, the student complains of the stresses of being a medical student – too little sleep, too much driving, too much studying, not enough time to eat. He feels like a slave doing scut work, and that his time is being wasted. Then the voice of the poem suddenly switches from that of the disgruntled medical student to those of pediatric patients. The stanzas continue to repeat the refrains that the student used to encourage himself: "Just hold on," "Make it," "A few more moments." This repetition serves to highlight the self-centeredness of the student's preoccupations compared with what is at stake for the patients. The narrator concludes: "Life is about perspective/Being grateful for what you have/Finding some shred of happiness in a sea of sorrow/Finding hope." He realizes that when his alarm clock rings again, he should wake up with gratitude. Here the student is able to put his complaints within a perspective of downward comparison to the real suffering of patients.

EXPLOITATION AND HUMILIATION
Chaos stories

One of the most problematic aspects of training is students' perception that they are exploited, disrespected, and even humiliated by their superiors. Almost uniformly, poems that address this topic are chaos stories, reflecting the students' shock and bitter disillusionment. When students write specifically about their interaction with residents, they report many negative events. Since, in practice, residents are responsible for much of the hands-on teaching in the clinical years, it is not surprising that they receive the brunt of students' stunned distress. It is likely that these cruel and demeaning interactions remain with these students longer than more positive exchanges. Nevertheless, it is highly troubling to read about them.

In a typical poem, the student makes an erroneous diagnosis. As a trick, residents lie to the student, confirming his diagnosis to see how he will react: "What? I was embarrassed and in shock. Thoughts were racing and my mind was locked." The student is humiliated by this experience. In this chaos story, the student is left with the feeling of having been demeaned and humiliated by residents. Another third-year student reports being made to feel dumb by residents and attending clinicians: "I remember being asked questions that were all pretty hard/And after I got all of them wrong, thinking to myself, I really am a retard/I remember some of the doctors thinking, 'This student's a fool'/ While residents would think, 'How the hell did he get into med school?'" The student feels that he is being used as a "scut monkey slave." Yet another student notes how attending clinicians and residents criticize and ridicule medical students. He would like to linger and talk with his patients, but he knows that the residents will evaluate him for doing so. The resident acts as an intimidating superego, forcing the student to behave in distressing ways towards the patient (waking them up, re-asking questions) in order to receive a better evaluation. The student feels trapped and helpless to change. On a pediatric clerkship, the senior residents are impatient and irritated with the student's lack of knowledge.

A haiku uses the simile of the medical student as a lawn that people are supposed to treat with care and respect, but which is instead trampled on. The poem conveys feelings of exploitation, helplessness, and even abuse.

On Call By: Elisabeth Erekson

Originally appeared in Body Electric *Anniversary Issue, 2005, p. 10*
first published in Body Electric *Vol. XVI, 2000, University of Illinois – Chicago*

I feel like a lawn
With a "Keep off the Grass" sign
Everyone still walks on.

A poem that apostrophizes the "short white coat" that medical students wear portrays it as a symbol of shame and embarrassment. It placed the student at the bottom of the medical hierarchy, where superiors could mock him and make fun of him, and he was helpless. The coat positioned him to be victimized by unfair evaluations, to endure worthless assignments, to prepare irrelevant presentations, and to do the residents' scut work. The coat was the repository of the student's "sweat and tears." The student's hatred of the white coat is palpable – it is a symbol of all the indignities that he has suffered, and of his insignificance at the hands of those who were supposed to guide and mentor him.

In another chaos poem, the narrator describes the process of pimping, in which an attending physician asks a battery of questions primarily for the purpose of embarrassing and even humiliating the student. The student feels blinded – a startled "deer in the headlights." The lower-case personal pronoun "i" stresses the insignificance of the student. Only in the last stanza does the student begin to claim his identity by expressing his yearning to be treated with kindness, and to be nurtured into physicianhood. The poem expresses distress both at the student's own suffering and at the unprofessional behavior of the attending physician whom the narrator had formerly admired as a venerable redwood tree.

pimp me By: David Chang
UC Irvine 2001

like Redwoods in the forest so aged to be wise
the attendings i feared, so began my demise

your questions so asked, i can't read your mind
no map no compass i feel like i'm blind

a deer in the headlights, i startle to fright
can't think, i'm stunned, did i get that right?

you answer correctly and your world is fine
one slip, then another . . . now . . . end of the line

absent words, a mumble, a simple "i just don't know"
are words, not meaningless, but not a good show

second thought, second chance, maybe i'd be alright
one chance, now gone, is this just for spite?

Oh great one! Oh leader! Is this how we learn?
humiliated, i stumble, ruminating after my turn . . .

I came here to grow, I came here to learn
Absent kindness I'll forget, for knowledge I yearn.

Another student complains about an attending physician who won't even speak to him about a particular patient, despite the fact that the student is knowledgeable and well informed about the patient's status. The poem exudes a feeling of helpless anger and resentment at the attending physician's indifference to and ignoring of the student.

In a final illustration of this phenomenon, a student describes his experience during a surgery on his obstetrics-gynecology clerkship. The poem is ironically presented as the transcript of a conversation between a medical student and an attending physician. Although we hear only the student's voice, the poem makes it easy to imagine the physician's remarks. The attending physician is portrayed as insulting, humiliating, and patronizing towards the student, and callous, cruel, and insensitive towards the anesthetized patient. The poem is an expression of helpless rage against an insensitive and cruel attending, who could bully the student with impunity. Within the context of the operating theater, the student has no recourse but to scrape and grovel in response to the vitriol of the surgeon. His only revenge is a poem.

A "Transcript" of my Conversations with OB/GYN Surgeons By: Bobby Rostami
Originally appeared in Plexus *2004, p. 36, UC Irvine School of Medicine*

Yes sir doctor, I am a third year. Bobby Rostami, sir.
Thank you for allowing me to watch this procedure, doctor.
Yes sir, I did scrub for 5 minutes.
Yes sir, I tried to learn the names of the instruments.
Well I don't know, sir, I guess I didn't learn them well enough.
Yes sir, I am stupid.
Thank you for telling me how to do it correctly.

Yes sir, I agree, I hate patients, too.
Yes sir, it is their fault for getting the cancer, sir.
Yes sir, I also deserve to get a tumor, sir.
Well sir, I don't know why the standard approach for uterine cancer is like this.
You're right sir, this is further testament to the fact that
     medical students are getting stupider and stupider as the years go by.
Yes sir, I wish I were dead, too, sir.
Yes, thank you for sticking that bloody scalpel in my face sir.
I now know how to use one.
Well sir, I'm not used to waking up at 3:20 AM
     and standing on my feet for 9 straight hours.
Yes sir, it does show what kind of a pussy I am.
Yes sir, you're right. I should pray for my own death.
Thank you for praying for it as well sir.
Well yes, sir, I do enjoy the sweet savory smell of cauterized flesh.
Yes sir, you can cauterize my intact flesh.
Mm mm that smells great.
Yes sir, I agree. I should drop out of med school and become a shoe salesman.
Thank you, sir, for allowing me to watch this procedure, sir.
Ha ha ha . . . thanks for tripping me on the way out of the operating room, sir.

When they are not downright punitive and ridiculing, the attending clinician is frequently seen as aloof and distanced from the student. However, there was very little evidence of racist, sexist, or otherwise discriminatory behavior from attending clinicians towards students, although one gay student believed that he was both pimped harder and not given certain training opportunities because of his sexual orientation.

NEGATIVE PERSONAL CHANGES
Chaos stories

Many students worry that the medical school experience is changing them in negative ways. These poems are often chaos stories. For example, in a poem that is primarily a cry for help, the author notes that upon entering medical school she was innocent and ignorant. Slowly, however, she undergoes a process of transformation, becoming almost unrecognizable to herself. The experience is bewildering and frightening. She hopes that as she becomes a physician she will not lose her essence as a person: "If and when I am transformed, I hope that I still recognize my reflection." She wonders how to locate the "self" of the physician when it is so successfully hidden behind the white coat.

In similar chaos poems, another student refers to "becoming a doctor and losing myself." She remembers a patient's "shaven groin" but has forgotten his name and face. She now functions like a robot "to fit the white-coat role." Her new self, shaped by medical school, is becoming hardened and unyielding. Yet another student describes her initial feelings of elation, joy, and relief when she was accepted for medical school. Now the implication is that medical school might not have been worth the eager wait. The author sees herself as going on automatic pilot. She clings to vague memories, rapidly fading, of a normal life. Her life has become chaotic and disconnected. She asks, "Can body suffer malnutrition of mind's ideals?", suggesting her disillusionment with the medical school experience. Another poem explores loss through the metaphor of a neglected plant. The student laments that seven months ago (the start of the academic year?) the plant had "no cares, green healthy", but now it is shriveled and it is too late to revive it. The narrator tries to nurture the withered sprig, but she only imagines new shoots. Sadly, she concludes that "It's time to let go," suggesting that she must let go of her former, pre-medical-school self.

In a different example, while confronting the family of a patient who has died, the student first reflects on four years of incessant, unremitting training. The phrasing of the lines creates the expectation that all of this education will somehow have prepared the student to deal with whatever "this day" has in store for her. Like earlier cited poems, this one also laments all that has been lost of normal life, the terrible price that has been paid and which is continuing to be paid. Yet, instead of compensatory wisdom, the student observes that what she has learned over the past four years is only that her own tears are ". . . unacceptable . . . a sign of my own / weakness and mortality." As a physician in training, she has come to believe that her role is to "be unbreakable / for this broken family." The student has been broken down and reconstituted so that she cannot cry. The poem implies that much of her humanity and vulnerability has been destroyed.

Four years By: Heather Hinshelwood
Originally appeared in Panacea *Summer 2005 p. 13*
University of Florida College of Medicine

This day
has been four years in coming.

The books and the paper
we memorized even in our sleep.

The tests we took
after days of little sleep.

Proving, justifying
our presence in this place.

And what we lost
we can never measure.

The friends we didn't talk to,
the weddings we missed,
the funerals that impinged on our tests.

For we are learning to heal
so sickness and death should not happen to
us.

And now, the patients
that we memorize even in our sleep.

The sleep that is disturbed
by memories and thoughts of them.
For this day is

four years in coming.

I have paid my price,
and I will continue to do so:

The sweat rolling down my breasts
from the heat in the trauma OR.

The burning muscles that
scream with each chest compression.
(Please live!)

The blood . . . Oh, God. The blood.
All bleeding stops eventually.

And the tears flowing freely from the family.
Mine are unacceptable . . . a sign of my own
weakness and mortality.
For I must be unbreakable
for this broken family.

Four years.
Am I a doctor yet?

Transcendence stories

Once in a while, poems exploring these negative personal changes take on a transformational quality. One student reflects on how he commenced his medical education
feeling idealistic and elated, and regarding medicine as a noble profession. He remembers that the White Coat Ceremony encouraged him and his classmates to be not only
scientists and clinicians, but also humanitarians. Now, confronted with a terminally ill
patient, he chastises himself that he "stood strangely inadequate on that isthmus of an
uncertain strait / Stripped of the science of curing / Why had he felt bereft of the art of
healing? / Had it been a moment of self-test, an evolution within the physician's soul?"
As he contemplates his silence in the face of the patient's fear and pain, he knows that
he could have done better.

Up to this point, the story is a chaos story. Then, however, the encounter becomes
an opportunity to move closer to the doctor he wants to be. The student realizes that
physicians can always reach out to patients with empathy and compassion, "with
heightened awareness / To heal the intangible pain." Armed with this insight, the student
returns to the patient's room, and she calls him "son." "That word would ever echo
through his soul." "Both patient and physician had shifted gears / To reveal a tender,
vulnerable side / That would make whole the healer and the healed." At this point, the
narrator begins to acknowledge the patient's humanity. By the conclusion of the poem,
the narrator has reached a place of transcendence, recognizing the common bonds of
woundedness between patient and student, and also the potential for mutual healing.

Another poem begins with the student losing his love of "little things" – all that is
left is brooding, helplessness, numbness, fatigue, and an obsession with giving the right
answers and impressing the attending clinician. He has lost touch with his family, and
is disconnected from himself. He ridicules the five-minute case presentation that he
is simultaneously trying to prepare as inadequate to "present" the factors involved in
child abuse, meth addiction, abandoned babies, and dying patients. However, in the

concluding stanza the poem takes a transcendent turn, as the student accepts alterations, and is inspired to alleviate the pain that he finds around him: "There are no answers to human suffering/Just my chance to help/create sunrises when there is only darkness/ and sing lullabies to life's forgotten children."

SUMMARY

In poetry that explores the theme of becoming a physician in multiple manifestations, students cover the developmental spectrum from medical school applications and interviews to the transition from preclinical to clinical years. Primarily, they struggle to understand the all-important but intangible and, to them, somewhat opaque concept of what doctoring is all about. Their poetry validates findings in the literature that document the emotional stresses and pressures exerted on students by the medical school experience. Many focus on the difficult transition from "normal life" to the life of a medical student. The stresses of medical school are also enumerated and examined in numerous cries for help, including lack of sleep, studying, and confinement in an artificial and seemingly indifferent world. Related themes include loneliness and personal sacrifice, fear, exhaustion, and being overwhelmed. Some students feel beleaguered by the all-consuming nature of the physician's role.

Students' poetry also validates the existence of a troubling gap between what they imagine their training will be like and how they often actually find it to be. Many of their poems speak to the existence of a hidden curriculum that is punitive, demoralizing, and disillusioning. Students write at some length about their humiliation and exploitation at the hands of residents and attending physicians. Encounters with residents appear to be particularly distressing to students, probably because of the emotional and instrumental proximity in which these two groups work. These emotionally traumatic interactions often produce chaos stories of humiliation, despair, and anger. However, students are equally concerned about the negative changes that they perceive in themselves which they attribute to the experience of medical school. They see themselves becoming emotionally distant and detached, and losing their identity. Only occasionally are these deleterious alterations in self transformed by the student's commitment to medicine.

REFERENCES

1 Draper C, Louw G. What is medicine and what is a doctor? Medical students' perceptions and expectations of their academic and professional career. *Medical Teacher* 2007; **29**: e100–7.
2 Ozolins I, Hall H, Peterson R. The student voice: recognising the hidden and informal curriculum in medicine. *Medical Teacher* 2008; **30**: 606–11.
3 Papadimos TJ. Voltaire's Candide, medical students, and mentoring. *Philosophy, Ethics, and Humanities in Medicine* 2008; **2**: 13.
4 Fischer MA, Harrell HE, Haley HL, *et al.* Between two worlds: a multi-institutional qualitative analysis of students' reflections on joining the medical profession. *Journal of General Internal Medicine* 2008; **23**: 958–63.
5 Dyrbye LN, Harris I, Rohren CH. Early clinical experiences from students' perspectives: a qualitative study of narratives. *Academic Medicine* 2007; **82**: 979–88.
6 Rucker L, Shapiro J. Becoming a physician: students' creative projects in a third-year IM clerkship. *Academic Medicine* 2003; **78**: 391–7.
7 Good BJ, Good MJD. "Fiction" and "Historicity" in doctors' stories: social and narrative dimensions of learning medicine. In: Mattingly C, Garro LC (eds). *Narrative and the Cultural Construction of Illness and Healing.* Berkeley, CA: University of California Press; 2000. pp. 50–69.

8   Haidet P, Stein HF. The role of the student–teacher relationship in the formation of physicians: the hidden curriculum as a process. *Journal of General Internal Medicine* 2006; **21**: 516–20.

9   Hafferty FW. Beyond curriculum reform: confronting medicine's hidden curriculum. *Academic Medicine* 1998; **73**: 403–7.

10 Adler SR, Hughes EF, Scott RB. Student "moles": revealing the hidden curriculum. *Medical Education* 2006; **40**: 463–4.

11 Branch WT Jr, Kern D, Haidet P, *et al*. The patient–physician relationship. Teaching the human dimensions of care in clinical settings. *JAMA* 2001; **286**: 1067–74.

12 Suchman AL, Williamson PR, Litzelman DK, *et al*. for the Relationship-Centered Care Discovery Team. Toward an informal curriculum that teaches professionalism: transforming the social environment of a medical school. *Journal of General Internal Medicine* 2004; **19**: 501–4.

13 Smith KL, Saavedra R, Raeke JL, O'Donell AA. The journey to creating a campus-wide culture of professionalism. *Academic Medicine* 2007; **82**: 1015–21.

14 Aultman JM. Uncovering the hidden medical curriculum through a pedagogy of discomfort. *Advances in Health Sciences Education* 2005; **10**: 263–73.

15 Brainard AH, Brislen HC. Learning professionalism: a view from the trenches. *Academic Medicine* 2007; **82**: 1010–14.

16 Cohen JJ. Linking professionalism to humanism: what it means, why it matters. *Academic Medicine* 2007; **82**: 1029–32.

17 Seabrook MA. Intimidation in medical education: students' and teachers' perspectives. *Studies in Higher Education* 2004; **29**: 59–74.

18 Lempp H, Seale C. The hidden curriculum in undergraduate medical education: qualitative study of medical students' perceptions of teaching. *BMJ* 2004; **329**: 770–3.

19 West CP, Shanafelt TD. The influence of personal and environmental factors on professionalism in medical education. *BMC Medical Education* 2007; **30**: 29.

20 Marta J. Toward a bioethics for the twenty-first century: a Ricoeurian poststructuralist narrative hermeneutic approach to informed consent. In: Nelson HL (ed.). *Stories and Their Limits: Narrative approaches to bioethics*. New York: Routledge; 1997. pp. 198–212.

21 Das V. Suffering, legitimacy and healing: the Bhopal case. In: Das V (ed.). *Critical Events: An anthropological perspective on contemporary India*. Delhi, India: Oxford University Press; 1995. pp. 137–74.

22 Dyrbye LN, Thomas MR, Shanafelt TD. Systematic review of depression, anxiety, and other indicators of psychological distress among U.S. and Canadian medical students. *Academic Medicine* 2006; **81**: 354–73.

23 Dahlin ME, Runeson B. Burnout and psychiatric morbidity among medical students entering clinical training: a three-year prospective questionnaire and interview-based study. *BMC Medical Education* 2007; **7**: 6.

24 Dunn LB, Iglewicz A, Moutier C. A conceptual model of medical student well-being: promoting resilience and preventing burnout. *Academic Psychiatry* 2008; **32**: 44–53.

25 Niemi PM, Vainiomäki PT. Medical students' distress – quality, continuity and gender differences during a six-year medical programme. *Medical Teacher* 2006; **28**: 136–41.

26 Dyrbye LN, Thomas MR, Shanafelt TD. Medical student distress: causes consequences, and proposed solutions. *Mayo Clinic Proceedings* 2005; **80**: 1613–22.

27 Stratton TD, Saunders JA, Elam CL. Changes in medical students' emotional intelligence: an exploratory study. *Teaching and Learning in Medicine* 2008; **20**: 279–84.

28 Dyrbye LN, Thomas MR, Huntington JL, *et al*. Personal life events and medical student burnout: a multicenter study. *Academic Medicine* 2006; **81**: 374–84.

29 Dahlin M, Joneborg N, Runeson B. Stress and depression among medical students: a cross-sectional study. *Medical Education* 2005; **39**: 594–604.

30 Humphrey HJ, Smith K, Reddy S, *et al.* Promoting an environment of professionalism: the University of Chicago "roadmap." *Academic Medicine* 2007; **82**: 1098–107.

31 Enns MW, Cox BJ, Sareen J, Freeman P. Adaptive and maladaptive perfectionism in medical students: a longitudinal investigation. *Medical Education* 2001; **35**: 1034–42.

32 Tyssen R, Dolatowski FC, Røvik JO, *et al.* Personality traits and types predict medical school stress: a six-year longitudinal and nationwide study. *Medical Education* 2007; **41**: 781–7.

6 It's Not Only What's In Your Brain, It's What's In Your Heart: Becoming a Physician – Part 2

The quest to understand the nature of physicianhood is a complex one. After the initial shock at the overwhelming nature of medical school, and a sense of grievance at how they are treated and how they are changing, students often expand their attempts to answer the question "How do I become a doctor?" Some common themes explored in students' poetry include struggling with their insecurities about their lack of knowledge, and then, as their knowledge increases, attempting to understand the true nature of what one needs to know to be a good physician, and finally coping with the realization that, regardless of knowledge, medicine is limited and uncertain. As their understanding deepens, many students are able to reconcile the value of content information with more ineffable qualities of compassion, caring, and service, and learn to balance the art and the science of medicine. Contemplating their journey towards physicianhood, some privileged students achieve a kind of transcendent perspective, often guided by their religious faith.

Roses are Red, Violets are Blue By: Sabin Motwani
Originally appeared in Plexus *2003, p. 11, UC Irvine School of Medicine*

Roses are Red
Violets are Blue
Why does it seem every physician has a different view?

To many patients, we garner respect because of the white coat
As we try to find the perfect antidote.

Are we really striving for preventative perfection
Or are we merely treating a symptomatic deception?

In medical school, we admit the best of the best
So that they can survive, test after test.

After two years of cerebral regurgitation, stenosis begins
the pressure builds, the third year begins

We are finally allowed to critique and think
Even after retracting without a blink, smelling a stink, or sleeping a wink.

Fourth year: it's time to decide what kind of patients do you want to see?
Kids that are stung by a bee or older patients who are unable to pee.

You've graduated, two more letters, a longer coat

and some pocket change to pay rent on your humble abode.
To the patient, nothing has changed; except maybe their ICD9 code

All this training, but do patients care?
Oh, quite contraire, they want to be heard, be treated fair.
Not learn some esoteric fact about the half life of Voltaren.

Are physicians occupied too much with the A and P rather than the H and P?
Can't our reward be a person's smile of glee
Rather than a paycheck full of G's?

Compassion and empathy will take us physicians far.
Yet when death comes unexpected, we drown our sorrows at the nearest bar.

It's all about efficiency and speed. Where is the time?
Do we turn away disheveled, dysenteric patients with all this grime
that can't afford to pay a dime
And then admit a drug-seeking addict for no reason or rhyme?

Medicine is full of patterns and paradox.
Patients inherently ask "Can we make sense of it?"

The answer is no, but we do our best learning patient by patient
bit by bit trying to make the pieces fit.

In the end, medicine's not an exact science, it's an art.
It's not only what's in your brain, it's what's in your heart.

In this poem, a young doctor is trying to sum up his training, and in the process is touching on many of the issues and concerns that comprise the focus of many student works addressing this theme. The poem represents a review, in rhyming couplets and trios, of the four years of his medical education. In a chronological narrative, the narrator briefly references the harsh adjustment, delineated in detail in Chapter 5, of entering medical school as "the best of the best," only to be reduced to survival mode. He then gives a nod to the intellectual and memorization demands of Year 2, suggesting that as a result there is a stenosis (a narrowing process often associated with cardiac disease) of his heart. Next come the stresses and pressures of Year 3, reiterating the sense of being besieged we saw in Chapter 5. Fourth year brings decisions about choice of specialty, and finally, the long-awaited graduation with the ironically impressive accoutrements of a longer white coat, accumulated credentials, and the promise of a paycheck.

The poem explores the relationship between content knowledge attainment and learning to becoming a physician. In the very first stanza, the narrator tackles the issue of uncertainty, and implies that he has come to realize the limitations of knowledge and the separation that exists between knowing information, data, research and clinical practice. The narrator admits to aspirations to perfection, which may have seemed achievable at one point through study of textbooks and attendance at lectures, but he has learned that doctoring is an imperfect pursuit.

Later, the narrator recognizes that although didactic training is of course necessary and important, what patients care most about is not the esoteric information absorbed by the student, but being heard and treated with respect, empathy, and compassion. In the end, the narrator accepts that medicine is full of "patterns and paradox." This phrase, too, is partly a reference to academic training, in that clinical reasoning is often taught through a process of pattern recognition. It is also a reference to its limits, in that clinical surprises inexorably come along that violate the pattern. As the poem ends, its author circles back to the question of uncertainty. Patients want to know the answer to this question: can their doctors make sense of what is happening to them? The answer in the largest sense must be no, despite all the learning, memorizing, lectures, and examinations. The most that doctors can do is to make sense of pieces here and there, and do their best to fit them together. The poem ends by acknowledging that the best learning comes not from textbooks, but slowly, painfully, patient by patient. In the end, the student comes to learn that although mastering content knowledge is essential, equally essential is the quality of one's heart.

The poem also explores, at the deepest level, why one becomes a doctor. Comparing the A and P (probably a reference to the market chain) to the H and P (patient history and physical) is shorthand for the materialistic, consumer focus that can all too easily overwhelm a physician's concern for the patient's well-being. This is substantiated by the lines that follow, which talk explicitly about the rewards of doctoring, and how these should be defined not only in monetary terms but also in human terms. In related themes, the poem raises important questions about how physicians cope with the death of patients (*see* Chapter 12 for an in-depth examination of this topic), and how inequities of access and care exist (*see* Chapter 11). Both of these issues challenge physicians (and the student himself) to have the courage to confront death and injustice, rather than turning away. Witnessing to such concerns with an open heart, it is intimated, constitutes the art of medicine.

LACK OF KNOWLEDGE

The acquisition of knowledge sometimes appears to be a way of overcoming role confusion. Yet students' relationship to learning the requisite information, facts, and data of their medical education is complex. Students worry that they do not have enough knowledge, yet they often resent having to acquire such vast quantities of information. They feel that the constant testing and evaluation turns them into passive machines that absorb and then spew out facts. Eventually, they begin to feel that they are succeeding in their mastery of knowledge, and they even begin to reflect on the nature of the knowledge that will truly transform them into physicians, challenging and enlarging what kinds of knowledge matter in medicine. Students address this issue through a variety of narrative types.

Chaos stories

Students often feel confused about their role as a medical student, with more knowledge than the patient, but not nearly enough to really be a physician. One student observing a surgery contrasts her own bewilderment with the surgeon's arcane expertise. To the novice student, the surgery seems like a dance, "choreographed by years of experience," with the dancers speaking "an unknown tongue."

In another poem, the student prepares for her first day as a doctor, white-coat pockets stuffed with the equipment and trappings, accessories meticulously selected to convey competence and professionalism. She tries on the metaphor of being a superhero, and knows that she has the knowledge. But then "the chill" – the reality of her situation – sets in, and she feels only insecure and uncertain. She is "not ready."

First Year By: Monya De
Originally appeared in Plexus *2002, p. 9, UC Irvine School of Medicine*

The instrument's in place
Draping my shoulders like a superhero cape.
Mirrors blind me as I behold the white. My hands, at the sides
"Open, friendly."
Glasses, now. More distinguished-looking.
Even a wedding band! Just to calm the nervous
Mabels and Pollies, and Thomases too.
The knowledge is there, in the corners
Of my eyes, and in
Those three horizontal lines.
The pen, Mont Blanc; heavy, wise.
My memory, purged of rubbish
Brimming with molecules and lives
Five alarms. Extra scrubs.
Pager, nerves, and Stedman's.
Pharmacopoeia, Vivarin.
The best of the best of wishes.
And still —
The chill —
I am not ready.

Another student perceives himself as "bumbling . . . fumbling." He expresses his exasperation at having to ask his patients so many questions over and over, even as he recognizes that he has to "cover all the bases." In another poem, a student who is supposed to perform a pelvic examination describes himself as nervous and uncertain. He reflects on the irony that, while the patient is "all done," he is "just beginning," sobered by his awareness of the long road of training ahead. Another student on pediatrics brags that he is "without fear" in the face of a baby's crying. Later, however, he begs the infant for help because "I have no clue / Of what to do." Another poem poses a list of questions that a medical student might want to ask, but cannot for fear of being perceived as stupid, insecure, or uncertain. The student-poet is looking for answers. She seeks the truth, but wonders how to recognize it. The poem ends on a plaintive note: "Is that all there is?"

In a different poem, a student struggles to define his role in relation to a seriously ill patient. He reflects on the precise moment at which an old World War Two veteran becomes his patient, when the student has to break bad news to him. The student realizes that there would be no Yanks coming to rescue this "old soldier." The student is daunted ("My mind became incontinent") when he realizes that the only reason why the patient's grin is "no longer absurd" is because the patient is counting on his new "doctor" (the student) as his last hope. The student is terrified because, unlike the patient, who "knew nothing of limitations," he is aware of how little he can offer this patient. He is also terrified because he is about to become responsible (morally, if not medically) for this dying man. This poem contains both elements of chaos and elements of journey. The student accepts responsibility for the patient, a first step on the journey to physicianhood, but he is overwhelmed and unprepared for assuming the responsibility of functioning as the patient's "doctor."

In a humorous poem that expresses both chaos and at least the hope of restitution, the narrator is studying diligently when he falls into a thrilling fantasy of a man choking in a restaurant and the student, the "doctor in the house," trying to remember how to save his life. But then the narrator realizes that he isn't a doctor yet, he's just a little "mouse," studying at his desk. He knows that one day he will find his place and have "a tall white coat to hide the tail." However, in the meantime he must stop dreaming and keep studying. The poem gives voice to both the student's heroic aspirations and his current ignorance.

Desktop Daydream By: Rishi Doshi
Originally published in Body Language: Poems of the Medical Training Experience *edited by Neeta Jain, Dagan Coppock and Stephanie Brown Clark, 2006, p. 32 Reprinted with the permission of BOA Editions, Ltd,* www.boaeditions.org

Xeroxed wisdom
Flips in slippery pages through paper-slit fingers
And quivers in the beam of a desk lamp
To hit these pupils
Before my lids slam shut the night
Angered by the insistence of the carbonated
And the carbon-copied paper
Resting threateningly on my notebooks

Somewhere
A man falls in a densely packed restaurant
Clatter of plates reverberates to tell me
It is time
Yes, there is a doctor in the house
I lie/tensely beside him
His pulse a drizzle next to my own storming chest
Wrestle with remembered modes of
Resuscitation/vaguely studied information
Curious crowd gathers in loud gasps
Fingers clasped I pound my fist
To crack open memory/but why can't he
Breathe?

Back to reality
No doctor in this house
Just a lazy town mouse experimenting
Atop a fence of frustration
A first-year imitation with a vision
And a new desk lamp
That makes the carbon shine
Just dimmer than a daydream
He's back at the Xerox machine
Paying for knowledge with common cents

And one day he'll find his place
With a tall white coat to hide the tail
It's all the rage/but till then
Stop the dream/open your eyes/take the copies
Turn the page.

In a poem that has elements of both chaos and journey, another third-year student is both mocked and helped by his resident "guides." He desperately hunts for physical causes of a patient's disease, only to realize eventually that the source of the problem was the patient's broken heart. He had not known enough yet to consider a psychological explanation, but instead investigated all sorts of complicated and rare biomedical possibilities. However, through diligence and being tested, he acquires greater insight and understanding.

LEARNING AND ACQUISITION OF KNOWLEDGE
Witnessing (resistance) stories

Studying and preparing for examinations constitutes a large part of becoming a doctor. Although some of these stories are cries for help (one student writes about the "first aid" of coffee to help him keep awake to study), most of these poems assert resistance to this aspect of medical education. For example, in the poem just mentioned, by referring to his textbooks' physician-authors as "embalmed," the poem evokes images of death (or deathly boredom), staleness, and irrelevance. In general, students can see little redeeming value in the test-taking, and write witnessing counter-narratives. One student complains about having to memorize irrelevant material for exams. He asserts that he has good skills with patients, "But I don't get points for past acts of empathy." In this poem, the author challenges the conventional wisdom of the crucial importance of exam scores, and trusts the excellence of the physician he knows himself to be. The student attempts to keep faith with the vision he brought with him into medical school, and resists the more dominant view of what constitutes a successful medical student.

Transcendence stories

Some poems about knowledge attainment are stories of transcendence. A tired student forcing herself to study suddenly has an epiphany – knowledge is about more than passing exams or appeasing professors. Ultimately, it is about the patients who will one day depend on her. In this case, the student's frame of reference shifts suddenly and unexpectedly. At first, the student feels burdened by the constant studying required in medical school. Then she moves to a different level of connectedness and devotion by realizing that the aim of this studying is not to pass exams or to placate professors, but to assist patients. This allows her to place learning in a more generous and altruistic context. Another student reflects that all this learning must come from the inside out. She realizes that she is learning about life and death, and that it is important always to take the time to keep learning. In the end, all this learning is to serve people who need hope for healing, which physicians can provide. In a similarly transcendent poem, the narrator also challenges the definition of learning. What is learning all about? What is important in the learning process? The student acknowledges the crucial importance of lifelong learning not to perform well on tests, but to serve patients. These poems all have an element of transcendence, in that ownership of the learning process is occurring, and the definition of knowledge is deepening.

INCREASING KNOWLEDGE, SKILL, AND CONFIDENCE
Restitution stories

As students advance through training, they move from ignorance to some measure of confidence. These are partly journey stories, in that they move the student towards greater ownership both of patients and of the profession. However, on the whole they are most like restitution stories, because the student's familiar confidence and competence have been restored. These poems are often less about personal growth and evolution, and more about acquisition of skills and consequent reclamation of status. One student symbolized this evolution by saying that, just as the white coats are transformed from clean to dirty during anatomy lab, so the first-year student evolves from lack of knowledge to expertise. Such poems emphasize the achievement of knowledge as a kind of secret power. In these cases, the student-physicians develop special "abilities" to see past the surface of people into their inner core, often detecting weaknesses and vulnerabilities in the process. This new-found power to know more about people than they necessarily know about themselves or than others know about them is viewed as one of the advantages of specialized training.

In contrast to the poem noted above, in which the student's short white coat was a symbol of humiliation and degradation, a different "Ode to a White Coat" sees the coat as a "badge of knowledge." Although the coat is "starched, impersonal," it is "still my friend." It carries everything that the student needs, and provides some much needed status. She is confident that, in the process of becoming a doctor, it will grow with her. One third-year student doing his pediatric clerkship acknowledges feelings of boredom, tiredness, and frustration: "it's easy to view each patient as another tedious examination." However, as the clerkship progresses, he realizes that a better approach is to look at each encounter as an opportunity to learn something new, or to finally use what has been presented in textbooks in a real-life setting.

Journey stories

Some poems that focus on students' evolving attainment of learning and competence are true journey narratives. In a poem that documents her journey to physicianhood, one student compares herself to "a lump of potter's clay, waiting to be formed." By Year 3, thanks to wise mentors, "The clay now has a shape." Although she still has doubts about her choices and skills (the demons and monsters with which she struggles), when a patient calls her "doctor", she begins "to see a shadow of a form on the wheel." By the end of the poem, she cannot predict the outcome, but restates her commitment to medicine and to lifetime learning.

In another journey poem that adopts the rhythms of the charming holiday poem "'Twas the Night Before Christmas," the student starts the all-important clinical clerkship year confused and unprepared (the reluctant hero). She dreads the hassled residents and the scut work that they will assign her (monsters and obstacles). After a month, she is ready to retire. However, by the end of the year, she realizes that she had had great teams and grateful patients (both her wise guides), was finally able to "connect the medical clues," and had learned to set aside her fears. She has learned and grown (wisdom gained), and is now closer to being a real doctor (returning to the world to assist others).

'Twas the Night Before Clerkship By: Nita Doshi
UC Irvine, 2002

'Twas the night before clerkship, I couldn't sleep a wink
Even with Ambien, I stayed up to think.
My white coat was hung in the closet with care,
In hopes that a cute doctor the next day would be there.
My patients "to be" were restrained in their beds
So much to look forward to, I thought in my head.
And the residents so bitter, and I so naive
I was not looking forward to the scut up their sleeves.
The next day finally came, my brain was a scatter,
Given my board scores, third year probably did matter.
Up from my bed, I arose way too quick
Orthostatic hypotension, boy did I feel sick.
I went back to sleep, but forgot my alarm
Fifteen minutes, I thought, wouldn't do any harm.
When what to my wondering eyes and bad luck
7:45 on the clock, I thought, oh f#ə%!
With my toothbrush and iron, and then a loud rip,
My pants tore on a corner, so much for my cute outfit.
More rapid down Campus Drive I came
The slow commuters passed as I cursed out names.
Left on University, then left on the 73,
Who knew that it was soon to be second nature to me.
To the top of the stairs in good old med ed
Noon conferences and vignettes so soon for me to dread.
Out in the heat, we all had to extinguish a fire
Code red, code yellow, code blue, I already wanted to retire.
When down the hall, I heard beepers beeping
I knew right away it had to be Dr. Amin.
"Who wants to fail?" he asked with a smile
Then Tara came in with our folders in a pile.
20 write-ups, a shelf, and an oral exam
There had to be a way out, I'd think up a scam.
Four weeks through it and at the VA
Sixteen admissions on our first call day.
Soft, non-tender, but severely distended I'd write
More veins missed than draws I got right.
How could I get stuck with Fred for 8 weeks
And why did my first paracentesis spring a leak.
Sixteen weeks later, and five pounds lighter
The light at the end of the tunnel was brighter.
I thought to myself what great teams I had had
Aside from my CPX, nothing went bad.

The patients' gratitude and numerous thank you's.
Being able to finally connect the medical clues.
No need for the cute outfits, and no need for the fear
Ladies and Gentlemen, Welcome to 3rd Year.

Witnessing (resistance) stories

Some students doubt whether they improve with training. These are counter-narratives to the prevailing narrative of an upward trajectory of competence and success. They bear witness to a more complex future that includes pretense and mistakes. One such poem suggests that as the medical student gains experience, he becomes emboldened and must appear more competent and brighter, although he has not really become wiser or stronger. In another poem, the narrator notes that her white coat, once pristine, has over time become stained and yellow, a testament to all that she has learned and experienced. However, four years later there is "the same stuff underneath" – the same person with the same doubts and fears. The student feels the same confusion and chaos that she felt at the beginning of her medical training, but now must also deal with repression of her uncertainty, and the pretense of knowledge. In a similar vein, another medical student apologizes in advance to the unknown patient for an error he has not yet committed. He recognizes that making a mistake is inevitable. Although his intentions are to help, he knows that he will never achieve sufficient knowledge and skill to avoid harming some patients.

DEVELOPING AN UNDERSTANDING OF DOCTORING
Restitution stories

Some poems that reflect on what it means to become a doctor wax more philosophical, trying to consciously determine their views of the nature of medicine and doctoring. In the preclinical years, students often adopt a positivist view, framing disease as evil (the enemy), and medicine as healing, strengthening, and life-affirming. Medical treatment has a happy ending, where the patient is free of suffering and ready to return to life.

Journey stories

When students reach the clinical years, their poems become more nuanced and complex, often representing more of a journey in the sense that ownership of their knowledge and skills is developing, as well as recognition of limitations and ambiguous information. These authors have altered their view of what makes a successful physician, and put knowledge and competence within a humanistic framework. One such poem, which is cited in full in Chapter 10 ("The clinic"), recognizes the limitations of the physician role, but also concludes that if the student listens to the point of view of patients, they will always say something of value. Another student comes to realize that although "each patient has a story," these stories are incomplete and "patchy," not black and white as the student first expected, but mostly shades of gray. A student on a pediatric clerkship struggles with the pain that he feels listening to the cries of children, but after many encounters concludes that the rewards of the profession lie in their smiles: "it makes your heart feel light again."

Transcendence stories

In another type of reflection on the nature of doctoring, the student uses an extended metaphor of hundreds of starfish washed up on a beach after a storm. The narrator starts throwing them back into the ocean when a jogger stops to point out the futility of this act. The narrator does not disagree, but nonetheless he continues his ultimately impossible task. Ultimately medicine is like throwing back the starfish – you save a few, many die, and in the end they all die. Over the course of his training, this student has arrived at a deep understanding of both the impossibility of ultimate success, and the necessity of providing succor. His observations suggest that the value of medicine is found in the act itself, regardless of the outcome. The narrator has meditated on and come to peace with the knowledge that it is part of the human condition that ultimately death will always win. The poem is one of transcendence rather than witnessing, because the student is not only acknowledging this harsh reality, but also in the face of this witnessing makes a commitment to provide comfort and assistance to the best of his ability.

A few students literally cry out to God to help guide their evolution from student to physician. These poems are always transcendent in that they release their fears, limitations, doubt, and frustrations to a higher power; and in return find the consolation of spiritual healing and the support of faith. In one representative poem, a second-year student thanks God for providing blessings, support, and strength. He prays for guidance in good times and bad, and beseeches God for help to sustain him. He uses the biblical phrase "Here I am" (*hineini* in Hebrew), often used to convey readiness to accept God's will.

A prayer in weakness By: Gabriel Herscu
UC Irvine

Thank you Lord
for blessing me
with everything I need and more
for bringing me here
for giving me strength for direction for perseverance for peace, for peace
I could never do this alone

Help me Lord
to look to you
when things go wrong when things go right as I study
your creation and marvel
at your works
as I learn to follow as I make my way yours

Guide me Lord
in my purpose in your purpose
stay with me as I make my decisions in weakness
Here I am

In Jesus' Name.

Another student prays to God to help him to love, to care, to be giving, and to provide help to others. He asks to live in peace, to be a healing presence, and to be meek, forgiving, and tolerant. With God's help, he seeks to serve his patients with compassion.

In a different poem a student also asks for divine support and guidance to be a healer. The first section of the poem is a paean to the miracle of life itself. Next, the author recognizes the potential "derangement" that can afflict the physical body, while also recognizing that we have the intellectual capacity to cure as well as the "spirit to heal." The student then asks for help in seeing beyond the laboratory results, the machines, and the diagnosis to "the sufferers, the human being." He goes on to ask for gentleness and calmness, patience, passion for his profession, strength for continual learning, and an "endless supply of love," and admits "I could never do this alone." He prays for God's guidance in making decisions, and to make God's way his way and God's purpose his purpose. He reminds himself that although the doctor may be perceived as a god, God is the true physician.

The prayer of Ben Rogoway By: Ben Rogoway
Based upon the work of the RAMBAM
UC Irvine, 2003

Almighty, you have created the human body with infinite wisdom
You have seen fit to endow us with legs that run, lungs that breathe
a heart that pumps, and a brain that thinks
You have given us a soul that feels, a spirit that soars
and an essence that yearns for fulfillment

Every time I look through a microscope, I can see the wonders
of your living world
I am so easily reminded that such complexity must not be by accident
Carbon, Oxygen, Hydrogen — all elements have their place
Working in undetectable, infinitesimal space
Laws of physics and chemistry to power life

Random? Free will? Predestination?
Is there a designer for this design, an architect of this building
a planner of this plan?
Are we a sum, or just a collection of parts?
The complexity of harmony between its ten thousand organs, vessels, ducts, foramen, notches, hitches, trochanters, arches, and
Neurons combine to act unceasingly to preserve the whole in all its beauty
The body acts to envelop the immortal soul
They act, without thought or effort in perfect order to agree to keep us alive

Yet, sometimes frailty of matter deranges this perfect order
and forces clash between body and spirit
Yet, sometimes our greatest intentions and efforts and technology that are used to thwart this process are to no avail
Sometimes, despite its perfection in agreement and accord, the body crumbles
into the primal dust from which it came

You have blessed the Earth, rivers and mountains with healing substances
You enable creatures to alleviate their sufferings and to heal their illnesses
You have endowed man with the wisdom to relieve the suffering of his brother
You have allowed us to recognize disorders, and extract the healing substances
You have allowed us to discover powers to suit every ill
You have given me hands to touch and eyes to see
You have given me ears to hear and a heart to feel
But you have given me even more — a spirit to heal

In your eternal providence, you have chosen me to watch over
the life and health of your creatures
I am now about to apply myself to the duties of my profession
Support me in these great labors so that I may benefit mankind
For without your help not even my greatest effort will succeed

Inspire me with love for my art and for my patients
Do not allow me to thirst for profit or ambition
Let not desire for renown or admiration cloud my judgment
to interfere with my profession
These qualities are my enemy and can lead me astray
in fulfilling the great task of attending to the welfare of your creatures

But medicine is hard
I am tired so frequently
I frustrate and get angry
I feel incapable, unworthy and alone
I often know not what I am doing
I fail in treating myself with the respect
I so desire to treat others

Preserve the strength of my body and of my soul that they ever be ready
Allow me strength to cheerfully help and support rich and poor
good and bad, enemy as well as friend
Let me see beyond the x-ray, beyond the lab
beyond the blips and the bleeps of the machine
Let the sufferer be more than just a collection of symptoms
Please let me see only the human being

Illumine my mind that it recognizes that which may be hidden
Let me not fail to see what is visible
Yet, do not permit it to arrogate by seeing what cannot be seen
Let me never be absent-minded
Let me be not lazy or forgetful
Let me be not hasty or indecisive
Let me be prudent
Let me do what is right
May no strange thoughts divert my attention at the bedside of the sick

Grant that my patients have confidence in me
May they follow my directions and my council

May they trust that I do for them as I would have done unto me
Let not a needed medication go unfilled or a needed procedure go undone
Let not another cigarette be smoked or bottle of beer be drunk
Remove all charlatans and cruel people
who arrogantly frustrate the wisest purposes of our art

Almighty, send me a teacher
Should those who are wiser than I wish to improve and instruct me
let my soul gratefully follow their guidance
Let me one day be in their shoes
Vast is the extent of our art

Imbue my soul with gentleness and calmness
When older colleagues, proud of their age, wish to displace me or to scorn me or disdainfully to
teach me grant me patience
May even this be of advantage to me
They know many things of which I am ignorant
but let not their arrogance give me pain
For they are old and old age is not master of the passions
I also hope to attain old age upon this earth, before Thee, Almighty God!

Let me be contented in everything except in the great science of my profession
Never allow the thought to arise in me that I have attained to sufficient knowledge
Grant me the passion to continue to love what I am doing
Grant me the strength to continue to learn until the end of my days
Grant me an endless supply of love that I can shower
on all people until the end of my days

You have given me an awesome responsibility
Grant me the humility to know that I am not the cause nor am I the cure
I am only the vessel, the tool, the machine by which you work
Grant me the power to fix what I can, and the serenity to know
that which I cannot
For in my life, may I always remember the true healer is You.

SUMMARY

In their poetry, clinical students not infrequently describe a sense of uncertainty and inadequacy. The accumulation of knowledge seems a natural way of clarifying this confusion, as suggested by research (cited in Chapter 5) which found that knowledge was regarded as the prime determinant of becoming a doctor. However, although many students worry about their lack of knowledge, they also express resistance towards the quantity and nature of the learning process, feeling it to be both oppressive and overwhelming. In this way their poetry challenges the emphasis on knowledge acquisition and examination performance that appears to be central to the informal curriculum. As they proceed through training, they document increasing knowledge and confidence in restitution stories. Yet some students witness to a countervailing story that challenges the positivist view of an upward trajectory of increasing mastery and competence. When students attempt to reflect on the deeper meaning of doctoring, they sometimes attain a transcendent comprehension, especially if they are supported by a spiritual perspective.

7 Oh Doctor, Doctor, What Can I Do? Becoming a Patient

In the mid to late twentieth century, literature about patients' subjective experiences, usually written by patients themselves or by family members, mushroomed. It is impossible to discuss this phenomenon in detail here, but from its inception it emphasized a phenomenological approach[1,2] that examined the subjective, particularistic, and emotional experiences of patients, from the perspective and priorities *of the patient*, not the physician, who previously had been in control of the patient's presentation (usually in a professional context, such as medical rounds). An underlying theme of this body of work is the value of reclaiming the individual patient's voice and of documenting and sharing personal, subjective experience. The study of pathography, or stories of illness,[3] has identified various narrative genres, such as were mentioned in Chapter 3.[4] Other conceptual analyses have also been proposed.[5] In addition, scholars have identified certain underlying phenomena in the experience of illness, such as loss, including loss of control,[6,7] disintegration of the non-ill self,[6] the absence of order and coherence,[8] randomness, destabilization, and isolation and alienation,[9,10] but simultaneously, at least at times, the possibility of role flexibility and empowerment.[11]

This literature (published in both popular and academic venues) cannot be characterized in a single way, in that various works reify dominant narratives about illness (cure and restitution), while others offer counter-hegemonic accounts. Some do both within the same document.[12] Some focus on individual growth and transformation – how an encounter with serious illness has made them better people. Others refuse to accept a purely personal understanding, and instead take on societal and political aspects of becoming a patient.[13,14] It has been pointed out that non-patients, in the world of the well, prefer to hear restitution stories, which obviously have a reassuring effect while diminishing the perceived distress of patient and family resulting from illness.[15]

Interestingly, little of this voluminous literature has entered the formal training of medical students as a tool for assisting them in understanding the subjective experiences of their patients. It is commonplace to include empathy training in communication proficiency courses.[16–18] Empathy, of course, is the primary way in which we apprehend the experiences and perspectives of others. Necessarily, this skills-based approach emphasizes behavioral, observable dimensions of the expression of empathy, such as verbal skills of paraphrasing and clarifying. Most research shows that these interventions are at least somewhat effective in improving behavioral empathy in medical students, although significant methodological limitations make this conclusion tentative.[19,20] As with most formal coursework in medical school, this training usually occurs during the preclinical years, *before* students have had much significant exposure to patients. In the last decade, medical educators have also engaged in numerous creative and bold curricular experiments to bring the subjective, particularistic experience of patients closer to the awareness of students. A handful of these are described below.

Increasingly, we are seeing courses or other curricular offerings in narrative medicine, or other novel patient-oriented encounters, whose primary purpose is to bring medical students into contact with the unmediated voice of people who are experiencing illness, or at least to move them closer to the experience of these patients. Some of these learning activities go back decades – for example, the practice of having students or residents admitted as "patients" to the hospital where they will be practicing as part of their orientation.[21] Other activities include shadowing patients over time,[22] making home visits,[23] and arranging conversations between beginning medical students and patients suffering from chronic illnesses.[24,25] Yet other approaches include engaging in dramatic enactments of medical encounters,[26] often using patients' own words,[27] writing first-person narratives from the perspectives of patients[28] or cadavers,[29] writing letters to doctors from the patient's perspective,[30] using reflective writing to have medical students describe personal illness experiences, and then sharing this writing with other students,[31] and reading literature and poetry written by patients or written from the patient's point of view.[32-4] Another curricular project used a variety of creative media to help third-year students on a medicine clerkship to better understand the patient's experience of illness.[35] The aim of such initiatives is to bring the medical student closer to the patient's experience without, of course, having to endure the actual distress of *being* a patient. However, students and physicians who have had the misfortune to become ill themselves or to experience serious illness of a loved one indicate that, as a result, their empathy has been heightened.[36]

These and other pioneering efforts hold great promise. In general, when they are evaluated, the findings indicate that participating students develop a deeper, richer understanding of the complexity of illness phenomena, incorporating familial, cultural, emotional, and spiritual dimensions as well as biomedical dimensions. Exposure to patient stories is effective in challenging students' assumptions about what it is like to have a particular disease or to care for people with that disease, and is successful in helping students to see the world of sickness from other perspectives.[25,32,33,37] Yet even now such curricula are rarely considered central to training, and they are often either offered on an elective basis, or in other ways positioned on the margins of the mainstream curriculum.

This is perhaps not surprising, given that the idea of learning directly from patients threatens the supremacy of the physician as sole source of knowledge (and therefore power) by placing him or her more in the role of guide and interpreter of information and experience exchanged between patient and student. A groundbreaking medical school in the UK has adopted the radical approach of prioritizing the formation of a direct, collaborative relationship between student and patient across multiple learning contexts, emphasizing the production of collaborative knowledge between student and patient.[38] Other scholars have pointed out that the traditional method of taking the patient history and establishing the chief complaint in many ways discourages patient self-disclosure and the kind of patient-centered medicine that allows patients to share their real concerns and give students a glimpse into their lives.[39] Rita Charon has provided a strong theoretical argument as to why narrative medicine should play a central role in medical training,[40] and recently Kumagai has contributed additional theoretical work drawing on both theories of empathy and moral development to expand these arguments.[24] I have also attempted to theorize as to why it is necessary to change or at least expand some of the philosophical premises on which medicine is based in order to make empathy a more accessible response for learners.[41]

What must be emphasised is that, at present, almost all of these promising curricular initiatives occupy a fairly marginal position in the formal, mandatory curriculum. Therefore, although they have exciting potential, they only suggest what might be, and not, unfortunately, what is. As a result, students often do not receive much formal training in understanding what illness looks like from the patient perspective. We know that in the presence of patients, students can learn about what it is like to be a patient, as well as about patients' emotional responses, ranging from fear and sadness to optimism and transcendence.[42] We also know that, as in all aspects of medicine, an understanding of the patient's experience is often inhibited by the hidden curriculum, which can convey objectification of the patient, prioritize efficiency over empathy, and encourage students to engage in practices that "subject patients to discomfort and indignity in order to learn."[43] In the face of this inconsistent curricular guidance, medical student poetry is particularly instructive in helping us to understand how they think about, explore, and wrestle with what it means to be a patient.

Students seemed to understand instinctively the importance of attempting to penetrate the subjective experiences of their patients. In the face of patient suffering, some students told chaos stories through their poetry, and some told restitution stories, perhaps to relieve their own sympathetic anxiety. However, the majority of these students seemed able to see clearly the chaos experience of their patients, and generally positioned themselves in the role of bearing witness to their suffering. These students appeared to be intensely aware of the ways in which patients are sometimes turned into the "unacceptable other", and chose to take a stand in solidarity with the patient, not the medical system.

Heavy Questions By: Rebecca Smith
UC Irvine, 2001
What makes you think you can waltz in here
With your long, clean, white coat
A stethoscope draped elegantly around your neck
Chart and pen in hand
And tell me what kind of person I am?

Who says you can tell me
My cholesterol is too high
My BMI says I'm obese
My blood pressure is uncontrolled
And that I need to change my "lifestyle"?

Who are you to doubt me when I say
"I've tried every diet, I exercise daily
I eat healthy
But I still can't lose weight"?

How can you say
That it's not my thyroid
That I don't have a slow metabolism
And that it's not in my genes?

How can you look at me with disdain, as if I deserve
Shortness of breath when I exercise
Constant pain in my joints and muscles
And that annoying rash under my breasts?

Where do you think you earned the right
To think twice about my honesty
Wonder about my determination
And to question my will power?

How can you really think
That Jenny Craig works
That Weight Watchers is easy
And that the Atkins is the perfect solution?

Why don't you address
My troubled childhood
My loveless marriage
And my dead-end job?

Why can't you see
My loss of interest
My depressed mood
And my suicidal thoughts?

Why don't you look inside
Beyond my fat arms
Swollen ankles
And double chin?

Have you ever been overweight a day in your life?
Have you ever struggled to lose a single, solitary pound?
Do you think you can really understand me?
Can you really understand what I feel?

Well, doctor
Although you may not understand me or my problem.
And although you may
Not deem obesity to be a real "medical problem"
I deserve the compassion, respect, and dignity
That you treat all of your other patients with.

And please, doctor
When you are treating those who are like me
And you catch yourself
Judging, doubting, and questioning
Recall what you have learned from me
And remember that heavy people have feelings too.

This poem is typical in many ways of the poems that students write when they are trying to understand the experiences of their patients. This author chooses to use the first-person voice, so she is writing from the point of view of the patient. In this poem, the patient confronts her doctor, who is silent throughout. It is quite possible that the narrator is only speaking inside her own anguished head.

In the discourse, we learn a lot about the doctor, who is portrayed as judgmental and supercilious. In the first stanza, the doctor hides behind the accoutrements of the role – white coat, stethoscope, and chart. This description of the seemingly in-control, well-organized, "elegant" professional serves to underline the gulf that exists between him or her and the patient, who, at least initially, appears to be overwhelmed, depressed, and suicidal. The patient chronicles her many resentments against this doctor, which include the tendency to tell her what to do, rather than dialoguing with her, the assumption that her lifelong struggle with weight can be solved easily and simply, and the skepticism and judgmental attitude concerning her efforts to improve her health, and even about her honesty.

The patient invites her physician to look deeper, to take the time and have the interest to develop personal knowledge about the patient as a human being, which would include awareness of her difficult marriage and dead-end job, and her feelings of depression and despair. (The reader is struck by the fact that all of these aspects of the patient's life would apparently be new information to the doctor.) The patient pleads for empathy and understanding, but worries that the gap between her and her doctor cannot be bridged.

Then, after 11 stanzas of questioning, unexpectedly and even somewhat miraculously this patient steps forward and asserts herself: "Well, doctor." What follows is a strong chastisement directed at the physician. The patient forgoes her longing to be authentically "seen" and understood by her doctor. Nevertheless, whatever his or her personal stereotypes or lack of interest in the patient, she reminds the doctor that it is a professional requirement – an ethical bottom-line, so to speak – to treat her just like "all your other patients," with "compassion, respect, and dignity."

This poem is notable for the way it champions an often stigmatized group of patients (those who are obese) and gives this particular woman a voice that she may have had trouble finding for herself. It shows a patient who is initially lost and desperate, but who by the end of the poem is not only advocating for herself, but also speaking out on behalf of other obese patients who have experienced similar belittling and humiliating treatment from physicians. It provides an example of a medical student being willing to stand with the despised, marginalized patient rather than with the high-status doctor (who is also probably her supervisor and evaluator) and, through a profound act of empathy, to see her shame and frustration. However, the poem goes beyond this level of witnessing to active advocacy. By refusing to accept the shabby, insensitive treatment of this patient, the student demands change in the way that medicine is practiced by too many physicians.

PATIENT PLEAS FOR EMPATHY AND COMPASSION
Chaos stories

Students recognize that patients need caring and emotionally connected physicians. At times these poems do not extend beyond a chaotic cry for help. In one poem written from the patient's point of view, the distressed patient demands "another doctor, one / who suffers with me." The patient's current physician is too emotionally distant and uninvolved. This patient with chronic pain longs for a physician who is not afraid to empathize with her suffering.

Witnessing stories

Most of these poems engage in authentic witnessing of the patient's hopes and emotional desires. These student-authors are unafraid at least to hear the vulnerable longing of the patient. In a typical poem written from the patient's point of view, the patient tells the physician that she has placed her trust in him and reminds him that it is a privilege to care for another human being. She explains that she shows him her sickness and shame, weakness, and hurt in exchange for the hope of healing and compassionate, humane treatment. The patient beseeches the doctor to be an ally and protector; and prays that he will see the person of the patient first, and the disease second. She hopes that the physician will never forget "how delicate and precious the miracle of life is."

In a similar poem, again the patient is addressing the physician. He implores his doctor to see that behind his anger, indifference, and joking attitude are fear and concern about his survival. He speaks about the importance of caring: "I hope that you take the time to share / To open your heart though at times it's a scare / You need to have strength because at times it's unfair / And will feel like more than you can bear / But keep in mind how precious and rare / It is to have this opportunity to care." This poem acknowledges the difficult emotional demands on the physician, but does not swerve from prioritizing the patient's need for caring, humane treatment.

A bleaker poem, also written from the patient's perspective, shows the anonymity, detachment, and coldness of the hospital, which is filled only with silence, rustling papers, faces that appear and disappear, muffled voices, and pens writing. There is no human warmth or comfort to be found. In this poem, the yearning for someone who cares is implicit, but palpable.

PATIENTS' FEARS AND SUFFERING
Restitution stories

Patients are usually portrayed in student poetry as worried and fearful, which certainly reflects the emotions of many patients, but is a perception that also resonates with the students' own feelings. In response to this perception of patients' concerns, students' poems frequently tell restitution stories. In one such poem, a hospitalized patient both hopes and fears. He focuses on all that he does not want to do – show fear in front of his children, ask too many questions, or cry. He recognizes all that he cannot control and will not enjoy about the surgery that lies ahead. However, he concludes that what he "will enjoy [is] getting better." The message of this poem is that the patient must undergo suffering in order to achieve the ultimate goal of recovery.

In one poem, a patient with diabetic retinopathy has lost his vision and pleads with the physician to restore his sight. He describes the way that blindness has "surrounded my soul and left in my heart a huge, vast hole." Blindness is perceived as a physical, psychological, and spiritual catastrophe. Although in the past the patient had acted "tough and bold / pretended like the disease will forget about me," he now regrets not taking his disease more seriously, and vows to faithfully follow all physician instructions if only his sight can be restored. This is a bargaining story, in which the patient pleads for restitution, and promises to be a model patient. It is probably an (anti)-restitution story in the sense that, although it sympathizes with the patient, it also blames him, and implies that his sight could have been saved if he had been compliant and obedient.

In the following poem, the student uses the patient's voice to tell a restitution story in which the patient's fear of her deteriorating medical condition is ameliorated by a kind and caring physician. The poem empathically documents the patient's distress. Fortunately, this is more than balanced by a physician who addresses the patient's "every need." The patient is probably facing a prolonged and difficult dying process, but remarkably she feels "lucky" because her doctor "cares" about her. Although a compassionate physician can be a great boon to a patient, the poem perhaps overestimates the impact of such a physician on the patient's experience in an effort to address the student's own anxiety when confronted with a seriously ill patient.

I am not sure By: Michelle Harako
UC Irvine, 2003

I am not sure what's going on with me
I wake up at nights and cannot breathe
    Very scared, scared I am
I want to know what's happening to me

    Doctor, what's wrong with me?
You sat and listened to all my problems
You carefully examined my every need
You did not rush off, brushing me aside

    Although you say that my heart is failing
I have all the confidence that you'll do your best
    Although my condition seems to be severe
      I feel lucky to have a doctor that cares

In a similar poem that is even closer to a restitution story, the patient undergoes delicate heart surgery for an aortic aneurysm, but is saved by a heroic physician. Told in the voice of the patient, this poem hails the physician as a "life saver." The patient seeks both to "relax and reassure" the "timid" medical student by sharing a positive story of cure and restoration. The images of a loving family surrounding the patient reinforce the satisfying glow of death evaded, and normalcy and order regained.

Empathy: A Patient's Point of View By: Ali Razmara
UC Irvine, 2003

I'm so tired, a little dizzy, a little hot.
Did I make it? Am I awake? I guess so.
I can see the ceiling.
A little fuzzy.
I can see mom in the corner.
I can feel Hilary's warm hand on mine.
Ah, my chest, so heavy, so weak, so uncomfortable, but no pain.
I hope Scott and Sarah are alright . . .
I hope Hilary told them their daddy will come home soon.
Ah, I can see Dr. Bea, my life saver.
Who's that with him . . . a student . . . what a surprise!
So proper and clean, a white coat, UC Irvine.
He seems to be nervous, somewhat timid.

I'll try to relax and reassure him.
These tubes all over me won't bite.
I'll tell him my story.
Thank God I survived!
Thank you Dr. Bea!
I hope your student will one day save life like you!

Witnessing stories

Other poems are examples of what I call chaos/witnessing. The patient's perspective is represented as one of chaos, but the role of the student is to witness the chaos and suffering of the patient. In one poignant poem, the student writes about the patient's feelings of fear, powerlessness, and being overwhelmed. The path ahead seems uncertain. The poem abounds with metaphors of thunder and fire – crushing, relentless forces of nature, much like the patient's disease. The patient faces an ominous foe, "impending doom," and fears for his very existence.

Fear By: Reuben Chen
UC Irvine

My head is screaming.
I walk down the street and there is a thunder in my mind.
I cannot walk forward, and my feet shake from the weight on my shoulders.
My mind is overwhelmed and unfocused, and I can't do anything but tremble at
      my thoughts.
The path ahead seems shadowy, like a cloud over my face.
There is fear for myself and my very existence.
My life is flashing before my eyes.
My mind is on fire.
I have no power, and fear is all about me.
What is happening to me?
I have never faced a foe like this; one so ominous and fearful that it causes the sweat to drip
from my brow as I face impending doom.
I fall, and I fight, and there is nothing as my eyes sting
anticipating the battle ahead.
And I fear.

In another poem, the patient is filled with feelings of uncertainty, fear, and loss of control. He charts the course of his disease from "feeling fine" to "Now my body feels as if it isn't mine." Another patient experiences confusion, fear, and pain as a result of illness. A patient with an undiagnosed condition experiences pain, discomfort, hopelessness, isolation, and endless waiting. Although the physician is portrayed as sincere, he has no answers, and the patient remains frightened and alone. A young woman with cerebral palsy fantasizes about a perfect world that seems completely beyond reach. In all of these poems the student faithfully records the patient's sense of being overwhelmed by and in despair about the ravages of their illnesses.

Another example of a witnessing poem takes the form of a eulogy, ironically called a "memo" in the impersonal and efficient language of medicine, for a doctor (perhaps a mentor or role model) who has recently passed away. First, the narrator, speaking directly to the deceased person, imagines what it was like to receive the devastating news. The first two stanzas of the poem emphasize the "silence" that engulfs the patient once he knows that he is dying, a silence that inevitably isolates and separates. The narrator continues resolutely to imagine perhaps the greatest loss when the flesh disappears – the loss of a lover's physical intimacy, the mystical union of two bodies in one. Now the student wears a doctor's coat, "weighing heavily on [his] shoulders." The narrator asks himself if the doctor wondered whether he was "leaving the world in capable hands." The student knows that he is assuming a daunting mantle, but leaves unanswered the question of whether he can truly fill these shoes, so that the doubts and fears of the dying man remain unresolved.

A Final Memo to Dr. Carlo Urbani By: Gregg Chesney

Originally published in Body Language: Poems of the Medical Training Experience
edited by Neeta Jain, Dagan Coppock and Stephanie Brown Clark, 2006
Reprinted with the permission of BOA Editions, Ltd. www.boaeditions.org

You must have sat there like an awkward
silence
hanging heavy in the air.

The Doctor will see you now.

You were silence with a message, the silence
that made sound stop
turning it from noise into music.
You were the thicket of thistle and burr
clutching fabric at arm's length – you held me
there, uprooted and choked as
you spoke, jaw unmoving though words came out
notes dangling in suspended hesitation
the world awaiting your crescendo.

Your eyes were resigned to the fact that you would
never again be touched
or swallowed by the arms of an unconquered lover
floating into your bedroom on a supple
August breeze, standing disrobed before you
at the foot of the bed. She leans over
and brushes against your cheek before lifting the
sheets and drowning herself in you.

You must have lain there in your hospital bed, swaddled in white
sheets reminiscent of your white laboratory coat
that now I wear, altered and weighing heavy on my shoulders.

When you rolled over at night, did you ever wonder if
you were leaving the world in capable hands?

In another witnessing poem, an ill patient prays to God that he will not wake, so as not to return to endless suffering. In his dreams he is healthy, young, and free. It is only in dreams that he "can deny my inevitable fate." He has lost the will to fight, and wants only peace. In yet another poem, the patient's pain is getting progressively worse, and she cannot remember a pain-free day. She can only communicate "in nods/grimaces/painful silence, gritted teeth." Another poem describes the medical team trying to place a nasogastric tube. During the procedure, the patient suffers greatly and confronts the student's role in contributing to this pain by looking directly into her eyes. These poems all look into the faces of patients in anguish and do not turn away.

In another poem, a patient starts talking to the doctor about her pain. Then she tells more of her story. She is a Vietnamese immigrant, and her husband died during the war. She has post-traumatic stress disorder and has tried to commit suicide. She experiences both physical and emotional pain, and neither can be relieved. In another poem, the patient complains about the absurdity of the pain scale, inadequate as it is to reflect her true misery. In yet another poem, a patient describes chronic pain as a constant in her life. It pervades not only her body, but also her soul. The patient is anguished and asks "Why me?" All she can hope for is that the pain will end soon.

Another patient, perhaps a drug user undergoing withdrawal (from black tar, a form of heroin common in the western USA), is wracked with pain. He cries out for Jesus and for ice-cream – anything that will soothe his suffering. He survives breath by breath, unable to see beyond each unendurable moment. His anguish is contrasted with the pastoral image of a solitary bagpipe player in a meadow, and a solitary fish in the vastness of the ocean (perhaps pictures in his hospital room?), both of which suggest the benign indifference of the universe to his misery.

Haiku moments By: David Finley
UC Irvine, 2003

morning mist
on wind barren meadows
kilted bagpiper plays to cows

the whole ocean
in a tropical pool of blue
one fish

evil tar
the dark night crow
in my gut

tied to the bed
can I have some ice-cream
oh Jesus, oh Jesus

morning
I breathe each breath
one at a time.

The common feature of all these stories is unrelieved suffering on the patient's part, with no end in sight, and no solutions apparent from the medical world. The witnessing component is present because the student is willing to acknowledge and to see this situation, and does not rationalize it or shy away from it.

STIGMATIZED VOICES
Chaos stories

In addition to the burden of illness, some patients, such as those who abuse drugs and/or alcohol, homeless people, the mentally ill, obese patients, noncompliant patients, patients who speak different languages and those from different cultures, are further stigmatized by attributes or characteristics that, in the minds of some healthcare providers, justify attitudes of disrespect or condemnation. The students in this sample made an effort to listen to and try to understand the voices of these patients. Occasionally, students were overwhelmed by the patient's circumstances. Their poems emerge as chaos/anti-restitution narratives, characterized by helplessness and patient blaming. A typical poem in the form of a dialogue between an alcoholic patient and his doctor represents differing but equally despondent viewpoints. The patient blames his genetics and social environment, and recognizes that he lacks control over his problem. The doctor knows about the complex forces that influence alcoholism, but finds it easier to focus on the chart notes than on his patient's dilemma. The alienation in this poem is complete – the patient is in denial and the physician does not know how to help him.

Some students write similar poems about psychiatric patients, in which the chaos of the student parallels that of the patient, unmitigated by any hope of understanding or healing intervention. A patient with borderline personality disorder in conversation with her doctor demonstrates her impulsivity, relationship disturbance, and lack of self-esteem, and her desperation to maintain an ephemeral relationship with a junkie whom she is convinced she loves. The doctor has no solutions to offer. Another poem chronicles a tragic turn of events in a psychiatric ward, where a young woman with persecutory delusions who seemed "grounded" and ready for discharge instead commits suicide. There is no resolution, no explanation, and no understanding possible in this grim poem. Having tried to penetrate the psychic world of this patient, the student feels that he has failed.

Witnessing stories

Most of the poems that represent the voice of stigmatized patients adopt a stance of witnessing, going beyond labels and stereotypes to find the human side of these patients. These poems often have an element of resistance in terms of rejecting the dominant conceptualization of such patients as self-destructive, noncompliant, and not "deserving" of care. For example, in one poem, the patient who is speaking is a drug addict with multiple medical problems, including AIDS. The patient is attached not only to his drugs, but also to his disease – both are his friends, because both distract him from the loneliness. He is "ready for the fall" (ready to die). He dares his medical team to answer the question "Are *they* ready for his death?" This poem embraces the patient's perspective, and challenges the doctors to have the same courage as the patient does to accept his inevitable demise.

In another witnessing poem, an obese patient wants to lose weight, but does not appear to be motivated to exercise or diet. While her doctor and her husband variously hold out incentives of improved diabetes control and new clothes, it is the student who sees beyond the patient's apparent noncompliance and realizes that she is afraid even to try. These poems are a witnessing of the devalued patient's perspective and an aligning with the medically identified Other.

In a more light-hearted account, a "noncompliant" Latina patient laments the conflict between her prescribed diabetic diet and traditional Mexican foods, which are symbolic of familial/communal sharing and connection at Christmas time. Here the student-author attempts to understand the conflicts that a dietetic intervention can pose with one's family and culture. This is an example of witnessing discrepancies in doctor–patient perspectives. The doctor in the poem, although not unkind, has a scientific approach to explaining "proper diet." What the student perceives is that to the patient, her traditional foods have strong emotional, familial, and cultural ties, and are not easily relinquished – a point that the physician misses.

VULNERABILITY/COURAGE OF CHILD PATIENTS
Restitution stories

Poems written from the point of view of pediatric patients are especially poignant. Sometimes these poems adopt a restitution narrative. In one poem, a healthy baby reflects on his developmental milestones from 0 to 12 months, concluding that up until now he has accomplished all that he needs in life. In this poem, baby and doctor work in concert to achieve a happy, healthy existence. In an enchanting poem, a student describes the birth of Jesus Christ as "a delivery that is natural, spontaneous, vaginal," although "mom had no prenatal care . . . paternity has been quite questionable." Despite a humble start, there are no complications, and the Christ Child is delivered – the ultimate possibility of redemption and salvation.

In a classic restitution tale, a student-athlete sustains a serious injury to his knee. He undergoes surgery, physical therapy, and an additional operation, and finally recovers. The poem describes his initial naivety about his injury, which changes to shock, disappointment, mistrust, skepticism, helplessness, and frustration as he discovers the severity of his problem. He addresses the physician with increasing anger and frustration. However, the story has a happy ending because ultimately it is medical skill and knowledge that restores the patient to athletic glory.

Several authors imagine sick children addressing their parents (usually the mother) directly, assuming a parental role, reassuring them and thanking them for their devotion, recognizing their sacrifices, and noting that the family's love and support have made a huge difference to the quality of the patient's life. The role reversal imagined for these children may reflect the students' desire to "make things right" under unbearably painful and tragic circumstances. In a similar manner to some cadaver restitution poems, the sick/dying child reassures their parents (and presumably also the medical student) that all is well. In one such example, a 16-year-old boy who is dying of Duchenne's muscular dystrophy details the course of his disease, including the progression of symptoms and loss of function. He acknowledges that the support and love of his family have made all the difference to the quality of his life. These are restitution stories in the sense that the children's gratitude and acceptance are able to restore family integrity.

Witnessing stories

The majority of the poems that explore children's experiences of illness take the form of witnessing. The narrator-poet bears witness to the child's suffering and the chaos with which illness has infused their life. In one poem, the dominant feeling is one of fear – nothing seems familiar, the child is afraid of being alone, and fears that she will die. Another poem is written bilingually with the repeated refrain of "No me pique!" ("Don't stick me!"). This little boy does not understand the medical procedures to which he is being subjected, and rejects the idea that the medical student is his friend. He ends with a poignant question: "When can I go home?" In another example, an infant who has been hospitalized since birth, despite her parents' distress, has come to terms with and adapted to her condition. She calmly hopes for the best. One poem describes a pediatric hospital as "an undersea world" and "no place a child should be." All the superficial cheerfulness cannot mask the fact that this "is a place very different than home," and the poet notes the suffering in the "sharp cries, soft cries, cries without tears . . ." Yet at the same time it is filled with the "brilliance . . . of love, the life of youth, of good work well done."

Another poem depicts an infant peering out of the incubator at the faces of the healthcare team. The student-poet tries to understand what life in a fishbowl must be like – security, comfort, complacency inside "this kingdom," but also the awareness that this is not much of a life. An infant with a digestive disorder ends up having recurrent hospitalizations. The poem represents her dislike of the hospital, her discomfort and pain, and her need to please the healthcare team. Her only protection against indifference is her smile. During an ostensibly "well-child" check, another child is afraid and wants to hide. It turns out that he is obese and embarrassed about his physical appearance, which leads to his being teased and hit by his peers. He longs to be hidden and unseen.

In the following witnessing poem, the student addresses the patient in the second person, attempting through this one-sided dialogue to enter into the worldview of this distant other. We are initially presented with an image of freedom and elegance – the one-legged boy (we never learn how he lost his leg – possibly Ewing's sarcoma or an accident?) swimming, gliding, released from the encumbrance of his metal limb. However, the past tense suggests that this escape is no longer available. The images of the poem are disjointed and incoherent, perhaps suggesting the child's own confused state. Next we learn of the mother, who is trying to normalize the intrusion of this artificial limb into her family's world. Then we see the child drawing a car with uneven wheels. Subsequently we learn that the boy has lost his faith in superheroes – the mainstay of most young boys' imaginations – dismissing them as "so fake." He hates falling down, which it seems he does often, and he longs for a carpeted world, perhaps to buffer not only his physical falls, but also all the harshness of life that he experiences. The only person who can possibly empathize is a stranger at a fast-food restaurant, who has also lost a leg, who comments gruffly on the difficulty in caring for the stump.

Poem for Joseph By: Sarah Mourra
Originally appeared in Plexus *2006, p. 13, UC Irvine School of Medicine*

You used to swim
    gliding deep to the smooth pool floor
       elegant
holding your breath
    watching your boy shadow

the strange steel limb gone

left behind for the moment
in an empty locker room

Every morning your mother
puts a sock over that cold metal

A drawing of a red car
in crayon and marker
(you drew one wheel different
from the other)

Superheroes don't exist, you declare
matter of factly
They're so fake
When they fall, they get up right away
You hate the sound of your body falling
steel hitting asphalt
You wish for streets and sidewalks of
soft silent carpet
like here, you say

The only person in the world
that you've ever seen
who looks like you
(other than your cat who died)
was a man in line at McDonald's

He said
It's tough to take care of
    ain't it
        Boy?

Transcendence stories

Sometimes, by paying close attention to a patient, a student's views of the patient's experience are radically changed. In one such poem, initially the student feels only pity for a pediatric patient with spina bifida, and focuses on the limitations imposed by the disability. The child, however, accepts his condition as natural and sees himself as capable. The patient teaches the student that real joy is found in effort and commitment, not in winning, and that real courage is not related to size or physical prowess. This is a poem of transformation in which the student's assumptions are dramatically altered.

PERSONAL EXPERIENCES OF ILLNESS
Chaos stories

Occasionally students write about their personal experiences of illness in members of their family or themselves. Perhaps because of their emotional proximity to the material, these poems are chaos stories, or have significant elements of chaos. One student writes about the illness, pain, and increasing physical limitations of her mother. Even as she challenges the reader to feel her mother's pain, she admits that she, her daughter, cannot empathize fully and concludes: "And I wonder / Who is the diseased?"

Another student becomes a patient and undergoes a diagnostic procedure. She is afraid, lonely and in pain. She experiences first-hand the vulnerability and humiliation of nakedness covered only by a hospital gown. Irrationally, in response to the routine questions, she worries that she might be pregnant. The next minute she becomes convinced that she has cancer, and the doctor was simply too afraid to tell her. The nurse who is assisting is unsympathetic, does not enquire about the student's anxieties, and ignores her tears. The student-patient, alone, without family or friends, is abandoned in her suffering.

Stream of Unconsciousness By: Jennifer Jolley
Originally appeared in Plexus *2003, pp. 16–17, UC Irvine School of Medicine*

It felt like 10 miles
It was probably 50 feet
The nurse didn't look up
The form goes here
Your signature goes here
Your clothes go off
No jewelry
No pacemaker, right?
No comments please
The cold crawled across my bare skin
Why did it have to be in my middle?
If it was just my arm
Then all I'd have to take off
Is just my shirt
All I get is this little gown
Don't they realize it's freezing in here?
One of the ties is broken
I bet they don't even care
Which way to the front
Which way to the back
I'm not ready yet
Hop up here, she says
You're not pregnant, right?
No, no way
But wait, what if I am?
I don't know
But if I tell her I don't know
I have to go back
But if I am, what would that mean?
Med school would be harder
My parents would be worried
And the baby will have two heads
All because I got this x-ray
No, not pregnant
No, no jewelry
Yes, a lot of fear

But wait, you didn't ask that
This table is freezing
My stomach is aching
What is the doctor even looking for?
I haven't taken Path yet
So many things that it could be
It must be cancer
He just couldn't tell me
He knows how med students react
There are so many organs in there
It could be any one
I hope it's not my colon
I don't want one of those bags on the side
It's probably something rare
That would be just my luck
But then I couldn't study for Biochem
One good thing about being sick
The lights are dim
The air is cool
The nurse told me to lie down honey
She slapped on the lead pads
Protect your ovaries and thyroid
What's the thyroid?
If this pad doesn't protect it
What will that do?
And oh great
Now I really won't be able to have kids
Without two heads
The door closed behind her
My eyes closed tight
I know this won't hurt
But what if it does?
It makes a whirring noise
Does anyone even know that I am here?
No one does
My parents are far away
My boyfriend too
My sisters are at school
My friends are busy
My classmates are in class
No one knows that I am here
No one knows that there's something wrong.

In another example, the medical student-patient comments sardonically that, from the patient's perspective, physical examination is much less of an "art" than it is for the physician ("Maybe in YOUR eyes it seems like an art"). Although on the whole the patient is satisfied and hopeful that the prescribed medication will work, still he gets in one last dig, and promises the doctor that next time *he* will be the one who is late! Although this poem ultimately tells a restitution story – medicine holds the solution to the student's problem – there is a leakage of chaos. The student is unwillingly seeing a little through the eyes of the patient, and defends himself against this by employing hostile humor.

SUMMARY

Student poetry about patients demonstrates clearly just how possible it is for students to learn to see through the eyes of their patients and listen to their voices. Almost without exception, their poems provide examples of narrative empathy. This is often a broader and deeper empathy than the behavioral, skills-based empathy that is emphasized in most medical school curricula. Students are successfully able to identify difficult patient emotional experiences of isolation, fear, suffering, loss of control, and loss of order and coherence, and they replicate well Frankian categories of illness narratives. The poems show that students are eager to learn, and in fact do learn directly from their patients, and not only about sickness and pathology, but also about an infinite range of patient experiences in the face of illness. The poems also show that students are well able to form their own conclusions about how patients are treated within the healthcare system.

When students try to comprehend the experience of illness from the patient's perspective, they occasionally tell chaos stories in which the student is overwhelmed by the patient's distress, focuses on the helplessness and futility of the patient's situation, and cannot summon the strength or wisdom necessary to contain the patient's suffering. They also sometimes craft a restitution story, in which the patient's experience of suffering and sickness is resolved through the skilled intervention of the physician.

However, the dominant narrative typology for poems that attempt to understand the patient's experience of illness and suffering is witnessing. In these works, the student perceives the patient's situation as a chaos story, and the role of the student is to witness to this chaos. This both expresses solidarity with the patient's pain and suffering, and often expresses resistance to what students perceive to be the dominant narrative about patient experience. In these poems, the student invariably aligns him- or herself with the patient in an act of empathy and in an attempt to preserve the patient's self-respect. Sometimes these poems focus on stigmatized patients, such as drug-abusing individuals, or patients whose diseases are judged to be self-inflicted by the dominant medical community, and the poems find unexpected depth and dignity in these individuals. Most of the poems that are written in the voice of child patients tell restitution or witnessing stories. Some students want to believe that children are at peace with their suffering, but more often they are willing to stand as witnesses to this suffering. When the student becomes the patient, the resultant anxiety tends to produce stories of chaos.

REFERENCES

1 Toombs SK. *The Meaning of Illness: A phenomenological account of the different perspectives of physician and patient.* Dordrecht: Kluwer; 1993.

2 Schwartz MA, Wiggins OP. Scientific and humanistic medicine: a theory of clinical methods. In: White KR (ed.). *The Task of Medicine.* Menlo Park, CA: Henry Kaiser Foundation; 1988.

3 Hunsaker-Hawkins A. *Reconstructing Illness: Studies in pathography,* 2nd edition. West Lafayette, IN: Purdue University Press; 1999.

4 Frank AW. *The Wounded Storyteller: Body, illness, and ethics.* Chicago: University of Chicago Press; 1995.

5 Anderson CM. Me acuerdo: healing narrative in Stones for Ibarra. *Literature and Medicine* 2006; **25**: 358–75.

6 Cassell EJ. *The Nature of Suffering and the Goals of Medicine.* New York: Oxford University Press; 1991.

7 Kleinman A. *The Illness Narratives: Suffering, healing, and the human condition.* New York: Basic Books; 1988.

8 Hawkins AH. Pathography and the enabling myths: the process of healing. In: Anderson CM, MacCurdy MM (eds). *Writing and Healing: Toward an informed practice.* Urbana, IL: National Council of Teachers of English; 2000.

9 Rimmon-Kenan S. What can narrative theory learn from illness narratives? *Literature and Medicine* 2006; **25**: 241–54.

10 Stein M. *The Lonely Patient.* New York: William Morrow; 2007.

11 Hunt LM. Strategic suffering: empowerment among Mexican cancer patients. In: Mattingly C, Garro LC (eds). *Narrative and the Cultural Construction of Illness and Healing.* Berkeley, CA: University of California Press; 2000. pp. 88–107.

12 Drew S. The Delta factor: storying survival and the disjuncture between public narratives and personal stories of life after cancer. *Storytelling, Self, Society* 2005; **1**: 76–102.

13 Diedrich L. *Treatments: Language, politics, and the culture of illness.* Minneapolis, MN: University of Minnesota Press; 2007.

14 Lorde A. *The Cancer Journals.* San Francisco, CA: Aunt Lute Books; 1980.

15 Wagner AT. Re/Covered bodies: the sites and stories of illness in popular media. *Journal of Medical Humanities* 2000; **21**: 15–27.

16 Wagner PJ, Lentz P, Heslop SD. Teaching communication skills: a skills-based approach. *Academic Medicine* 2002; **77**: 1164.

17 Boyle D, Dwinnell B, Platt F. Invite, listen, and summarize: a patient-centered communication technique. *Academic Medicine* 2005; **80**: 29–32.

18 Fernandez-Olano C, Montoya-Fernandez J, Salinas-Sanchez AS. Impact of clinical interview training on the empathy level of medical students and medical residents. *Medical Teacher* 2008; **30**: 322–4.

19 Satterfield JM, Hughes E. Emotion skills training for medical students: a systematic review. *Medical Education* 2007; **41**: 935–41.

20 Stepien KA, Baernstein A. Educating for empathy: a review. *Journal of General Internal Medicine* 2006; **21**: 524–30.

21 Markham B. Medical students become patients: a new teaching strategy. *Journal of Medical Education* 1979; **54**: 416–18.

22 Henry-Tillman R, Deloney LA, Savidge M, *et al.* The medical student as patient navigator as an approach to teaching empathy. *American Journal of Surgery* 2002; **183**: 659–62.

23 Muir F. Placing the patient at the core of teaching. *Medical Teacher* 2007; **29**: 258–60.

24 Kumagai AK. A conceptual framework for the use of illness narratives in medical education. *Academic Medicine* 2008; **83**: 653–8.

25 Sierpina VS, Kreitzer MJ, Mackenzie E, Sierpina M. Regaining our humanity through story. *Explore (NY)* 2007; **3**: 626–32.

26 Dow AW, Leong D, Anderson A, Wenzel RP and VCU Theater-Medicine Team. Using theater to teach clinical empathy: a pilot study. *Journal of General Internal Medicine* 2007; **22**: 1114–18.

27 Rosenbaum ME, Ferguson KJ, Herwaldt LA. In their own words: presenting the patient's perspective using research-based theatre. *Medical Education* 2005; **39**: 622–31.

28 Charon R. Reading, writing, and doctoring: literature and medicine. *American Journal of the Medical Sciences* 2000; **319**: 285–91.

29 Reifler DR. "Poor Yorick": reflections on gross anatomy. In: Hawkins AH, McEntyre MC

(eds). *Teaching Literature and Medicine*. New York: Modern Language Association of America; 2000. pp. 327–32.

30 Siemińska MJ, Szymańska M, Mausch K. Development of sensitivity to the needs and suffering of a sick person in students of medicine and dentistry. *Medicine, Health Care and Philosophy* 2002; **5**: 263–71.

31 DasGupta S, Charon R. Personal illness narratives: using reflective writing to teach empathy. *Academic Medicine* 2004; **79**: 351–6.

32 Shapiro J, Duke A, Boker J, Ahearn CS. Just a spoonful of humanities makes the medicine go down: introducing literature into a family medicine clerkship. *Medical Education* 2005; **39**: 605–12.

33 Shapiro J, Morrison E, Boker J. Teaching empathy to first-year medical students: evaluation of an elective literature and medicine course. *Education for Health (Abingdon)* 2004; **17**: 73–84.

34 Hawkins AH, McEntyre MC (eds). *Teaching Literature and Medicine*. New York: Modern Language Association of America; 2000.

35 Rucker L, Shapiro J. Becoming a physician: students' creative projects in a third-year IM clerkship. *Academic Medicine* 2003; 78: 391–7.

36 Woolf K, Cave J, McManus IC, Dacre JE. "It gives you an understanding you can't get from any book." The relationship between medical students' and doctors' personal illness experiences and their performance: a qualitative and quantitative study. *BMC Medical Education* 2007; **7**: 50.

37 Kumagai AK, Murphy EA, Ross PT. Diabetes stories: use of patient narratives of diabetes to teach patient-centered care. *Advances in Health Sciences Education: Theory and Practice* 2008; 31 May. [E-publication ahead of print]

38 Bleakley A, Bligh J. Students learning from patients: let's get real in medical education. *Advances in Health Sciences Education: Theory and Practice* 2008; **13**: 89–107.

39 Benbassat J, Baumal R. What is empathy, and how can it be promoted during clinical clerkships? *Academic Medicine* 2004; **79**: 832–9.

40 Charon R. *Narrative Medicine: Honoring the stories of illness*. New York: Oxford University Press; 2006.

41 Shapiro J. Walking a mile in their patients' shoes: empathy and othering in medical students' education. *Philosophy, Ethics, and Humanities in Medicine* 2008; **12**: 10.

42 Dyrbye LN, Harris I, Rohren CH. Early clinical experiences from students' perspectives: a qualitative study of narratives. *Academic Medicine* 2007; **82**: 979–88.

43 Allen D, Wainwright M, Mount B, Hutchinson T. The wounding path to becoming healers: medical students' apprenticeship experiences. *Medical Teacher* 2008; **30**: 260–4.

8 A Friendly Touch Would Have Done So Much: The Doctor–Patient Relationship

Although the doctor–patient relationship is assumed to be driven by altruism, caring, and compassion, there are other less benevolent elements at work as well. Starting with Mischler's pioneering work on doctor–patient communication contrasting the voice of medicine with the voice of the lifeworld,[1] numerous scholars have noted what Hunter referred to as the "narrative incommensurability" between doctors and patients.[2-5] These philosophers of medicine argue that doctors and patients are much more likely to perceive the patient's situation differently than similarly, including differences in meaning, signification, and implication. This makes it likely that doctors and patients will have trouble understanding each other at a deep level. Few scholars have been willing to examine the essential otherness of the patient in the eyes of many physicians and learners,[6,7] but when they do so, they recognize that differences between doctor and patient can lead to the unconscious activation of responses of fear, hostility, and consequent distancing on the part of the physician.

In addition to the assumption of a doctor–patient relationship based on caring, there are other inbuilt assumptions to the relationship that can also create difficulties. For example, many learners (and some physicians) take it for granted that because physicians are trying to help patients, patients should reciprocate by expressing gratitude towards their doctors. Frank is one of the few who have challenged this model,[8] but in the absence of alternative viewpoints, seemingly ungrateful patients can be used to justify physicians' expression of resentment and disdain. In another example, despite numerous curricular innovations in recent years that have brought the patient's voice into greater prominence (*see* Chapter 7), much of medical education still assumes that the doctor–patient relationship should be primarily a vertical rather than a horizontal one.[9] This separation is reinforced and accentuated, at least from the student's perspective, by the prioritizing of attitudes of clinical objectivity, detachment, and distance on the part of physician role models.[10] This is not to say that power should be expressed in the doctor–patient encounter in an entirely egalitarian manner, or that rationality and empiricism are not crucial elements of the physician's thought process. It is to say that it is sometimes hard for students to grasp how even their best physician role models move between and blend various sources and types of knowledge in their interactions with patients. The result may be an overly simplistic view of what the doctor–patient relationship should be about, what it should include, and where its emphases should lie.

Students are eager to learn from their physician role models, who include both residents (physicians who have completed medical school and are pursuing advanced training in a particular specialty) and attending physicians (more experienced, board-certified doctors). Students are generally idealistic and hopeful, anxious to learn how to "properly" engage with the patient. They want their role models to be compassionate as well as competent, and to model devotion to their patients: "They want us to teach them how to care for patients as well as how to treat them."[11] Much of the time, this is precisely what happens. Especially during the preclinical years, students tend to have positive views of the physician role models that they encounter. However, as they make their way through the clinical years, too often students become increasingly aware of a considerable gap between theory and practice in terms of the way that the doctor–patient relationship is actually manifested.[12]

Both medical educators and students themselves have pointed out that students frequently witness unprofessional acts by their supervisors for which these individuals are not held accountable.[13,14] One study found that over 25% of second-year students and 40% of senior students did not agree that their teachers behaved like humanistic caregivers with patients or were good role models in teaching the doctor–patient relationship.[15] In a similar study, only 46% of clinical students agreed that their teachers displayed the humanistic characteristics of interest. They were especially critical of their teachers' apparent lack of sensitivity, with as many as three out of four students declaring that their teachers seemed to be unconcerned about how patients adapt psychologically to their illnesses.[16] A recent study indicated that students still perceived lack of respect for the patient as a significant impediment to bedside teaching.[17] As Wear has noted,[18] when students observe physicians who interact empathetically with patients at the bedside or in the exam room, and then speak disrespectfully and demeaningly about these same patients in the corridor, or when they see attending physicians doing nothing in response to residents making jokes about patients, they become first confused, and then disillusioned and cynical. Often they join in the humor in an attempt to become part of the high-status, powerful in-crowd of residents and doctors.

Residents and attending physicians are well aware that they are serving as moment-by-moment role models for medical students on hospital wards and in clinics. Medical educators have stressed the criticality of this bedside/clinic role-modeling, especially in terms of developing humanistic qualities, in which students have the opportunity to observe what the physician is actually doing, as opposed to what the physician is talking about doing.[19,20] In these learning situations, it is especially important for physicians to manifest "inner qualities" as well as specific behaviors,[19] so that students do not form the impression that relationship is developed exclusively through mechanistic methods.[21] However, neither group receives significant preparation for how to function as effective role models. Medical students identify residents as their most frequent and important teachers,[22] yet most residents receive little training in teaching,[23] and especially in teaching humanistic aspects of medicine. There is some evidence that without specific training, residents experience reduced enjoyment of teaching, become easily frustrated by time constraints, and often express lack of empathy, as well as attitudes of cynicism and blame, towards learners.[24]

Other research suggests that physician teachers pay little attention to the way in which they serve as role models, and do very little either to highlight and analyze positive patient interactions, or to analyze and interpret problematic interactions.[25] In particular, they rarely address the human dimensions of patient care overtly with learners. Even excellent role models have a range of ability to reflect on and communicate to learners exactly why they are so successful in their interactions with patients.[26] For example, without formal training in narrative medicine, even physician role models who are able to imagine, interpret, and recognize the plights of their patients[27] may lack the skills to translate such insights in ways that are understandable to learners.

In one of the few studies to focus directly on how doctors teach about the doctor–patient relationship,[28] attending physicians were found to have difficulty describing situations or behaviors in which they specifically modeled relationship-building with patients. At times their own negative feelings about their patients interfered with their ability to address this topic. In another example of the gap between theory and practice, these teachers expected their students to maintain higher relational standards with patients than they themselves held. Even when physicians become patients themselves, the recommendations that they make in terms of improving the doctor–patient relationship are rather basic (e.g. bedside charting, attention to patients' nonverbal cues). These recommendations are disappointing both in that these physician-patients did not have greater insight into what is lacking in their own doctor–patient interactions, and also in that their doctors were not demonstrating even these basic skills.[29] Conversely, evidence exists that when the process of role-modeling is made more conscious and transparent, both role models and learners benefit.[30,31]

Scholars and medical educators like Inui and Frankel have recommended a revival of "Samaritan medicine," in which physicians model how to form connection with "otherness" or difference in patients[6] (*see* Chapter 7). Dobie[32] has called for a paradigm shift in which the doctor–patient relationship in all its complexity receives sustained and systematic attention during training. What is abundantly clear is that a therapeutic, ethical, and altruistic doctor–patient relationship is not a given, and that much more effort needs to be devoted to devising effective and creative ways of role-modeling this relationship for learners.

Attending physicians and residents are students' primary source of experiential learning about what it means to be a physician. They are the behavioral and attitudinal role models on whom the students will pattern themselves. During the preclinical phase of their training, students' poetry tended to tell restitution stories through their poetry. Doctors, with whom they still had relatively little contact, were perceived as heroes and life-savers. Later, however, their views of the doctor–patient relationship became more complicated. Students paid careful attention to what was going on around them, especially what they saw their putative role models doing, as opposed to what they were telling learners to do. What students learned about doctors and patients was sometimes troubling, but often uplifting.

Never Imagined By Michael Liu
UC Irvine, 2003

PATIENT
I see you once a day
Let me tell you all about my pain
But you just walk away
I cannot eat, and this is making me crazy

DOCTOR
I see you once a day
I try to be nice, but you complain to me
anyways
I'll give you PCA
Please understand, I haven't slept since

Yesterday

PATIENT
My worst nightmare
You think you know it all, but you just don't care
These lines I cannot bear
I'll rip them out and show you it isn't fair

DOCTOR
My worst nightmare
You stress me out with your crazy dares
You need me or you will die
Then on whose shoulder are you going to cry?

PATIENT
You're the only one
I depend on you, but you hurry up and run
I have everything to lose
I feel worthless, I am the fool

DOCTOR
You're not the only one
There are 40 others that I need to follow on
You're selfish, you think you're king
You'll probably sue for all I can bring

PATIENT
I am begging you to hear my voice
I am desperate for your touch
I am lonely, I need you
Won't you remember me, please don't abandon me

BOTH DOCTOR AND PATIENT
Don't you see what I go through?
I'm tired, I can't move
Believe me, what I say is true
Our dignity, we both lose
I never imagined this day

This poem sums up the difficulties that doctors and patients can experience with each other, and how hard it is for them to deeply understand each other's worlds and lives. It also shows, ironically, how much they actually share in common, and how through imperfect but persistent interaction, a small hope emerges that eventually they can come together with mutual sympathy and understanding. An unusual feature of this poem is that its author is able to simultaneously recognize the disparate voices of patient and doctor. However, the poem does seem to imply that, although both are suffering, it is the physician's responsibility to put aside her* own wretchedness, and to prioritize the needs of the patient.

---

* To avoid awkward gender-neutral constructions, I have arbitrarily designated male pronouns to refer to the patient and female pronouns to refer to the physician.

The patient opens the conversation with an attack on his physician. He frets about the infrequency of her visits. The physician finally does arrive, but before the patient can even present his distress and his problems, she has left. From the perspective of the patient, the doctor is rushed and insensitive to his torment, which is so intense that it makes him feel as if he is losing his mind. However, the doctor (perhaps a resident) has a perspective of her own, and ignores most aspects of the patient's concerns, although she does offer to help with pain management. She insists that she "tries to be nice" (a rather feeble term in the face of the severity of the patient's suffering), and implies that "once a day" contact should be quite enough to satisfy him. After this superficial acknowledgment, the physician retaliates by pointing out how difficult it is to continually hear the complaints of the patient. Finally, she grumbles about her own exhaustion.

Next, in order to get his physician to "hear" and "see" him, to engage with him, the patient takes a greater risk in terms of what he is willing to reveal. He provocatively asserts that his "own worst nightmare" is the physician herself, whom the patient accuses of being an uncaring and indifferent know-it-all. However, when the patient threatens to rip out his intravenous lines, he is not only being simply annoying and "crazy" as the physician suggests in the next stanza, but is also desperately hinting at the deeper feelings that he harbors – "it isn't fair." What is he referring to? Having such an arrogant doctor? Being sick and in the hospital? Is he perhaps referring to life itself? Maybe he contemplates this dramatic action as a way of punishing this unfeeling doctor, so that she too will experience a brief moment of life's unfairness.

The doctor still cannot, or will not, listen to her patient. She seems unable to witness to the pain underlying the acting out. She does not bother to ask "What isn't fair?" Instead, in a sad, pathetic moment reminiscent of playground name-calling she informs the patient that *he* is *her* worst nightmare. She tells him that his threats and crazy behavior are making her stressed and miserable. Furthermore, she reminds the patient that his life itself is on the line, and she points out that he needs her and the expertise that she brings in order to avoid death. This statement seems to contain an implied threat. If the patient does not behave, will she abandon him? In the face of the patient's suffering, the doctor continues to focus on her own suffering, and uses the unequal power of the doctor–patient relationship, the inherent reliance of the patient on the physician for health and healing, to intimidate him. Beaten down and completely demoralized, the patient admits the truth of what the physician is saying. He feebly returns momentarily to the theme of the doctor's hurrying and unavailability, but acknowledges that she is "the only one." The physician has exerted her power, and the patient is crushed. He blames himself: "I am the fool."

Even at this moment of the patient's abasement and humiliation, the physician continues to drive home her advantage. She accuses him of being selfish and demanding, while reminding him that she has a large patient load in addition to him. Mocking his language of concession, she tells him bluntly that he is *not* the only one in her professional life, thus further differentiating between her high-status, important self and her lowly, dependent patient. To add insult to injury, she accuses the patient of being a prima donna, deflecting on to him the various attributes that have so offended him about herself, and goes so far as to position him as her enemy, by speculating that he will probably sue her. By now, the patient has been reduced to a quivering mass. He throws himself at the mercy of the physician, stripping himself bare – he is lonely and in need. He begs the physician to listen to him, to touch him, to remember him, and not to abandon him. The gap between physician and patient has become a chasm. It is a painful process to witness.

Yet, in the final stanza, we encounter an astonishing development. These two people, who seem to hate each other, who bully and harass each other, who do not seem capable of listening to each other, and who become, in a sense, perpetrator and victim, suddenly speak as one. The voices of the patient and the doctor, which were previously so disparate, unexpectedly merge so that they are indistinguishable. There is little doubt that the author, while recognizing the challenging, demanding nature of the patient's behavior, reserves his harshest judgment for the physician. The portrayal of the physician is almost beyond redemption, violating virtually every stricture of professionalism. And yet . . . Patient and doctor both cry together about their shared suffering, exhaustion, and loss of dignity. They both confess that they could never have imagined reaching the state in which they now find themselves. It seems that they have both reached the very dark bottom. But they have reached the bottom together, and by sharing the same words, they acknowledge that they are not different from each other, not enemies, but fellow sufferers, both overwhelmed by circumstances beyond their control. And it is in this commonality, in this shared suffering, that we may find a glimmer – just a glimmer – of hope.

PRECLINICAL OBSERVATIONS ABOUT THE DOCTOR–PATIENT RELATIONSHIP
Restitution stories

Especially during their second year, students tended to form highly positive impressions of physicians whom they observed during tag-alongs and other clinical exposure. In a poem typical of this phase, a patient facing cataract surgery encounters a physician who is friendly and smiling, with a warm and soothing office, and a reassuring, gentle staff. The patient feels grateful. In another example cited in full earlier (*see* Chapter 7, "Empathy: A Patient's Point of View"), a patient recovering from major cardiac surgery views his physician as his "life-saver," and expresses gratitude both for his survival and for his excellent surgeon. Another cardiac patient with arrhythmia is helped by "miracle drugs" that "gently heal." The doctor in this situation reaffirms his Hippocratic Oath to do no harm and to practice his art.

Yet another poem imagines various patients calling their doctor the "Master of My Health," saluting him as an educator, a restorer of health, and a miracle worker. In these vignettes, the physician improves quality of life with "magic pills", and restores another patient to "perfect form and shape" through surgical intervention. The physician is invariably engaged, empathic, ready to extend himself "to any length" to help the patient, and impervious to biases based on culture, socioeconomic status, or gender. (The poem also cleverly incorporates a doctor–patient communication model based on the "5 E's" of engagement [with the patient], empathy, [patient] education, enlistment [of the patient in her own healthcare], and extending [oneself and the healthcare system to maximize benefit to the patient].)

Master of My Health By: Michael Brewer
UC Irvine

I come to him when I am down and out
When health is gone and nothing's left but doubt

With great engaging interest in my strife
He vows to boost my quality of life

I come to him with unremitting pain
When all have tried to help, but tried in vain
His empathy outweighed just by his skill
He finds an efficacious magic pill

I come to him when things have grown awry
Enlisted by the hope to rectify
He sculpts me back to perfect form and shape
A gifted artist, scalpel blade embraced

I come to him when I have lost all hope
I can't go on, I can no longer cope
He takes me by the hand and gives me strength
For me he does extend to any length

He is my doctor – master of my health
He cares not of my status, race, or wealth
Not only does he help when health is squelched
He educates so I can help myself

These restitution stories posit disturbance in the patient through disease, in which physical or at least emotional recovery is made possible by the healing skills of the physician.

POSITIVE VIEWS OF THE DOCTOR–PATIENT RELATIONSHIP IN THE CLINICAL YEARS

As students proceeded in their training, some continued to tell restitution stories that confirmed or restored assumptions about a "just universe." However, for many other students, their views of the doctor–patient relationship became more nuanced, and tended to take on characteristics of journey or witnessing.

Restitution stories

Examples of restitution persist in the clinical years. In one example, a woman who has been scheduled for a pelvic examination trustingly sees her physician as a "broad white shield." This poem "restores" the patient's security through the protection that the physician provides. In a similar depiction, a nervous, embarrassed Latina patient who needs a breast examination has a good outcome. Thanks to the attention and concern of the doctor (and the medical student), by the end of the examination the patient recognizes that it is better to be embarrassed now than sick later. This is a restitution poem because the patient is initially portrayed as embarrassed, mistrustful, and uncommunicative, but subsequently, due to the physician's wise guidance, she becomes a "better" patient.

A different poem, which is quoted in its entirety in Chapter 9 ("They sit at attention"), portrays residents as positive role models. They deliver bad news and listen to their patients' desperate reactions. They are able to touch scars and wounds without fear or shame. They are able to gaze on the worst suffering without turning away, "steady and strong." "They ask the hard questions and make/the hard decisions . . ." They are wise: "I know they see much more than I." In this poem we see heroic residents, who are capable of handling all problems competently and calmly, balance out the intimidating nature of medical practice.

In another poem, a female patient who has been raped by her boyfriend is initially reluctant to confide in a male physician. However, the physician is intuitive, perceptive, and persistent, and is finally able to get the patient to open up. By the end of the poem, she sees the physician as "Healer and Friend." This narrative is closer to restitution than witnessing, in that the patient's "problem" seems to be solved through the sensitive ministrations of the physician. In another poem that describes a patient's close encounters with death, the physician is described as gentle, wise, compassionate, and comforting. The physician is the rescuer who saves the patient from the vacuum of the void of Silence and Death. In this poem, the physician acquires an almost god-like role. The poem tells a restitution story in that an apparently omnipotent physician who stands against death restores the patient to health.

Journey stories

In a typical journey poem, a heroin user, battling the demon of addiction, has experienced sadness and loss. Filled with emptiness and longing, she embarks on a quest and discovers that her doctor, a wise guide, is there to help. When the patient implores the doctor "to make things as they once were," he listens, and forms an alliance with his patient. The discerning physician knows that "Drugs are not the answer," and from this point on there must be no going backward. "Together searching," they try to discover the next step.

She cries out in pain By: Matt Holve
UC Irvine

The sadness consumes her soul
Her husband is gone

Methadone only masks
Emptiness and her longing
to be held once again

Help comes in many forms
Doctor listens to her needs
Together searching

She asks the doctor
To make things as they once were
Drugs are not the cure

In a somewhat different version of the journey story, a pregnant patient with a brain tumor is determined to breastfeed once her infant is born. The doctor at first says this is impossible, but then, sensing how important this is to her patient, she negotiates a schedule of radiation, breastfeeding, and chemotherapy. The doctor is supportive, and the patient feels less alone. The shift from authoritative control to humane negotiation occurs after initial resistance on the part of the physician, who is then able to see how important the patient's desire is to her. Like the addict and her doctor, they have started on a journey together, unsure of its conclusion, but united in the face of uncertainty.

Witnessing stories

Many poems become a respectful act of witnessing the healing power of an affirming doctor–patient relationship. For example, in one poem a patient is worried about chest pain, and her fears about her health preoccupy her. The physician listens carefully, and is reassuring, thorough, and "far beyond kind." The patient takes comfort in the caring of the physician. Another poem in the outpatient setting chronicles a series of difficult patients with out-of-control diabetes, obesity, and hypertension, and praises their doctor as someone who, although he "... might not be able to cure ... was overflowing with care."

In another example of witnessing, a seriously ill cancer patient is recovering from surgery, surrounded by her sons. A surgeon and "fifteen white coats" enter. The surgeon is kind and poised. He speaks in a soft tone and knows his patient's body "from within." He recognizes his limits, and he admits to the family that he has been unable to remove all of the tumor. He holds the patient's hand, and compassionately tells her sons that she will recover in the short term, but "will soon be gone." The physician is able to acknowledge the patient's suffering and recognize the limitations of medicine and the inevitability of death, all within a context of tenderness and concern.

In the following poem, a doctor pauses outside his patient's room. He realizes from her lab results that she is very ill. He is moved to the point of tears by his patient's fate. In a striking visual image (the hidden beauty in a trompe l'oeil picture), the physician wishes for happier news, but as he prepares with little personal ticks to open the door, he knows that he is powerless. Raising his hand to knock (the ironic inappropriateness at this moment of a knock-knock joke, to which everyone already knows the answer, does not escape the poet), he notices the wedding ring and, in a moment of counter-transference, thinks of his own wife – her beauty, her aliveness, her preciousness. When he breaks the bad news, he reassures the patient that he will be there for her, and then holds her hand as she starts to cry. This poem witnesses a moment of connection between physician and patient, as well as a physician who is present enough to hold both his patient's and his own suffering.

The Conversation By: Pelin Cinar
UC Irvine, 2003

He got the lab report
Stared at the numbers
Looked at it until his eyes got blurry.
He wished it was a 3-D picture;
Just when he gave up
He would see that magical flower or bird.
But his vision wasn't misleading him.
Then he looked at the chart
Hoping to find a better bone scan.
No sir, wish all you can
You won't find any good news here.

Why do I feel so tired again?
Just when I thought I was getting better.
She looks at the magazine
But does not see the pages.
I wonder if the results are back
He should be knocking on the door soon.

A hopeless sigh
A slight combing of hair with his palm
A pause
And a sudden rise.
An outwardly slow pace
With an inwardly fast-moving locomotive engine.

He noticed the ring on his finger
As he raised it to knock on the door.
He saw his wife before him
Looking more beautiful than ever before.
Knock knock
We know who's there
His cold hand touched the handle
Turned it with complete care.
He stepped in the room
And saw her there.

My, he doesn't look so good
Please doctor tell me the news
No more pauses
No more uncertainties
I know I'm still fighting
But tell me who is my rival

"I'm afraid I've got bad news
It has not gone away
But, I will be here for you
You can be sure of that"

I have lots of questions
Don't know how to start
Then he held my hand
And I started to cry.

All of these poems witness to the beneficial effects that compassionate, humane attitudes and behavior can have on patients.

POSITIVE VIEWS OF PEDIATRICIANS

I single out pediatrics for attention because, far more than for any other specialty, students described these doctors in a positive light. Many of these poems tell restitution stories, usually resulting in successful treatment for the pediatric patient.

Restitution stories

Contemplating an infant in the neonatal intensive-care unit, hospitalized since she was born, with a mother who is a "homeless hooker" with two other kids and AIDS who appears to have abandoned her infant, the student describes the medical team who stroke the baby, take care of her, and talk with her, as the real "family." The voice of the infant speaks: Although they "prod and poke/But at least they're kind/They hold me, they rock me, and ease my mind." This infant feels "loved and needed" by her doctor and the hospital staff. In this restitution story, the infant's "hooker mother" has abandoned her, but the pediatrician and nurses step in to recreate a better family.

In another restitution poem, the pediatrician is described as a "protector of innocence," "a bodyguard of angelic faces," and an expert whose skills allow children the good health to continue to explore life and achieve their potential. In a different poem, the pediatric patient views his pediatrician as really there for him, and the only person who's promised not to harm him. The doctor has personal knowledge of her patient's life, as well as anything that might put him in danger. The patient marvels at how much the doctor understands him, inside and out. The doctor is gentle, caring, reassuring, and contrite when she has to inflict pain. She has kept the patient healthy and disease-free. In another poem, the young patient perceives the "white coats" as friendly and as knowing his name. The patient's final estimation of his doctor is that "He is so cool." Another pediatrician is portrayed as warm, calming, gentle, and reassuring. He educates and reinforces a young, first-time mother with regard to care of her infant. He is wise and compassionate, and wins the mom's gratitude. The kind and knowledgeable doctor restores the worried mother's confidence in herself and her parenting abilities.

NEGATIVE VIEWS OF THE DOCTOR–PATIENT RELATIONSHIP IN THE CLINICAL YEARS
Chaos stories

In their poetry, students often observe and comment on negative doctor–patient relationships. Occasionally, poems about negative doctor–patient interactions express a sense of chaos on the part of the student. In one such poem, the patient expects a compassionate physician, "But indeed what I got was a geek." This doctor lacks any semblance of social skills, bombards the patient with questions, and then announces that he has gout, which shocks and confuses the patient, who thinks this is a disease of old men. The end result is that the patient rejects the diagnosis – and the doctor. This chaos story becomes a cry for help when the patient (the narrator) discovers that he cannot rely on the physician who is supposed to comfort and support him. In another example, mentioned previously, a dialogue between an alcoholic patient and his physician shows the alienation between a patient who is in denial and a physician who does not really know how to help his patient. Neither the patient nor the physician knows how to reach the other. The situation is out of control and uncontained. In a final chaos poem, a close friend of the medical student-author is severely injured in a motor vehicle accident. The student visits his friend in the surgical intensive-care unit: "With tears in my eyes/I listen to the team/discuss you, debate you, speculate about you." The student is filled with feelings towards his friend, but the team is logical, objective, and detached. Whereas he sees his friend, they see only a puzzle. When medicine becomes personal, this student realizes its emotional shortcomings.

Journey stories

In a typical poem, a patient with rheumatoid arthritis undergoes a painful draining of his knee. The ER resident is kind, apologetic, and concerned, but does not value the patient's expertise about his own body, and does not appear to be too competent. The first time, he is unsuccessful in performing the painful procedure. The second time around, the resident is chastened and listens to the patient's advice, and all goes well. This poem represents a journey for the resident, in that he does not initially recognize the patient's greater knowledge of himself, but due to the patient's willingness to educate the resident (and thus become a wise guide), the resident becomes wiser and enlightened.

Witnessing stories

Occasionally, a poem reflects on the limitations of the training that produces doctors who are often bewildered by and afraid of their patients' emotional needs. One such poem recognizes that the patients want care, but the educational system teaches only harshness. Physicians are trained to identify, treat, and defeat the cause of disease, "But they [the patients] want more, they always will / They need support, instead we offer them a pill." "They need to see a friend in us, advisor," but doctors don't know how to fill these roles. This poem witnesses the physician's inadequacy and lack of preparedness in the presence of the patient's need for support, guidance, and friendship.

Most of the poems that address problematic relationships and interactions between physicians and patients are examples of witnessing, and align themselves with the patient against the doctor. For instance, in the poem "Heavy Questions" (quoted in full in Chapter 7), the physician is arrogant and uncaring. He makes assumptions about the patient based on her weight. He regards the patient with disdain, and questions her honesty, determination, and will power. He proposes solutions to her weight problem that seem simplistic to the patient, and he ignores the other aspects of her life. The poem witnesses both the patient's pain and her resistance. In another poem that examines a similar situation, a callous ER doctor chastises a patient who has had a heart attack and a positive history of heart disease because of his unhealthy lifestyle. The author criticizes the physician for being a "health hypocrite," punning on the name of the father of medicine, Hippocrates, for not healing the patient but instead condemning her.

In another poem, "Manger" (French verb meaning "to eat"), an obese patient with heart disease talks to her resident. However, the latter is "hearing impaired" in the sense that she does not listen to the patient's concerns. On behalf of the entire medical team, the student begs the patient's forgiveness and explains that the resident's head "has chomped her Ears / into bitter ribbons." In a witty but poignant play on words, the author suggests all the different forms of eating that are going on. The patient, whose body seems to be consuming her, may have eaten her way to early death, the patient's heart is now literally devouring her life, and the resident's intellect and biomedical orientation have eaten up her capacity to empathize with the patient's quandary. The student witnesses insensitive treatment on the part of the resident, and chooses to identify with the stigmatized and scorned other (the patient). However, she also acknowledges her own culpability in being more concerned with the patient's interesting medical condition than with her humanity.

Manger By: Sarah Mourra
UC Irvine, 2005

It appears that your
Neck has swallowed your Chin, Madame.
Your Legs devouring Ankles
Arms engulfing Elbows
A Stomach masticating on flopping Breasts.

Your Thighs have taken your Knees
Into their mouths
And refused to let go.

You speak.
Red wires for hair
Watery cantaloupe eyes
Lips like bursting blisters

But the Resident is hearing impaired.
Please forgive.
Her Head
Has chomped her Ears
Into bitter ribbons.

Forgive us, Madame. I, too
Cannot forget the photograph
(Black and White)
Of your hungry Heart
Silently chewing its way
across your Chest.

On a psychiatric clerkship, a student encounters a friendly, happy patient who loves life, God, and basketball. The supervising psychiatrist, however, can see only the patient's diagnosis of bipolar disorder, labels him as "crazy," and warns the student not to fall into the trap of thinking that these patients are "normal." The student rejects this view and challenges the doctor: "I want to know / what's wrong with being happy all the time?"

Yet another poem presents a patient with abdominal pain waiting for his doctor, waiting for "good or bad news." When the doctor finally arrives, the patient begins to explain his pain, but almost immediately the doctor prepares to leave. The patient protests: "Why are you getting up? / Why are you leaving so soon? / I know you are busy and / have other people in the rooms / but don't let me be / this pain is too much to bear." Here, taking the patient's perspective is an act of witnessing the patient's helplessness and suffering. The patient is filled with anxiety, fear, and eventually anger (which he only dares express to the medical student), but the doctor is focused only on her schedule, and pays no attention to the patient's suffering. This poem rejects the physician as an anti-role model, and demonstrates identification with the abandoned patient.

Ouch, this pain By: Daniel Chun
UC Irvine

Ouch, this pain in my abdomen. What will the doctor say?
Will she give me good or bad news? I wish I knew right away.

The pain I thought would go away after 5 days
But it never did.
What did I do before then?
Was it something I ate?
Did it get worse or

Was it always the same?

I hope the doctor can help me
It's hard to wait.
Ten minutes feel like thirty.
I just want to know
Please don't let me stand here and contemplate
About the things this pain could be
Cancer possibly.
No. It can't be that. It won't be that.
I don't believe it can be.

Hi doctor. The pain is here
Why are you getting up?
Why are you leaving so soon?
I know you are busy and
have other people in the rooms
but don't let me be
this pain is too much to bear
I need to know now
I'm running out of air.

I wish I could let her know
My anxiety and fear, but I understand
I don't want to be a burden.
I'll just try to sit comfortably here.

I notice the medical student
sitting with me in the room.
I smile, avoid his glances.
Will he notice my trembling hands?
I have to hold on to these.
Tightly I grasp them
Keeping still.
Time is passing and I can't resist
I try to politely ask
"Will you please get the doctor, I'm getting kind of pissed!"

Sometimes the entire medical team is perceived as insensitive and superficial. In one poem, the patient has a problem that is not obvious. The team ignores the patient's emotional and mental state, and focuses only on the physical findings. Expressing a similar theme, a patient with chronic pain longs for "another doctor, one/who suffers with me." The implication is that the patient's current doctor is just the opposite – someone who does not empathize with and does not care about the patient. Both of these poems witness the suffering of the patient in an act that "resists" the callousness of the medical team.

Physician insensitivity is also targeted in a poem about a medical team who "poked and prodded, examined and recorded . . . /jotted down their diagnosis and delivered their prognosis . . . /And having thus spoken, she [the patient]] watched them depart/ With a swish of sterile, white coats/As they filed out of her room, conferring most solemnly . . ." These doctors are impersonal, detached, and self-important. The scene epitomizes bad news delivered badly. "When they prodded and measured and recorded/ The spasms that invaded her heart/No time was taken to hear and listen/To empathize and understand/That the waves that battered her heart/Were but the ebb and flow of some silent storm deep within//A listening ear, a soothing voice, a friendly touch/ Would have done so much." The medical team is technically competent, but uncaring. The student chooses to identify with the patient, to notice the patient's suffering and fear, and to observe the medical team's indifference.

In another poem, a patient with cancer is despairing, afraid, and unable to ask the questions that she needs to ask. The doctors, for their part, are afraid to answer the questions that the patient cannot ask. The patient accepts that no one can really answer questions like these, but what wounds her is that her doctors are not even willing to discuss them. Unable to put her questions to rest, they "float around in the air around me/Sometimes I breathe one in and it encircles my body/I breathe it out and replace it with a new one." She hungers to be heard and listened to, but her doctors are not able to be present for her in this way. This poem is a witnessing of the patient's fear, as well as her physicians' inability to respond to her.

In a poem that is quoted in full in Chapter 12 ("Dream"), another dying patient rails against the doctors who won't let him die. He pleads "Let me go/Let me be free", but "The white coats bully me into doing what they believe is best." In this poem, the physicians' paternalism interferes with the patient's dignity. In another poem, the patient receives an unexpected diagnosis of terminal cancer. Yet in this emotionally critical situation, the medical team appears impersonal – professional, but indifferent. In yet another poem, a heartless physician is blasé about describing patients' causes of death. His indifference is contrasted with the student's compassionate thoughts.

A similar poem is written from the perspective of a young woman diagnosed with lymphoma. Initially, the narrative reads like a restitution story. The patient is young, she is ready to fight and endure pain, and "her prognosis was very good." Unexpectedly, however, the patient does not respond to treatment. As her condition deteriorates, and she experiences more and more assaults on her selfhood, the doctors want to continue intervention, but the patient has had enough. She wants only to die peacefully, but the doctors accuse her of "giving in, and then they begged her to fight."

They Told Her . . . By: Reema Basu
UC Irvine, 2004

They told her that she had lymphoma and to put her plans on hold.
She told them she was ready, and she would do anything that she was told.
They told her that they caught it early, and that her prognosis was very good.
She told them if anyone could survive, she was the one who would.
They told her that she may experience some pain
and would probably lose her hair.
She told them that she would wear a wig, and to bring on the treatment
she didn't care.
They told her that they were trying their best, but something was wrong
she was losing too much weight.
She told them not to worry, and she promised them by the end of next year
they would watch her graduate.
They told her that she had to go another round, because she wasn't getting well.
She told them that she would do it, but was getting tired of this hell.
They told her that she couldn't breathe, and so they needed to make a hole.
She told them that she had to keep her body in one piece
or she would lose her soul.
They told her that she was suffocating and that she had to be tough.
She told them that she did everything that they asked her to
but now she had had enough.
They told her that she was giving in, and then they begged her to fight.
She told them that it was finally time to go
and that she wanted to sleep in peace that night.

In these poems, the narrator witnesses and validates the patient's right to die, empowering the patient through empathy in the (indirect) presence of powerful but uncaring physicians.

Another student experiences his first code on an 82-year-old patient with aspiration pneumonia. The student is shocked, disbelieving, dumbfounded, and numb. However, the residents begin to joke about the patient while the chief resident counsels the bewildered student not to be offended. Here indifference and insensitivity are represented as simply part of the culture of medicine. A similar poem describes an encounter with a dying patient who is frightened and helpless. The residents, on the other hand, are blasé in the face of the patient's plight: "The residents have seen this many times before / But it's all new to me." These residents also make jokes about the patient, and the student is horrified: "But I cannot see the humor in his pain." These are both examples of witnessing through resistance. They represent rejection of normative behavior, indifference and insensitivity as part of routine, everyday practice and distancing humor. Like many of the other poems discussed in this section, they express identification with the "othered" patient.

Sometimes the witnessing is more complex. One poem shows the resident expressing compassion at the death of a patient, but also thinking about the next admission. The intern is merely annoyed by the additional paperwork necessary to process the body. In a poem cited in Chapter 6 ("'Twas the Night Before Clerkship"), the student starting her third-year clerkship initially perceives her supervising residents to be cynical taskmasters: "the residents so bitter, and I so naive/I was not looking forward to the scut up their sleeves." However, towards the end of the year, looking back she realizes that her teams overall have been responsible and caring. These poems illustrate more nuanced witnessing. These student-authors begin to see the complexity of resident roles – both the need to get on with business, and the efforts made to sincerely care.

NEGATIVE PHYSICIAN IMAGES IN PEDIATRICS
Witnessing (resistance) stories

Poems that question the dominant pediatrician–child patient narrative often adopt a humorous tone. In one poem, a pediatrician locks herself in the bathroom and moans about the monotony of pediatrics – the earaches, TSVs, ADHDs, and well-child checks: "In exchange for a heart murmur or a nice case of scrofula/I'd give my left arm or sell my organs to the Mafia." She clings to the fantasy that she must stay strong so that one day she will be able to save a "polite, demure" child who has a disease that only she can cure. The pediatrician composes herself, only to discover that her next patient has a terrifying "Overprotective Mother." "Junior sat there, all trembling, as his mother's voice boomed/And the doctor soon realized that she too was doomed/She'd grow old and gray in that room with those two/She knew in her heart she'd met her Waterloo." Here the physician secretly loathes her young patients and their overbearing mothers. Another poem reaches a similarly humorous conclusion. It pokes wry fun at the stereotype of the saintly ill child, and acknowledges that sick kids can be aggravating and annoying to the physician.

This morning By: Dorota Jakubowski
UC Irvine

I have seen
so many kids –
sick
confused
innocent.
I've been lulled.

Until this morning.

This morning
a terrible 3 y/o hurricane of a boy
(was it . . . just a boy?)
screamed up and down our hallway
Leaving strewn otoscopes
    crumpled masses of stickers
       torn books
         (violence).

This morning.
This one child.
I understood
finally

why fewer pediatricians
seem to have
children
that they call
their very own.
And (instead)
seem to own . . .
dogs.

One nonhumorous poem sees pediatricians as being more comfortable focusing on superficial matters, rewarding their young patients for routine behaviors, but being reluctant to delve into issues of domestic violence. This poem also expresses resistance to the normative story of pediatricians as warm, friendly people who love children, and rather criticizes them for being shallow and superficial in the care of their patients. In another poem, the doctors and nurses who are caring for a 17-year-old girl with AIDS appear to the student to be unsympathetic, unsupportive, and upset with the patient for being noncompliant with her medications. Another poem describes an 11-year-old with an unresectable brain tumor whose doctors only "see through" their patient, write about her, and "bicker" among each other about the nature of the tumor. Both of these poems witness to – and reject – the priorities of the medical team that put the medicine before the patient.

These poems are all examples of witnessing narratives that cast a critical eye on pediatricians' harshness and indifference – often masquerading as professional detachment – that turn the patient into a rejected other. The poems challenge the comforting stereotype of the physician as a nice doctor who loves kids. They are counter-hegemonic, an alternative narrative, and therefore an example of witnessing to other, less spoken truths.

PHYSICIAN ENCOUNTERS WITH PATIENTS' FAMILIES
Chaos stories
A few poems consider physician interactions with members of patients' families. These poems sometimes tell chaos stories. In a typical poem, the medical team promises the wife of a DNR patient, "Don't worry, your husband will be all right." But then the patient pulls out his ventilator, and since he is DNR, nothing can be done. The student is consumed by helplessness and the need to take action. As he watches the patient die, he thinks of how loving the couple seemed and how incapable he is of helping them. The patient pursues death, while the wife clings to his life, which the medical team carelessly promised her. The student is the observer of it all – the struggles, the thoughtless words, the enduring love. This poem expresses feelings of chaos about the way in which the team carelessly exercises its perceived power over life and death, trampling on the love between the couple.

Restitution stories
Sometimes these poems adopt the tone of restitution narratives, in which the physician takes the role of hero or, failing that, of knowledgeable and clear-sighted expert. In one typical poem, the medical student takes the role of observer. When a dying patient is transferred to "the safety of the CCU," she sees the family waiting, crying, and praying.

In this case, the resident is humane and gentle, although he must prepare them for their loved one's imminent death. As the student watches him, she flinches: "But I know it's true/The family knows it's true/But somehow they hope." The family is portrayed with compassionate sympathy, but also as somehow naive, unable to face the impending demise of their loved one. The resident, on the other hand, is the truth-teller. This poem is closest to a restitution story, in which the family is perceived as naive and childlike. The resident is the heroic expert who conducts himself with humaneness and gentleness, and who enables the suffering family to accept the truth.

Witnessing stories

Most of the poems that address this topic are closer to witnessing, often perceiving the partnership that can develop between physician and family member. In one such poem, the student is witness to a dialogue between the doctor and the wife of a dying patient. The student is learning about death, and how it interrupts a life. The doctor and the patient's wife agree on their assessment of the patient ("much improved," "much better"). The student agrees as well, but her private opinion is that the patient does not look good at all because he is dying. The doctor and the wife seem to have a partnership, a team approach to the husband. The student is outside this mysterious bond.

Hospice By: Heidi Cruz
UC Irvine, 2001

"He's looking good. Much improved."
I nod in agreement.
Despite the fact that I have never seen him before.
Despite the fact that he does not look good.
He lies naked in a hospital bed, dying.
Not in a hospital, but in his own bedroom.
Family pictures line the walls.
A half-empty laundry basket sits on the floor.
A dog barks from the kitchen.
A home. A family. A life.
And metastatic melanoma.
And me, a medical student.
The only noise, his labored irregular breaths.
His wife agrees with the doctor:
"Much better."

In other poems, physicians variously console, empathize, and explain or, less often, they ignore or detach. In witnessing poems, the students record these interactions with either respect or condemnation. Their primary purpose seems to be to acknowledge these encounters and prevent them from disappearing into the ephemera of transitory experience.

SUMMARY

Medical students are astute and attentive observers of their physician role models. They are eager to learn from those further along the road of physicianhood about the "proper" relationship between doctor and patient, and how to construct it. At the same time, they are quick to note the sometimes looming gap between theory and practice, between what they are taught about the relationship, and what they see unfolding before their eyes on hospital wards and outpatient clinics. They are surprisingly aware of the differences in perspectives between doctor and patient, which sometimes deteriorate into true narrative incommensurability. Although they willingly acknowledge positive examples of physicians, the majority of their poems focus on negative role models, whom they perceive to be distancing, judgmental, and unprofessional in their attitudes and behavior. In too many of these poems, we see the consequences of what happens when not enough physician-teachers put conscious thought into how they are guiding the daily informal learning of their students.

In general, preclinical students' poetry evaluated doctors' relationships with patients positively, and tended to favor restitution narratives. In the third year, a number of students continued to describe positive encounters, especially involving pediatricians. Occasionally students were impressed with technical competence, but more often they valued compassionate attitudes and behavior. Although some poems told simplistic restitution stories, many of these poems showed awareness of the power and importance of humane patient care.

However, the largest number of student poems suggested many concerns about the doctor–patient relationships described. The most frequent criticisms related to callous, detached, and disrespectful attitudes on the part of physicians, and their insensitivity, arrogance, and lack of skill in addressing psychosocial issues. Sometimes students expressed feelings of chaos when observing physician interactions with challenging patients. In these situations, patient, doctor, and medical student alike appeared to be overwhelmed. Occasionally, students would also see physicians as evolving in these circumstances, willing to participate in a journey towards greater closeness to and commitment to these patients. Students generally adopted a position of witnessing to the physician's shortcomings, and aligned themselves with the neglected, demeaned, suffering patient.

REFERENCES

 1 Mischler EG. *The Discourse of Medicine: The dialectics of medical interviews.* Norwood, NJ: Ablex; 1984.
 2 Hunter KM. Patients, physicians, and red parakeets: narrative incommensurability. In: *Doctors' Stories: The narrative structure of medical knowledge.* Princeton, NJ: Princeton University Press; 1991. pp. 123–47.
 3 Toombs SK. *The Meaning of Illness: A phenomenological account of the different perspectives of physician and patient.* Dordrecht: Kluwer; 1993.
 4 Kleinman A. *The Illness Narratives: Suffering, healing, and the human condition.* New York: Basic Books; 1988.
 5 Frank AW. *At the Will of the Body: Reflections on illness.* New York: Houghton Mifflin; 2002.
 6 Inui TS, Frankel RM. Hello, stranger: building a healing narrative that includes everyone. *Academic Medicine* 2006; **81:** 415–18.
 7 Shapiro J. Walking a mile in their patients' shoes: empathy and othering in medical students' education. *Philosophy, Ethics, and Humanities in Medicine* 2008; **3:** 10.
 8 Frank AW. *The Renewal of Generosity: Illness, medicine, and how to live.* Chicago: University of Chicago Press; 2004.
 9 Sweeney K. The consultation as Rubik's cube. In: Evans M, Finlay IG (eds). *Medical Humanities.* London: BMJ Books; 2001. pp. 83–100.

10 Wear D, Castellani B. The development of professionalism: curriculum matters. *Academic Medicine* 2000; **75**: 602–11.

11 Souba WW. Academic medicine and the search for meaning and purpose. *Academic Medicine* 2002; **77**: 139–44.

12 Nogueira-Martins MC, Nogueira-Martins LA, Turato ER. Medical students' perceptions of their learning about the doctor–patient relationship: a qualitative study. *Medical Education* 2006; **40**: 322–8.

13 Coulehan J. Today's professionalism: engaging the mind but not the heart. *Academic Medicine* 2005; **80**: 892–8.

14 Brainard AH, Brislen HC. Viewpoint: learning professionalism: a view from the trenches. *Academic Medicine* 2007; **82**: 1010–14.

15 Maheux B, Beaudoin C, Berkson L, *et al.* Medical faculty as humanistic physicians and teachers: the perceptions of students at innovative and traditional medical schools. *Medical Education* 2000; **34**: 630–4.

16 Beaudoin C, Maheux B, Côté L, *et al.* Clinical teachers as humanistic caregivers and educators: perceptions of senior clerks and second-year residents. *Canadian Medical Association Journal* 1998; **159**: 765–9.

17 Williams KN, Ramani S, Fraser B, Orlander JD. Improving bedside teaching: findings from a focus group study of learners. *Academic Medicine* 2008; **83**: 257–64.

18 Wear D, Aultman JM, Varley JD, Zarconi J. Making fun of patients: medical students' perceptions and use of derogatory and cynical humor in clinical settings. *Academic Medicine* 2006; **81**: 454–62.

19 Branch WT Jr. Teaching respect for patients. *Academic Medicine* 2006; **81**: 463–7.

20 Branch WT Jr, Kern D, Haidet P, *et al.* Teaching the human dimensions of care in clinical settings. *JAMA* 2001; **286**: 1067–74.

21 Wear D, Varley JD. Rituals of verification: the role of simulation in developing and evaluating empathic communication. *Patient Education and Counselling* 2008; **71**: 153–6.

22 Mann KV, Sutton E, Frank B. Twelve tips for preparing residents as teachers. *Medical Teacher* 2007; **29**: 301–6.

23 Bharel M, Jain S. A longitudinal curriculum to improve resident teaching skills. *Medical Teacher* 2005; **27**: 564–6.

24 Morrison EH, Shapiro JF, Harthill M. Resident doctors' understanding of their roles as clinical teachers. *Medical Education* 2005; **39**: 137–44.

25 Weissmann PF, Branch WT, Gracey CF, *et al.* Role modeling humanistic behavior: learning bedside manner from the experts. *Academic Medicine* 2006; **81**: 661–7.

26 Shapiro J. How do physicians teach empathy in the primary care setting? *Academic Medicine* 2002; **77**: 323–8.

27 Charon R. *Narrative Medicine: Honoring the stories of illness.* Oxford: Oxford University Press; 2006.

28 Côté L, Leclère H. How clinical teachers perceive the doctor–patient relationship and themselves as role models. *Academic Medicine* 2000; **75**: 1117–24.

29 Klitzman R. Improving education on doctor–patient relationships and communication lessons from doctors who become patients. *Academic Medicine* 2006; **81**: 447–53.

30 Jones WS, Hanson JL, Longacre JL. An intentional modeling process to teach professional behavior: students' clinical observations of preceptors. *Teaching and Learning in Medicine* 2004; **16**: 264–9.

31 Goldstein EA, Maestas RR, Fryer-Edwards K, *et al.* Professionalism in medical education: an institutional challenge. *Academic Medicine* 2006; **81**: 871–6.

32 Dobie S. Reflections on a well-traveled path: self-awareness, mindful practice, and relationship-centered care as foundations for medical education. *Academic Medicine* 2007; **82**: 422–7.

9 You Are My Patient . . . Let Us Take Flight! Student–Patient Relationships – Part 1

It is surprising that the professional literature on the medical student–patient relationship is rather thin, in contrast to research and theorizing about the doctor–patient relationship, which is voluminous. Just as medical students sometimes make the mistake of thinking of pediatric patients as simply "little adults," scholars may err in thinking of the student's relationship with patients as a watered-down, shadow version of the doctor–patient relationship. This is inaccurate in many ways. For example, most obviously, students have virtually no direct responsibility for patients, either in terms of decision-making or even in terms of care. Although of course they perform simple procedures on patients and check laboratory results, they do so under careful supervision. Furthermore, especially in hospital settings, medical students, especially third-year students, may in fact spend more time with patients than either residents or attending physicians. As was noted in Chapter 1, there are parallels in the student's and patient's experience that tend to draw them closer together emotionally than may be true for more experienced physicians.

What we do know about students' relationships with patients overall is generally positive. For example, one study[1] concluded that students in their clinical years recognized that forming relationships with patients was beneficial to an accurate diagnostic process. They further perceived that these relationships had the potential to bring both meaning and frustration into their own lives. Although the students in this study sometimes reported difficulties in setting appropriate boundaries and establishing a professional relationship because of their age or gender, they realized the importance of good communication, acting in a professional manner, and investing time in building relationships with patients. Another study also highlighted how students valued their ability to spend time with patients, and the privilege of being entrusted with intimate knowledge by people undergoing experiences that made them vulnerable.[2] These students reported feeling positive about their ability to make a difference to patients' lives, despite their limited knowledge and experience. The students in this study were also aware of the importance of focusing on the patient rather than on the diagnosis, and the dangers of stereotyping patients.

However, there is also cause for concern. One study[3] of first patient encounters portrayed these as intense, consuming emotional experiences for medical students. Students reported feelings of helplessness and uncertainty when faced with serious illness and death, while their initial attempts at physical examination were often described as anxiety-provoking and confusing. Of course, these reactions are understandable given the emotional enormity of the human dilemmas that confront beginning students. Of more concern are indications that in the third year of training, although students report patient contact as rewarding, they also often continue to feel anxious, stressed, and fearful of not being competent or not being able to answer patients' questions.[4] Other research suggests that student attitudes towards patients become more negative rather than less so as their training proceeds,[5] and a growing literature documents significant declines in student empathy.[6–9] Students themselves recognize that many aspects of their clinical training are not conducive to establishing empathic relationships.[10]

One study examined the role of emotional connection in students' care of patients, particularly empathy, caring, and compassion, and what might be acceptable limits to these emotions.[11] Students were worried whether they cared too much about their patients, or not enough. They generally identified with patients and felt their suffering acutely, but wondered whether this emotional sensitivity might overwhelm them and render them either unprofessional or ineffectual. Several students noted both parallels and conflicts between the student's and the patient's roles. They expressed confusion and distress when they realized that the patient's agenda (i.e. to receive care and cure) might sometimes be at variance with the student's agenda (i.e. to finish on time, and to look good in the eyes of the resident). These students expressed concerns about an encroaching desensitization, lack of humanity, and failures of empathy in themselves. They were deeply troubled by the idea that their experiences in medical school were making them less caring, kind, and compassionate human beings, and they fretted about how the diminution of such qualities would affect them as physicians. Confirming these fears, other scholars have argued that the medicalization of experience involved in students' training makes it increasingly likely that they will split off from their own emotional responses and become detached from the meaning of the events that they observe.[12]

Another study documented that, in addition to positive emotions, students can also experience feelings of aggression and dislike towards patients, as well as feeling humiliated by them. Furthermore, they tended to rationalize or justify these negative feelings as appropriate, given the patient's behavior.[13] Other scholars have expressed concern that students tend to be spectators rather than witnesses to their patients' suffering, and on the whole to appear insufficiently aware of the societal and cultural issues implicated in healthcare.[14] A radical experiment in medical education emphasizes the production of collaborative knowledge between patient and student rather than information reproduction by the student to the expert attending, prioritizing narrative as well as biomedical aspects of the patient's experience.[15]

Students spend a great deal of time thinking about their relationships with patients. In writing poems about these relationships, sometimes students were overwhelmed by patient demands, and distanced themselves through chaos stories. Sometimes students wrote journey poems, in which the lowly student becomes the unwitting "hero" of the scene, reaching out to bridge the gap between physician and patient, or to address the patient's emotional needs. The majority of the poetry consisted of witnessing poems that acknowledged connection, solidarity, and advocacy with patients. Some students were transformed through a particular patient encounter and elevated to a new and deeper understanding of the human condition.

Metamorphosis By: Michael Doo
UC Irvine

First contact —
    Via chart, presentation
    A refined conglomeration of
    Vitals and diagnoses

And physical findings
Described in the jargon of medicine
The abbreviations
Nigh impenetrable to those uninitiated
Humanity cloaked
By a diagnosis
With each word spoken in
Your own voice, each exchange whispered
And exclaimed, with each disclosure
A cocoon erupts.
Texture disrupts sterile pages
Intervene! Help me to look beyond
This chart with your life
Deny me the temptation to
Interpret you as a process, reduce you
To a treatment plan
Let me in on the irrelevant, the
Maybe-not-so-insubstantial
It is no mere conjurer's trick
To uplift print into humanity
Construct a being out of labs
Perhaps it is enough that
You are my patient – the
Discovery that I am as
Human as you
Perhaps it should not be
My fate to walk this
Future alone, in hand with
Just another case
Study or learning opportunity
Just another entry in
Some log
Perhaps it is all that ever matters
Let us take flight! –
And for even a visit
Maybe a lifetime
Face this world, foreboding, and
Hopeful, you and me
Together.

In a poem about the student–patient relationship that contains both journey and transcendent elements, a student talks about meeting his patient first through the chart (the "obstacle" or "demon"), as a diagnosis and set of physical findings. The medical jargon and abbreviations make the chart, and by extension the patient, "impenetrable," inaccessible, and unknown, despite the wealth of objective information that is spread before the student. Identifying a common phenomenon in the medical encounter, the narrator of the poem astutely realizes that the more he studies the chart, the further the patient's voice recedes. The voice of the patient is overtaken by the voices and language of medicine. Yet the student intuits that when the patient's whispers and exclamations reach his ears, the "cocoon" of medical objectivity bursts and the patient is revealed. Invoking a sensory tactile metaphor to complement the previously used visual and aural ones, the student discovers that in the patient's voice, instead of sterility, he finds texture and the humanity that he has been missing.

At this point, the student suddenly switches from the relative impersonality of the third-person voice to a direct appeal to the patient. He implores the patient to "Intervene! Help me to look beyond / This chart to your life / Deny me the temptation to / Interpret you as a process, reduce you / To a treatment plan." Despite his earlier insight, the student is well aware of the ethical and perhaps spiritual risks that he is taking. He is equally aware that he cannot manage connection and relationship alone, without the patient's help. This recognition both acknowledges and helps to birth (extending the cocoon metaphor) the patient's power in the Foucauldian sense that power does not reside in any one person, but circulates within the situation, available to all.

Continuing this counter-hegemonic turn, the student next contests the notion that the medical establishment alone holds the power to discriminate relevant and important information about the patient's situation from the tangential and immaterial. In the next lines, the student eagerly cajoles the patient to "let him in on" (a phrase suggestive of a prized secret) all those details of the patient's life which to others within the medical community may seem irrelevant and insubstantial. The student suspects that it is through the narrative's small and personal details that he will truly grasp the meaning of the patient's illness.

In the next section of the poem, the author hints at the transcendent nature of this process of relationship building. Surely the phrase "to uplift print into humanity" recalls "the Word made flesh." Furthermore, the protestation that "it is no mere conjurer's trick" cautions that we are not dealing with magic, but with a sacred act, a holy interaction. The student himself is humbled by realizing the enormity of "constructing a [human] being", and concedes that this may not be completely possible. Instead, he accepts (in a phrase with biblical echoes – *dayenu*, the Hebrew word from the Old Testament spoken in prayer at Passover to acknowledge the bounteousness of God's gifts) that "it is enough" to enter into relationship with this patient, and to honor the fact that they share a common bond of humanity.

And now we hear some of the student's own loneliness and longing. He tentatively extends a hope – it is *not* a certainty – that he will not have to walk this path alone, with only a two-dimensional case study for companionship. In this disclosure, the student perceives the essential mutuality of the relationship – his need for the patient's humanity is just as great as the patient's need for his humanity. The student even speculates that perhaps in the end "all that ever matters" is that sense of connectedness, the sharing of the journey.

Finally, the student invites the patient by saying "Let us take flight! / And for even a visit / Maybe a lifetime / Face this world, foreboding, and / Hopeful, you and me / Together." In this plea, the student completes the metaphor of the cocoon. With each other's help, patient and student alike can break free from the dormant state to which medicine has consigned them both, and instead rise in brilliantly colored, swooping and soaring flight. Together, they can rediscover their humanity. Together, they can face the vagaries that lie ahead. They embark on the reciprocal journey of patienthood and doctoring together.

CONNECTION WITH PATIENTS
Journey stories

Students generally express strong connections to their patients. Often they see themselves as fellow travelers, a theme that first emerged in some anatomy poems. A typical poem uses the metaphor of patient and student taking a journey together. In this analogy, the enemy is probably Alzheimer's disease, and ultimately death. The student is the reluctant hero enlisted by the patient to accompany her. For a time, the two companions will share hopes and goals: "Together we will/mesmerize the world." Knowing that her life is slipping away, the patient begs the student to truly know her, and help to preserve her memory (the formidable task entrusted to the hero): "Learn the song that is in my heart/And sing to me when I have forgotten." For the patient, the student's presence "has made all the difference." However, in this poem there is the recognition that the journey is finite, and that at some point the student and the patient must go their separate ways, the patient, in this case, towards dissolution of self and death, and the student towards the fulfillment of her mission, the goal of doctoring.

Walk in through the door By: Juliessa M. Pavon
Originally appeared in Panacea, *Summer 2005, p. 12*
University of Florida College of Medicine

The nursing home: I see you walk in through the door
An environment I have grown to know more.
Do not be afraid, for I travel with you.
Let us hope together, for our goals will become true.
Take me to the patio, lend me the sunshine of your smile.

The nursing home: I see you walk in through the door.
Talk to me, so that I may hear you.
Wave to me, so that I may see you.
Touch my hand, so that I may feel you.
You laughed with me when I needed to laugh.

The nursing home: I see you walk in through the door.
In this place, together we will mesmerize the world
the world that is truly my own world.
Learn the song that is in my heart
And sing to me when I have forgotten.

The nursing home: I see you walk in through the door.
And now that you have come
And now that I must go
Know that you came, and you sang to me
And that has made all the difference.

Another example of a classic journey employs a religious context. In this poem, the reluctant hero (the medical student) is faced with a treacherous journey through towering, snow-covered mountain peaks. Thirst and cold are the demons challenging the hero. However, the hero's comrade (her patient) is "cold and wounded." In this case, the student has the best and wisest guide – God the Father. Through his example, the heroic band (the medical team) lifts up the wounded companion. The "discomfort" of the student and the team is overcome by their closeness to each other and to the patient. The lessons learned are the incalculable value of warmth and love, compassion and devotion.

The Rocks of Ahwahnhee By: Co Truong
Originally appeared in Plexus, *2004, p. 28, UC Irvine School of Medicine*

Cutting through the great divide of the majestic Rocks of Ahwahnhee
I find solace and peace among the few chirping birds and trees
Snow-packed peaks lie to my west and
The drying thirst of demons lies to my east
It is no site to seek service and certainly not a time to give my fleece
But my comrade is cold and wounded
And I know of no other gift but my warmth
The Father is stronger and wiser and has seen it all before
He warms our beloved with fire and tells us we have a little more
Our comrade is lifted onto our leader's shoulder as we reach above the horizon
Lifting the pain and anguish from our team's disposition
We know our closeness overshadows our discomfort
For we are all doctors and patients and no matter where we are
Our lives are forever entwined and we must love each other
We will live our lives together whether in the mountains or the stars
I need no coat to understand the fear of my brother
But I will learn from my Father the meanings
Of compassion and devotion to my patients and my doctors.

Witnessing stories

The sense of connection that students feel in relation to patients is often manifested as a form of witnessing. For example, a poem about a pediatric cancer patient describes a moment of intimacy when the patient rakes the student's hair with her fingers. The student pretends to reciprocate, running her fingers above the child's bald head. Here, student and patient are united through a basic but deeply touching act of grooming. This is a witnessing of a bond between patient and student that adds a more profound dimension to the professional relationship as it is generally conceived.

A poem written in "skater" language to a child who has a shattered wrist as a result of a skateboarding accident is an impressive act of empathy because the writer enters so completely into the reality, values, and priorities of the patient. This student models how immersing oneself (at least temporarily) in the patient's wild and risky subculture can build trust and improve treatment. The poem is a kind of testimony to the value of empathy without judgment towards an alien way of life. In another poem, written from the patient's point of view, the narrator is initially suspicious of the "kid with a stethoscope." Although he yells at the hapless student, they eventually bond over their shared disgust with the VA hospital. In this case, the connection consists of their mutual rejection of the dominant hospital culture.

In a more complex poem, the student-poet explores the interdependency of student and patient through the metaphor of sand wearing on stone to describe the action of student on patient, and patient on student. Here the predominant idea is one of mutuality – that there is a necessary connection and bidirectional influence between patient and student. It is still common in the medical profession to see the physician as agent and the patient as acted-upon and influenced object, with effects traveling only in one direction, from doctor to patient. This and similar poems challenge this worldview in favor of a recognition of affinity. Here the emphasis is not on hierarchy and difference, but on underlying similarity: "we're the same . . . / from the same earth."

Sand on stone By: Andrew Sledd
UC Irvine, 2003

we're the same
but in different
circumstances

from the same earth
but worn differently
by the body of time

can we tell
the difference
between sand and stone?

Yet another poem recognizes that patients and student may never "unite" perfectly in their communication. However, the student knows how to listen, not only to her patients' words, but to all that their bodies have to tell her. She uses her stethoscope in "those silent, sacred seconds" to hear "their hearts giving life . . . and the rhythmic well of their breathing." The student is humbled by this deep connection with patients to listen to things that they themselves can't see or know. These poems are examples of witnessing the deep, although imperfect, connection to patients, the importance of listening on multiple levels to their words and their bodies, and the sacred trust implicit in the student–patient relationship.

IDENTIFICATION WITH THE PATIENT

Students sometimes felt not only connection but also an actual sense of identification with patients. In fact, in the first three years of training, students often identify more strongly with patients than with either residents or attending physicians. Despite the obvious differences between students and patients, these student-authors realized that they had a great deal in common with patients, including at the deepest level a shared humanity.

Witnessing stories

One poem highlights parallels between the experiences of the student and those of the patient in a very concrete way. They both wear clothes that don't fit (hospital gown, short white coat), people (nurses, residents / attending physicians) talk unintelligibly to them in a language that they cannot comprehend, and both are asked questions to which they only occasionally know the right answers. The shared experience is one of discomfort, confusion, misunderstanding, and ignorance.

In a poem previously quoted in full in Chapter 6 ("On hearing the news that you had lost your nerve"), the student observes surgery to reattach a body part. The student's simultaneous horror and attraction fill him with shame and indecision. He asks "What are you going to do now?" – a question that applies equally to him and to the patient. Both the medical student and the patient have "lost their nerve." In this poem, the student expresses identification with the patient – both have become victims, and for both the future is uncertain.

In another poem reflecting a similar reaction, the student participates in prepping for an amputation. Although the surgery is necessary, the student's gut "crumples" in sympathy with the grief in the patient's face. The poem captures well the necessary physical intimacy of surgery. Neither the patient nor the student can be fully anesthetized against the pain of the procedure. Both patient and student will be damaged by the operation, literally and figuratively. The patient loses a leg and is emotionally devastated, and the student ends up bruised by the weight of the amputated leg pressing into her hip. She suffers right along with the crying patient and her spouse.

When the Blood Fell Short of Her Toes By: Vinita Jain
Originally published in Body Language: Poems of the Medical Training Experience
edited by Neeta Jain, Dagan Coppock and Stephanie Brown Clark, 2006, p. 75
Reprinted with the permission of BOA Editions, Ltd. www.boaeditions.org

I would advise my mother the
same if the blood fell short of her
toes, the anesthesia doctor tells.

The useless leg, staining rouge, sits in
the crook of my arm. I brace it
the knee's right angle corners my
elbow in my hip
    which bruises later.

She cannot endure intubation
from the weakness in her beat
eyeliner straight-edged below
a cloudy clean cap. We search

at her ischium
with numbing sticks, rooting
to quiet the sharpness of nerves.

My gut crumples
    with her face.

I'll make you a nice wooden one
her husband catches their tears
on his big thumb.

From a somewhat different perspective, a student perceives parallels between herself and a patient who is dying of ovarian cancer. They are both "caught in the middle" – the patient between living and dying, and the student between layperson and physician, "both awkwardly trying to make sense of our new roles." In this case, the student seeks out common ground, focusing on their transitional status. Her poem emphasizes that both student and patient are at a critical juncture in their lives.

Another poem describes a series of patients with unappetizing diseases, no money, and a history of drug and alcohol abuse, setting up the expectation of an emotionally distancing rant. Then, however, the poem draws a parallel with the student's body also falling apart due to bad food, no sleep, no fresh air, and no exercise. The student concludes on an empathic note, "all patients just need / someone to care," and intimates that students would respond well to the same caring concern. The narrator makes a special effort to identify similarities between herself and these patients.

COUNTERTRANSFERENCE

In these poems, countertransference refers to the student's seeing similarities between a patient and a family member of the student. In most cases, these poems are examples of witnessing to this personal dimension that the relationship has assumed. However, when the countertransference is too personal, it can produce chaos stories as well.

Chaos stories

In one example, a student acknowledges a particularly acute level of emotional distress in response to a severely injured child because she is also a mother, and imagines her own child in similarly dire straits. Here, in this chaos narrative, countertransference interferes with the student's ability to care for her patient. In another poem, quoted in full in Chapter 11 ("He reminded me of my father"), a Latina student takes care of a Latino patient with smoking-related hemoptysis. The patient is "trusting, simple, solid / with rough hands stripped and broken by labor." He expresses gratitude for the student's care, but she feels guilty and helpless because she cannot solve his multiple insurance and medical problems. In this case, the student sees her father in a good, humble patient, but the bond established through shared language and culture leads to a shameful feeling that she has let him down.

Journey stories

In a poem similar in content to the chaos story by a medical student-mother described above, but with a different outcome, a student-parent with a young daughter is traumatized by encountering a similarly aged girl in the ER. She reflects that the situation was more painful for her than for other students on her team: "As a mother I took it harder." However, eventually she is able to move back and forth between her medical role and her family role, learning lessons from each. Looking at the little girl in the ER she appreciates her own daughter. She also recognizes how important it is to reassure the parents of the child that they are not to blame. In this case, the worlds of family and work are mutually enhancing. In this poem, ultimately the roles of mother and doctor complement and improve each other.

Witnessing stories

Witnessing poems that examine countertransference have a steadier emotional core that allows the student to move closer to the patient. When a student's grandmother dies, her death helps the student to realize that every time a patient dies he needs to ask "Whose Grandma (or mother, daughter, father, son) Is She?" By putting his grandmother's face on each patient, the student is able to personalize and humanize them. Here, countertransference is used to draw the student closer to the patient, so it serves as a kind of witnessing of connection. In a similar poem, a Hispanic male who is an HIV-positive drug addict with lung cancer tells the medical student that she reminds him of his daughter. Although the hospital staff find him obnoxious and rude, and doubt his pain level, to the student he becomes a mentor, teacher, and surrogate parent. The patient encourages and protects her, and tells her to be brave, not to worry too much, and to take care of herself. Here the parent-child identification enables the student to see past this patient's stigmatized status to accept him as a human being and appreciate his strengths. The student rejects the dominant view of the patient as difficult and manipulative, and instead sees him in a father figure role, welcoming him as her guide, mentor, and teacher.

Transcendence stories

Students are sometimes unexpectedly transformed by their encounters with patients. One such poem portrays a medical team that is technically competent but uncaring. They cannot empathize with the patient's plight. The student himself initially mirrors this indifference: "Why had he felt bereft of the art of healing?/Had it been a moment of self-test, an evolution within the physician's soul?" As the student remembers his own silence in the face of the patient's fear and pain, he knows that he could have done better. He realizes that even when the limitations of medicine are encountered, the physician can still reach out to the patient with empathy and compassion, "with heightened awareness/To heal the intangible pain." Spurred on by this recognition, the student returns to the patient's room, where she rouses and calls him "son." He writes "That word would ever echo through his soul." At that moment, the boundaries between student-physician and patient are blurred: "Both patient and physician had shifted gears/ To reveal a tender, vulnerable side/That would make whole the healer and the healed." This poem describes a moment of transcendent healing for both patient and student.

In another transformative countertransference encounter, a student finds herself alone with a very elderly dying patient who is calling for her mother. There is no mother there for the patient, and the student is at first resistant: "I am not her mother." However, in a final act of maternal nurturance, the student meets the patient's need: "I hold the downy head in my hands." The student moves from rejecting the possibility of acting as the dying patient's mother, to embracing this role and becoming profoundly altered as a result.

PATIENT AS TEACHER

Just as they did with cadavers, students frequently perceive patients as their most important teachers. These poems take various narrative forms. For example, in a chaos story with a humorous twist, a student on a pediatrics clerkship confronts a crying baby. At first he maintains that he is "without fear," but soon he begs the baby for help because "I have no clue/Of what to do." Occasionally, these poems have restitution components in that an important function seems to be to reduce the student's anxiety and restore a sense of normalcy to emotionally difficult situations. In one representative poem, a dying patient reassures the student with her humor, confidence, acceptance, and fulfillment. As the student says, "Ma'am, you make growing old look damn good." Although the poem witnesses to the patient's courage, it is primarily a restitution story, in that the patient's courage, acceptance, etc. serve to reassure the student in the face of suffering and death.

Journey stories

Patient-as-teacher stories can have a strong element of journey narrative, in that the patient becomes the wise guide who directs the student towards greater understanding and insight. In one such example, the student encounters a difficult yet perversely endearing patient. Initially the student is frustrated, but over time the patient teaches the student that the art of any profession consists of practice, nuance and passion. The student goes on a journey with the patient, who at first seems to be a demon/monster, but eventually conveys unique wisdom.

In a poem referred to previously with a similar journey flavor, the student expresses gratitude for the privilege of knowing a patient dying of ovarian cancer. She sees the patient as an example of grace, strength, and dignity in the face of death, and feels that she has changed for the better for having known this patient. From this patient the student has learned about friendship, the importance of touch, not postponing life, learning from losses, and working to accept all parts of life. The patient has willingly served as a guide and mentor, with the result that the student has become a wiser, more insightful physician.

Witnessing stories

In an example of witnessing to the power of the human spirit, an 80-year-old patient shares a painting that she has done of herself as a little girl. The student is awed by an act of imagination that creates "a phoenix" rising out of the ashes of decay, dementia, age, and time. What the student learns from this partly demented patient is that her essential humanity can still be found glimmering even in the darkest places.

In a poem about a VA patient with multiple medical problems, including bilateral below-the-knee amputations, the student thinks "there wasn't much left of him . . . or . . . /was there?" The more she gets to know him, the more she admires the patient's spirit, sense of humor, and friendliness. She revises her initial statement: "There wasn't much left of him physically/but boy was his presence/large." The poem concludes with an ironic yet respectful metaphor, recording the patient's courage and optimism in the face of imminent death. In the poet's view, this patient was able to maintain "one foot straddling life, the other death." The patient has become the student's teacher and inspiration, not only for practicing medicine, but for living life.

Mr. C. By: Maryam Bahadori
UC Irvine

Mr. C. weighed 80 pounds, measured 3 feet tall
all in all
After having bilateral BKA's
MI
PE
CHF
ESRD
Pneumonia
there wasn't much left of him . . . or . . .

was there?
Every morning I would see him
cruising the halls of the VA
in his motorized electric wheelchair
cap set at a rakish angle on his head
eyes twinkling with humor and delight
Mr. C. the VA resident social butterfly
There wasn't much left of him physically
but boy was his presence
large
I'll never forget his boyish smile
especially given his adverse circumstances . . .
One foot straddling life, the other death

The student can also witness the situation of the patient, while recognizing that she cannot fully penetrate the mystery of the patient's experience. In the following poem, through a series of questions, the narrator tries to understand the reality of a patient with severe multiple sclerosis. The student admires and respects the patient's courage, while simultaneously observing the continual deterioration of his quality of life and being aware of all that he has lost. At the end of the poem, the narrator still does not know how to feel towards the patient. Here, the student admits that she is not sure what lesson the patient is teaching her.

Joseph By: Karin Chen
UC Irvine, 2001

Hey Joseph, how are you today?
If you could talk, what would you say?
That you wished you didn't have MS?
That you could do more than just lie and rest?

Hey Joseph, I'm sorry about hurting you today.
Do you wish that I would just go away?
Do you express pain with a yawn?
But how would I even know the difference between a smile and a frown?

Hey Joseph, do you get hungry? Do you think of all the things you used to taste?
Now your sustenance is whittled down to a paste.
Fed lovingly by your mom, through a gastric tube.
You'll get some, even if you're not in the mood.

Hey Joseph, you have beautiful eyes.
Clear, dark pools in which 20 years of memories lie.
To think that 17 years have gone by
Since you last walked, talked, or cried
If only you could see your nephew
How much he looks like you.

Hey Joseph, I admire your courage, your perseverance.
And you have a family who has cared for you ever since . . .

Though your hands are gnarled and your toes curled
Your face is smooth and young.
Should I feel sorry for you or consider you a lucky one?

Transcendence stories

Finally, the student can experience transcendence as a consequence of contact with a patient. The poem "They sit at attention" starts with a tribute to the courage, compassion, and competence of residents. The second component of the poem focuses on the student's experience with a dying patient and his wife. The student is initially focused on the "numbers" of lab results that the patient is asking about. However, perhaps as a result of those numbers, she uses other numbers to place a call to his wife, who cannot come to the hospital because she has no transportation. Taking a spur-of-the-moment step outside her role of medical student, the narrator bridges the gap of distance between husband and wife by holding the telephone to the patient's ear. Here it is the love, vitality, and commitment of these two people that inspires the student. She enters the hospital that morning in dark and gloom, feeling ponderous and alone, but their love transforms her life from exhaustion and drudgery to hope, rejuvenation, and release. When she "surrenders" to the simultaneous joy and tragedy of the situation, "three birds escape." Perhaps these are the souls of patient, wife, and student, who have up until this point been bound by darkness, heaviness, and suffering, but are now set free, into the light.

They sit at attention By: Jennifer Kuangwei Yee
UC Irvine, 2000

I.

They sit at attention staring
At the drawn curtain which fails
To hide the sound of bad news
Being delivered.
And they listen, giving no illusion
Of privacy which was relinquished
Upon admission.
They throw open bed covers
Revealing every wrinkle, sore, scar
Touching each one without fear or shame
Gazes steady and strong, they ask
The hard questions and make
The hard decisions I ethically
And maybe avoidantly
Leave up to them.
They don't believe in magic, but
They talk openly of God.
And in the hospital room's dim light
I know they see much more than I
Standing outside shading my eyes
From all left stark and bare in daylight.

2.

It is dark when I arrive at the hospital
And it is dark when I am ready to leave
But I look at this piece of paper
Barely legible, that the patient has handed to me.

I think those are numbers written there, and
He thinks they could be wrong
But I find this home number in the chart
For this patient too sick to recall.

And I dial the number to find his wife's
Voice, warm, strong, and true
"Tell him my car's in the shop right now.
Will you tell him I love him too?"

I call her back at his bedside and
Holding the phone to his ear I see
Life in his eyes in cachectic face, and
Steady voice from tracheostomy.

For in this man who was called "rock,"
Poured much vitality
So much happiness in 20 years of marriage
That now carried him through physical tragedy.

And though that morning I arrived with
Footsteps alone and heavy
That evening I left rejuvenated
With hope, feeling free.

3.

When I surrendered
Window shutters flew open
And three birds escaped.

THE MEDICAL STUDENT AS ADVOCATE AND ALLY OF THE PATIENT
Chaos stories

Once in a while, an advocacy/alliance poem is a chaos narrative. In one such poem, the student starts out as the uninvolved intermediary between the patient and the medical team, which casually assesses, diagnoses, and treats the patient in a situation where there is much to alarm the patient but very little to be done to help them. The student parrots both the words and the detached tone of his superiors to the frightened patient. However, at the end of the poem, he suddenly realizes in panic that "I am they," and that he has an ethical responsibility towards this patient from whom, up until this point, he has remained so comfortably disengaged.

They By: Ted Clark
Originally appeared in Scope, Vol. XII, Spring 2005
Southern Illinois University School of Medicine

They don't really know the cause.
They think it might be in the genes.
The thing about that is . . ..
They recommend a yearly screen.

That test helps them decide
The way to treat your problem.
They say there is nothing that can be done
So why even bother.

It is a simple procedure, and
They have some evidence that shows.
They say it is about 10 percent
The way this disease goes.

I will check with them.
I will get back to you today.
Oh shit . . . I am they.

Restitution stories

Poems that express this theme tend most often to be restitution stories, in which the student assumes the mantle of champion of the patient. A typical poem describes a difficult patient. The medical team is frustrated, but persists in focusing solely on his physical problems, with the result that care is compromised. The medical student, however, takes the time to talk about the underlying issues. The patient's behavior improves and he becomes more pleasant. The student, normally relegated to a bit player in the medical drama, has become the hero. The student's sensitivity and perceptiveness not only improve the outlook for the patient, but also make the task of the team easier. The student is restored to a meaningful and valuable role.

In another restitution story that tackles the pervasive problem of language differences, a poem written in both English and Spanish describes the student realizing that she cannot fully understand what her patient is saying. Instead of continuing and risking misunderstanding (as many residents and attending physicians do), the student decides to get an interpreter. The patient is grateful to have a doctor who wants to know what he is saying. Here the student models appropriate behavior – the "right thing to do" – and is willing to go the extra mile, when others in the healthcare team might not. It is another reversal in which the student becomes the teacher and role model. The reward is the appreciation of the patient. The student, by choosing appropriate patient–doctor behavior, is able to avoid misunderstanding, do the right thing for the patient, and win the patient's gratitude.

A similar poem also addresses the problem of language and cultural differences, with a patient thinking one thing in Spanish (specifically doubts and fears), but saying something else (also in Spanish, but much more polite and acquiescent), and the medical student speaking mostly English interspersed with the few words of Spanish that she knows. At the beginning of the examination, the patient is nervous and embarrassed.

Thanks to the attention and concern of the medical student, by the end of the exam the patient recognizes that it is better to be embarrassed now than sick later. When the physician finishes, the medical student declines to do a pelvic examination, sensing that the patient has endured enough. The patient thinks gratefully, "Gracias a Dios" ("thanks be to God"). In this case, the student helps the patient to overcome her reservations about the examination, but is also sensitive to the patient's limitations and is able to successfully balance the patient's need for time and distance to absorb her encounter with the medical system with her own need to do a complete physical examination which she can then report to her attending physician. Again, this poem is a restitution story in which a difficult patient interaction is positively changed through the intervention of a skillful student.

Although in most of these poems the student compensates for the deficiencies of the doctor and/or healthcare team, occasionally the student fills other voids as well. In one restitution poem, the medical student is portrayed as trying to play with a pediatric patient who has been hospitalized due to lead poisoning and general neglect by an uncaring, indifferent mother. The student, not the parent, is the one who tries to bring a little happiness into the child's life. In this situation, the student becomes a surrogate parent, filling the gap between the child's reality and what she deserves.

Witnessing stories

Most of the poems in which students choose to ally themselves with the patient are closer to witnessing narratives. Sometimes the student is the only person who really empathizes with the patient. In one poem, an 11-year-old girl is diagnosed with an unresectable brain tumor. The doctors "see through" the patient and write about her in the medical chart, and argue about the diagnosis. Only the student worries about how the patient and her family will cope with the devastating news. And only the student wishes the little girl a happy birthday – the one "gesture" that she has available. The student is glad that it is not "too late." Of all the medical staff, she alone registers emotions of both grief and joy. The poem expresses the need to take action, which the student does. Witnessing the suffering of the patient compels a compassionate gesture.

In these witnessing poems, the student often identifies with the patient rather than with the medical team. In a previously cited poem, "Drifting Away" (quoted in full in Chapter 12), a resident makes a joke about a terminally ill patient. The student rejects this callous approach: "But I cannot see the humor in his [the patient's] pain." Feeling helpless, the student is nevertheless able to offer "a few kind words" – something that does not appear to have occurred to anyone else on the team. As in the previous poem, the student is the only member of the medical team who is portrayed as still being able to empathize with the patient's plight. This poem shows both the limitations of the team and the need to take some kind of action on behalf of the patient, even if it is only to offer consolation.

STUDENT/PATIENT/FAMILY RELATIONSHIPS

Students generally viewed the student–patient relationship as a dyadic one. It was only rarely that family members surfaced as the "ghost" in the room. As might be expected, students thought about family members most often in pediatric situations, where the parent is an integral part of the interaction. Student poetry also incorporated family members in death-bed scenes. It is worth noting that in both of these situations, the patient is often not fully competent as a decision maker, and input from significant others is necessary. Of the poems reviewed, only one, written by a future family physician, addressed the inevitability of the effects of significant illness extending to the family as well. This author concluded that, once the physician becomes concerned with "what lies beneath" the surface of medicine, "To treat a person / Is to treat a family."

Chaos stories

When students consider the complexity of their sometimes conflicting obligations and commitments to patients and their families, occasionally they are overwhelmed and write chaos stories. A poem about an anorexic adolescent portrays the relationship between patient, parent, and medical student as one of "dueling chief complaints." The girl thinks she is too fat, the mother knows that the girl is too thin, and the student is afraid that the explanation will be a medical "zebra" she has not yet imagined. Through metaphors of broken china and spider webs, the author communicates a sense of fragmentation and helplessness, and the inability of these people to work together to save the patient. This poem witnesses to the different perspectives of the adolescent patient, her mother, and the medical student, as well as the vulnerability and at-risk status of the patient.

Dueling chief complaints By: Mary Alice Kalpakian
Originally appeared in Plexus, 2001, p. 29, UC Irvine School of Medicine

Some of my patients tell me they want to grow up to be firemen.
Some want to be doctors.
Some want to grow up to become purple dinosaurs.
Not Angela.
Angela wants to grow up to look like the girls
    on the cover of Seventeen magazine.
Her mother tells me her chief complaint is that her daughter looks too much
    like those girls already.
Angela's chief complaint is that she does not look enough like them.

While Angela continues with her obsession to weigh less than air
I continue with my obsession – searching for zebras.
I pray that I can find some rare malabsorption disorder that could explain
    her cachectic state, but I can't.
Angela is a beautiful, smart young girl, who is unraveling
caught in the spider web of Madison Avenue's images
yearning to accomplish the unaccomplishable goal of perfection.
She's like a piece of fine china, teetering at the edge of a table, ready to
    fall.
I wish I could put her back together again
with a medicine or a band-aid or a purple dinosaur
    but I can't.
I feel incredibly powerless.

(Anti-)Restitution stories

There is also occasional hostility expressed towards family members, particularly parents of pediatric patients. In one such poem, the medical student encounters an arrogant parent. The poem is structured in part as a dialogue between the child patient, his overbearing mother, and the increasingly frustrated medical student. The mother is portrayed as overly controlling and protective. The student is polite, but decides that "one parent at a time he will rid the clinic of arrogant parents." In another poem, the author walks into a pediatric examination room, and as soon as she sees the mother she thinks pejoratively "Geez, I hope this won't be a mess." These poems are both examples of restitution in absentia. The student/doctor is the savior, the pediatric patient is the victim, and the parent is the obstacle to "fixing" the problem.

In a typical restitution poem, the student first holds her dying patient's hand, and then grasps the husband's hand as well. When at last she leaves, the husband thanks her "for helping [the patient] to heaven today." The student feels that these words "broke forth from within his soul." Here the student has an essential role in mediating between the dying and the living. The poem is a restitution story, in which the need for this connection is recognized and she is the only person available to provide it.

Witnessing stories

In a poem that is closer to witnessing than (anti-)restitution, a dialogue occurs between a mother who recounts her desperate efforts first to save her pregnancy and then to nurture her severely delayed infant, and the medical team's grim chorus that the child needs specialist help and "needs more than affection." The mother is portrayed ambiguously. On the one hand she is passionately dedicated to her child, while on the other she rejects the physicians' diagnosis and offers of help. This is a more nuanced view that witnesses to the difficulty in bridging the different perspectives of the mother and the healthcare team.

In another poem, a young man is brought to the ER dead on arrival as a result of a heroin overdose. When the family arrives, they are callous and cold, dismissing the deceased as a worthless junkie. However, when the student peers into the rapidly fading eyes of the patient, she glimpses his humanity, and at least in imagination, "the mire of pathways/along which your soul danced in salutary leaps/at one time/with meaning, at fearless speed." Here the student chooses solidarity with the discarded patient as a way to redeem him against the judgment of family members.

Transcendence stories

In one remarkable poem, the medical student is poised between the medical team treating a comatose near-drowning pediatric patient, and the parents who continue to hope for the child's recovery. Initially the student identifies with the doctors ("We look on in sadness"), whose knowledge of the grim prognosis trumps any hope they might have for the child. The team is simply waiting for the parents to "realize the truth . . . begin to grieve" (i.e. conform to the doctors' view of reality). However, at this point a moment of transformation occurs: "But when I take a moment to really look at you/To see you as a little boy/And not a near-drowning victim/I begin to see what your parents see." An epiphanic shift has occurred for this student, and she begins to see the patient through the parents' eyes. She retains her cognitive knowledge that the child "will never wake up," but she learns that one "can never give up hope." By the conclusion of the poem, she has joined with the parents: "And I am waiting for your parents to receive their miracle." This poem is an expression of solidarity with the parents, a choice of faith in the face of what reason dictates. Although the poem has elements of journey, and also witnesses the suffering of the parents, it is primarily about transformation. The student chooses a position of faith over (or at least in addition to) science. She has been transformed by opening to the suffering of the family.

EMOTIONAL CARING AND CONNECTION

Obviously connection and bonding with patients, as well as patient advocacy, ideally require a high level of emotional openness. Some students worry that caring and compassion will drain them emotionally as well as making them ineffectual providers. However, the embracing of patients emotionally can also be celebratory and transformational.

Chaos stories

Students want to be caring, but they are afraid of the emotional price that they will pay. Many of the poems that examine this theme tell chaos stories. Caring is perceived as overwhelming and dangerous. Relaxing the boundary between patient and student can be threatening. One student worries that she is bleeding compassion, and the image of blood running from her wrists intimates that in "opening" herself to the suffering of others she is flirting with suicide. Various clinical scenarios, presented by the emotionally distant attending physician, provoke her empathy and heartbreak. She considers trying to "heal" herself of this "loss," and is afraid that she will either be "consumed by grief" or end up "an empty shell."

Bleeding By: Sayeh Beheshti
Originally appeared in Plexus, *2002, pp. 12–13, UC Irvine School of Medicine*

If I have compassion running in my blood
Then I must have cut my wrist.

Lecture Slide Show

Here's one of a woman who went into cardiac arrest during labor
    The surgical interventions are described
    "Unfortunately she woke up without a brain"
        I hear the doctor say
    I think of the mother who never lived to see her child
    I think of the child knowing she lives at the price of her mother's death

No time to think of those
    We're on the next slide

I see a drop leave my punctured wrist
    will I miss it?

Next we have the boy with the cut trachea
    He was fifteen
    The slide must be showing something about the surgery
    But I can't take my eyes off his face

I see myself giving his parents the news
"I'm sorry" I say
    to the woman who cradled him and sang him lullabies
"we did everything we could" I say
    to the man who stayed up at his fever bed all night
I put on my happy face
    just in time for dinner with my own child

I must focus on the next slide

Another drop leaves me
    did I need that?

Next comes the young man who jumped off a bridge
    broken bones everywhere
    yet all fixed up and sent home in a week
    Why did he jump off the bridge?
        I wonder

No time, next slide

Drip, drop
    will anything in my marrow replace that?

Anatomy lab

This one has her glitter nail polish
This one wasted away to nothing
That one looks too young and in good shape
    Cancer
This woman has breast implants
    She died on July 4th I hear
    I think of the bitter Independence Day holiday
        For her family
    In the same breath I decide
        To cut her up and see the implants

Another drop hits the floor
    I pretend not to notice

Should I attempt to heal this puncture?
    If I do I will be consumed by grief
    If I don't I will end up an empty shell
        Why did she ever choose to become a doctor
    I hear them say

I can't think of that now
There are exams, you know
I don't see the next drop
    As it trickles out over my wrist
    Courses down my thumb
And it is gone.

In a similar chaos poem, the narrator wonders whether she would have chosen this profession "if I knew I would care so much I would bleed." She tries to "be indifferent", because caring is too painful. However, indifference is impossible to achieve when she sees the suffering of her patients. "But I must remain indifferent or I will implode again." She fears that her emotional connection to her patients is harming her, worrying more about her patients than they seem to worry about themselves. She complains that "they didn't teach me in medical school how not to care too much." At the end of the poem, there is still no solution to how to solve the dilemma of caring without being destroyed by that caring.

In a humorous poem that starts out as restitution but devolves into chaos, a student catches a miserable flu from a pediatric patient. When the patient is sick, the student treats the condition as routine and easily remedied. The student labels the child as "fussy . . . uncooperative," a "bad" patient. When the student experiences the same illness, she resonates emotionally with the plight of the patient, and is similarly grumpy and belligerent. In misery, she angrily rejects the facile advice which, only a few days ago, she bestowed on her young patient.

Empathy By: Jenny Murase
Originally appeared in Plexus, 2003, p. 29, UC Irvine School of Medicine

Fever, cough, and a rash
As I enter legs do thrash.
"Please hold still. Please be quiet."
Crying, screaming, jaws defiant.
Swollen glands, painful ears.
Stuffy nose, tears and tears.
"Child fussy, uncooperative.
But no distress and non-toxic.
It's nothing serious. Just a bug!
Have some soup and use this drug!"

First my throat – it's just a scratch.
Nothing a night's rest won't patch.
Tonsils form a soft white coat.
Burning down my tender throat.
Fevers come, and then return.
Legs do ache and eyes do burn.
It's nothing serious. Just a bug.
I'll have some soup and use this drug.

Fevers follow one another.
Chills and heat attack the other.
A raging battle starts inside
My body along just for the ride.
How much I want a hospital stay!
Get me closer to D-day!!

OH, WHEN WILL MY FEVERS BREAK?!!
WHEN WILL MY LEGS NOT ACHE?!!!

WHEN WILL MY THROAT NOT BURN?!!!!
WHEN WILL MY LIFE RETURN?!!!!!!!!!
NOTHING SERIOUS?! JUST A BUG!?!
YOU HAVE SOME SOUP AND USE THAT DRUG!!

Transcendence stories

Emotional connection has the potential to uplift and transform students. In the following poem, a student uses a simile, and the refrain of "drip, drip, drip," to tell a patient how her essence is suffusing the student: "Like rain seeping through the roof that houses my soul/Your essence is seeping through." The student, perhaps unwillingly, sees her last defenses crumbling: "The tiny bucket of my last defense is overflowing." The student's mind is "flooded" with thoughts of the patient: "I am drowning from the inside out/Your pain is now my pain, because we are now one and the same . . . /an epiphany for the humane." The student has attempted to put up barriers against connection, but in vain. She feels the suffering of her patient and realizes that they are inevitably joined. The reference to an "epiphany for the humane" suggests how emotional connection can transform the student. In "failing to distance," she has experienced a moment of grace.

Drip, drip, drip By: Heidi Wen Chen
UC Irvine

Learning how to detach:
failing to distance myself emotionally from a patient's suffering

Drip, drip, drip
Drip, drip, drip
Like rain seeping through the roof that houses my soul
Your essence is seeping through
A smile here, your sound there
Thoughts of you are storming in the confines of my atmosphere
Drip, drip, drip
Drip, drip, drip
The tiny bucket of my last defense is overflowing
Once again thoughts of you are flooding my mind.
I am drowning from the inside out.
Your pain is now my pain, because we are now one and the same . . .
an epiphany for the humane.

SUMMARY

The poetry of medical students often creates, imagines and/or records their relationships with patients. If anything, the students represented in these poems threw themselves even more wholeheartedly into relationships with patients than the literature would suggest. They ardently pursued connection with patients, and far from emphasizing differences between themselves and their patients, they were eager to acknowledge the similarities, correspondence, and parallels in their experiences. As the literature does indicate, after risking such intense bonds, students wrestled with how to manage their emotional engagement so that it would not overwhelm them. The literature suggests that students are aware of the privilege of being entrusted with the intimate details of other people's lives, and this attitude of respect and appreciation is also reflected in their poetry. Both student poetry and the scholarly literature confirm that students try hard not to see their patients reductively as diagnoses.

These poems show a wide range of narrative approaches to the sometimes surprising interconnection between medical students and their patients, most often relying on journey and witnessing. Sometimes these connections take the form of identification, in which students actually see themselves in their patients. Sometimes countertransference is involved, and students perceive patients as wise parents, guides, allies, advocates, or teachers. At other times students see themselves as the ally and advocate of patients, often telling restitution stories that cast them in a heroic role. Although emotional connection sometimes frightened students, they often allowed themselves to be touched by their patients and to develop relationships of emotional intimacy. Writing about patients was the category that yielded the largest number of transcendent poems. Students often understood doctoring in a radically different way as a result of opening themselves emotionally to patients.

REFERENCES

1 Dyrbye LN, Harris I, Rohren CH. Early clinical experiences from students' perspectives: a qualitative study of narratives. *Academic Medicine* 2007; **82**: 979–88.

2 Fischer MA, Harrell HE, Haley HL, *et al.* Between two worlds: a multi-institutional qualitative analysis of students' reflections on joining the medical profession. *Journal of General Internal Medicine* 2008; **23**: 958–63.

3 Pitkälä KH, Mäntyranta T. Feelings related to first patient experiences in medical school. A qualitative study on students' personal portfolios. *Patient Education and Counselling* 2004; **54**: 171–7.

4 Beca I JP, Browne L F, Repetto LP, *et al.* [Medical student–patient relationship: the students' perspective] *Revista Medica de Chile* 2007; **135**: 1503–9.

5 Papadimos TJ. Voltaire's Candide, medical students, and mentoring. *Philosophy, Ethics, and Humanities in Medicine* 2008; **2**: 13.

6 Newton BW, Barber L, Clardy J, *et al.* Is there hardening of the heart during medical school? *Academic Medicine* 2008; **83**: 244–9.

7 Chen D, Lew R, Hershman W, Orlander J. A cross-sectional measurement of medical student empathy. *Journal of General Internal Medicine* 2007; **22**: 1434–8.

8 Hojat M, Mangione S, Nasca TJ, *et al.* An empirical study of decline in empathy in medical school. *Medical Education* 2004; **38**: 934–41.

9 Stratton TD, Saunders JA, Elam CL. Changes in medical students' emotional intelligence: an exploratory study. *Teaching and Learning in Medicine* 2008; **20**: 279–84.

10 Nogueira-Martins MC, Nogueira-Martins LA, Turato ER. Medical students' perceptions of their learning about the doctor–patient relationship: a qualitative study. *Medical Education* 2006; **40**: 322–8.

11 Rucker L, Shapiro J. Becoming a physician: students' creative projects in a third-year IM clerkship. *Academic Medicine* 2003; **78**: 391–7.

12 Good BJ, Good MJD. "Fiction" and "Historicity" in doctors' stories: social and narrative dimensions of learning medicine. In: Mattingly C, Garro LC (eds). *Narrative and the Cultural Construction of Illness and Healing*. Berkeley, CA: University of California Press; 2000. pp. 50–69.

13 Torppa MA, Makkonen E, Mårtenson C, Pitkälä KH. A qualitative analysis of student Balint

groups in medical education: contexts and triggers of case presentations and discussion themes. *Patient Education and Counselling* 2008; **72**: 5–11.

14 Wear D, Aultman JM. The limits of narrative: medical student resistance to confronting inequality and oppression in literature and beyond. *Medical Education* 2005; **59**: 1056–65.

15 Bleakley A, Bligh J. Students learning from patients: let's get real in medical education. *Advances in Health Sciences Education: Theory and Practice* 2008; **13**: 89–107.

10 If They Don't Care, Why Should I? Student–Patient Relationships – Part 2

Connection with patients is complex, and there is a more troubling, darker side to interactions and involvement with patients. Students struggle with a lack of connection when they feel that they should be connected. Sometimes they feel trapped by their patients, and are both resentful of all they sacrifice and guilty about this reaction. At times they attempt to detach emotionally from patients, due to fear of becoming overwhelmed by their own feelings, as a self-protective strategy. Many also express the perception that detachment is the appropriate professional attitude that they should learn to cultivate. Nevertheless, most of the students continue to feel ambivalent or even skeptical about the value of emotional disconnection. Patients may also be threatening to students, because there is the omnipresent possibility of making a mistake that could harm the patient. Lastly, students must come to terms with the fact that they do not have complete control over patients, and must accept that patients sometimes have different perspectives and priorities to their own.

laughter, the best medicine By: Karen WH Chiu
UC Irvine

buried beneath a mountain of paper sheets
evals, logsheets, and H & P's
can't study 'cuz my brain is fried
can't schedule a hospice meeting 'cuz the patient died

can't take any more fungal feet
fifteen minutes, look at the insurance sheet
complaint list a mile long
now the HMOs just can't be wrong?

some patients just wanna hug
some patients say "gimme a drug!"
poor patients can't afford medication
maybe we all need a vacation

naw, doc, course I don't smoke!
I don't drink, I'm much too broke
no IV drugs here on the West coast
drug of choice is Starbucks' roast

my hands are cracked 'n' peelin'
my neck's got this stiff feelin'
I don't know much, but that's okay 'cuz
Medline's available night or day

my nice shoes and blistered feet
losing weight, no time to eat
drug reps just wanna do lunch
carry power bars for somethin' to munch

from stayin' indoors, my skin's too pale
it's sunny outside, but I don't wanna fail
hang my white coat back on the rack
I want my Birkenstocks and my weekends back

reality hits, medicine's not fair
all patients just need someone to care
I keep holdin' my head up and they'll all see
I'll survive 'cuz P = MD

Students often inject humor into their poetry to help them to cope, as well as to give them perspective. Karen Chiu's poem is a typical poem in this regard. Its light-hearted tone balances aggravation with warmth. It commences as a characteristic medical student lament – overworked, exhausted – and the use of lower-case letters suggests that the student does not even have time to capitalize her reflections. She is losing weight because she has no time to eat, her feet are blistered by running from patient to patient, her hands are cracked from constant washing, and her neck is stiff from craning over patients. Like the cohort of medical students in Chapter 4, she hasn't seen the light of day in weeks because all her free time is spent studying. Like many of the students whose poems we read in Chapter 5, she worries about her lack of knowledge. Like many of the student authors in Chapter 4, she just wants her normal life back. The jocular tone continues even in the face of the death of a patient, where the emphasis remains on the student's perpetual state of being behind – by the time she starts thinking about arranging a hospice visit, her patient has passed away!

The poem openly acknowledges the revulsion ("fungal feet") and implied pulling away ("can't stand") that some patients inspire in their doctors, as well as the frustration with patients who steadfastly deny obvious truths (those who will not admit their smoking, drinking, or drug use to their doctor). The narrator also notes the maddening systemic imperfections that beset the healthcare system, such as HMOs that require brief visits even for multiple, complex medical conditions, uninsured indigent patients who are denied care, and pharmaceutical representatives who have better access to the student-physician than these patients.

The final stanza provides the healing summary, hints of which we have seen throughout the earlier parts of the poem. "Medicine's not fair" – it's not fair for medical students, and it's not fair for their patients either. As the student-poet suggested in stanza 3, "maybe we all need a vacation." It is not too much of a stretch of imagination to speculate that the "all" in this line refers not only to the student and her peers, who need a break from the stresses of training, but also to the patients who need a holiday from illness, from hospitals, and in some cases from the stresses of their lives. Despite the frustrations and challenges, this student knows that all patients need "a hug" and "someone to care." That is her job, and she is ready for it, notwithstanding impending collapse, hassles, stress and strain. She is ready because, in the end she knows that "P = MD" – that is, patient equals doctor. Her patients are not the source of her problems, they are not her enemies. They are, in fact, her, and she and they are ultimately indivisible.

SEPARATION BETWEEN STUDENT AND PATIENT
Chaos stories

The dilemmas posed by trying to navigate the student–patient relationship can sometimes overwhelm the student. In one poem, the student struggles with fear that inhibits her connection with her patient. A patient is diagnosed with cancer, but the student is only able to tell her that she will have surgery the following day – she is unable to divulge the prognosis, or the big picture. The student whispers reassurance, but doesn't believe it: "How can I comfort your crumbling body?" In this chaos story, the student is unable to cope with the patient's diagnosis of cancer.

Witnessing stories

In most of these poems, however, students tend to adopt a position of witnessing, only now they bear witness to incomplete or transitory connection, or the inevitable separation between student and patient. For example, one student's poem uses the metaphor of students and patients as "neighbors," yet argues that each is really an island. Like the tides, patients go in and out, wax and wane. This poem concludes that connection is impossible – the other will always remain an island, and will always remain unknowable. The poem explores the reality that connection is temporary and also involves the ultimate separation that always exists between self and others.

In another poem, the role of student-doctor separates the author from her patient. At first the patient thinks that the student is a nurse, and jokes and laughs with her. When she performs a good blood draw, he thanks her and calls her "'kid." However, when he realizes that she is a student-doctor confronting him with frightening and painful treatment options – no longer a partner or playmate, but a dispassionate bearer of bad news – the patient withdraws into passivity and distance: "Whatever you say, Doc." The student is on one side of the chasm between the well and the sick – between those with the power to heal and those who can only pray for healing – and the patient is on the other. As in the previous poem, this poem witnesses the separation between self and patients that can arise when illness, suffering, risk, and fear intervene.

Patient Relationships   By: Britta Moilanen
Originally appeared in Plexus, *2000, p. 16, UC Irvine School of Medicine*

When we admitted you, you thought I was a nurse.
You told me to find a good-looking doctor and settle down.
You asked why I wasn't out dancing on a Saturday night
And I laughed, and said:
Those are good ideas.

When I woke you in the morning to listen to your lungs
You growled at me and hid under the blankets and refused to cooperate.
And I thought of rounding with the attending,
And the inevitable questions,
And what if, under the hot lights, I am not really sure . . .
So I pulled back your blankets, woke you up,

Insisted.

When I drew your blood with just one stick
And found another blanket to keep you warm . . .
When I made sure you got the right meds, you said:
Thanks, kid.
And I smiled.

But when I told you you needed a dangerous surgery
When I said:
This treatment might help, but it will hurt.
When I said:
These are the options, what would you like to do?
You said:
Whatever you say, Doc.

And I felt the space open up between us.

In a humorous poem that witnesses to other types of separation, the student explores
the different priorities of students and patients. Patients feel that the hospital is like hell,
and they cannot wait to escape from the incessant poking and prodding of medical
students. Students pray to get through their histories and physical examinations without
embarrassing themselves. In another poem, the medical student talks to a psychiatric
patient. The patient refuses help, but begs the student to understand. The student is
forced to confess, "I don't think I do [understand]", and the patient replies, "Neither
do I." In this case, the student engages in witnessing of shared chaos with the psychiatric
patient.

DETACHMENT
Witnessing stories

Student poetry mostly adopts a position of witnessing to growing emotional distancing with clear-sighted concern. As we saw in Chapter 4, the dissection experience in
anatomy leads many students to reflect on emotional detachment. As students enter
their clinical years, their preoccupation with detachment persists. In one poem, a student
cultivates objectivity. She observes and performs several gruesome procedures and witnesses various appalling medical conditions. After each encounter, she prides herself on
the fact that she does "not flinch," and sees each lack of emotional response as evidence
of her moving closer to her goal of becoming a physician. However, she pays the ultimate price in not being able to cry at the death of an elderly patient, or share in the grief
of his wife. The composure that she has so carefully cultivated leaves her feeling empty
and disconnected, unable to relate to her patients.

One student observes that doctors treat patients and help them to survive, but that
patients want more: "They need to see a friend in us, an advisor." This student perceives
her medical education as teaching ". . . us the harshness in advance/So when we face
this realm [of patient suffering], we would be stiffer." The point here seems to be that
patients want care, but the educational system teaches only harshness. Thus physicians
are disadvantaged. They are trained to identify, treat, and attempt to defeat the cause of
disease, "But they [the patients] want more, they always will/They need support, instead

we offer them a pill." In this poem, a mechanistic, technical approach to patient care is portrayed as deficient and as ultimately failing the patient's hopes and expectations. This poem is witnessing to the teaching of harshness, detachment, and the consequent disappointment of the patient's hopes.

Another student is shocked when she realizes that although the bad news she delivers transforms the patient forever, she herself cannot feel its sting and hurt. She witnesses the effect on the patient in the collapse of her shoulders, the pain that pools around her eyes, her trembling hands, and the beating of her heart. Yet when she says goodbye, she feels "numb, nothingness," even though this act of saying goodbye is both literal, in that the student is leaving the room, and a farewell to a dying patient whom she will not see again.

Another student, in the previously quoted poem "Four Years" (*see* Chapter 5), is reflecting back on her four years of medical education, and realizes that what she has learned is that her own tears are ". . . unacceptable . . . a sign of my own / weakness and mortality." Confronting the family of a patient who has just died, she feels that her role must be to "be unbreakable / for this broken family." In this case, the expression of feelings must be suppressed and a veneer of strength and resilience superimposed.

In a similar poem, a student is separated from her patients by her latex gloves that make it difficult to feel, both literally and metaphorically. She searches unsuccessfully for "sensation sufficient for poetry" – the depth of feeling that would justify a poem. The narrator is also cut off from family, friends, and normal social intercourse, and can only observe, rather than participate in, the ordinariness of life. "Tentacles" from the outside world tentatively reach out to her, but she is trapped "Inside" the hospital, her gloves, and medicine itself.

Inside By: Meghann Kaiser
UC Irvine, 2003

Searching for sensation sufficient for poetry
In the rear left-hand corner of a near-abandoned cafeteria
Scented tangibly of seafoam misty aerosol
Flaccid southwestern decor
And looming hours past my break.
The two ladies sitting catty corner across from me
Immerse themselves in caffeine and candor
And I in them.

Patients, family, friends, feelers from the outside world
Wriggle into my 33-hour shift
In through doors and backdoors
In through over-taxed admissions desks
And glassy ER portholes whirring sullenly shut
To trap each tentative tentacle with
Insensitive mechanism.
Hospital gowned.
Latex bound
My gloves catch and snap over fascinated fingertips
When I lean forward to touch them.

MISTAKES WITH PATIENTS
Witnessing stories

Students rarely talk about mistakes, or even the possibility of making mistakes, in their poetry. However, when they consider this topic, they most commonly do so in the form of witnessing. Chaos stories may not be prevalent because, at this level of training, the types of mistakes that students can make rarely place the patient at any physical risk. Most of the mistakes that they record are either failures of sensitivity and caring or hypothetical fears. By making a record of these events, the students seem to attest to the seriousness of these mistakes, and their commitment not to "forget" them. For example, one poem apologizes in advance to an unknown, still unencountered patient for an error he has not yet committed. The student recognizes with resignation that although his intention is to help, making mistakes is inevitable. The poem seems to be an attempt to integrate and accept this fallibility, and bears witness to the prospect of future fallibility.

In another poem, the student works up a patient for all sorts of rare and complicated disorders. Only later does the student realize that the source of the patient's "bleeding" should have been obvious – it stemmed from the patient's broken heart. Here the student chastises himself for focusing on physical explanations when he should have considered the suffering of the whole person. Another student talks to a homeless patient with alcohol and drug addiction. He doubts the patient's protestations that he wants to reform and make a new start. Initially the "Skeptic" in the student is disillusioned and disgusted. Then he realizes that the patient is sincere, insightful and motivated to maintain sobriety, resist temptation, and take control of his life. The student feels embarrassed – he realizes that he made a snap judgment based on cursory interpretations – and convicts himself of the mistake of not looking deeply enough into the heart and soul of his patient.

In another poem the student is having a good day – pleasant patients and lots of laughs. Then she encounters a stressed, tense man with a "full calendar" in the next exam room, who says morosely "This calendar will be the death of me." The student responds with a jocular remark, thinking that the man is joking. But he responds, "No, this is not funny at all/My wife is dying of breast cancer/My life is doctors and death." Here the student reflects that her mistaken assumptions led her to make a hurtful and insensitive remark.

In another previously cited poem, "Manger" (*see* Chapter 8), an obese patient is badly treated by the resident and medical team. The student proceeds to ask forgiveness of the patient for the entire medical team, including herself. The student's own culpability lies in the fact that the patient's "hungry heart/[is] Silently chewing its way/across your Chest." What has fascinated the medical student is not the patient's suffering but the X-ray image of this defective organ. The poem is an example of bearing witness to the insensitive, analytic medical gaze of the team and the student.

A final example is a poem titled "Unasked Questions," which explores the student's growing awareness that "to get an answer, I must first ask." The student admits to himself that he has been afraid to ask his patients the hard questions. He does a daily mini-mental status examination on a psychiatric patient, but never dares to ask him if he knows who he is. He is careful not to ask a deteriorating post-surgical patient if he knows that he is dying. Here the student faults himself for a lack of moral courage.

LIMITATIONS OF PATIENTS/LIMITED CONTROL OF PATIENTS

One of the most troubling aspects of students' evolving role with patients is their realization that, as physicians, they have only limited "control" over their patients' adherence to medical advice and lifestyle decisions. Most often this awareness surfaces when they are attempting to "enforce" lifestyle recommendations. Emotions of frustration and resentment sometimes arise in students when they come face to face with the limits of their influence and what some students label as patients' disinterest in their own healthcare.

(Anti-)Restitution stories

Blaming patients is a variation on the restitution story, in which patients who refuse to cooperate in their own restitution deserve the consequences of their illness and are not worthy of the student-physician's attention. Restitution (cure of the patient) is impeded by the patient's unreasonable demands, noncompliance, and generally difficult attitude. In a typical poem, a patient demands antibiotics for a "nose itch." The student cannot convince the patient that the medication will be ineffective for her complaint. In another, more serious poem, the student blames the patient for his alcoholism. He outlines the treatment plan in cynical, jaded terms, knowing that the patient will continue drinking. He concludes by saying, "Thus goes the tale of another alcoholic sucker." In this case, restitution (cure of the alcoholic patient) is made impossible by the patient's own addiction and unwillingness to change.

One student-physician observes, somewhat grudgingly, that some patients cannot or will not comply with his advice, no matter what he does. The student cannot coerce or force them, if the patients "won't listen" – a phrase that locates the locus of blame squarely with the patient. Briefly, the narrator wonders whether greater knowledge on his part would increase his persuasiveness, only to decide that "maybe they would believe me/but maybe they wouldn't." Ultimately, he concludes that although he can try his best, he may never know whether he has had an impact. This poem expresses both feelings of chaos at the inability of the student to control patient outcomes, and resentment that patients will not do as they are told, even for their own benefit.

Some people can By: Andrew Sledd
UC Irvine, 2003

some people can't
some people won't
others never will

I can't make them
I can't tell them
if they won't listen

I may never know
what's really wrong

if I could convince them
that I knew something
maybe they would believe me
but maybe they wouldn't

all I can do is try
and let them go, wondering if I've
ever made an impression.

In a somewhat bitter poem, the student-author actively blames patients for not getting better. He expresses hostility towards and frustration with patients who do not care about their own health, who are noncompliant with their treatment regimens, or who think that they know more than the student. In exasperation, he wonders why they bother to come back, since they are obviously not serious about improving their condition. The annoyed student threatens to withdraw his caring and his care unless the patients take their fair share of responsibility.

Don't Come to Me for Help By: Micheal Chao
UC Irvine

Diabetes, COPD, HF, renal failure
What awaits me behind the next door?
What chronic disease is next in line to control, but not cure?

Another non-compliant patient?
Another patient who doesn't care?
Or is it another who cares too much
And thinks he/she knows more than me?

Frustration builds and turns to ambivalence
What do I care?
Why should I care if the patient doesn't?
All I can do is give my professional opinion
But why do they keep coming back
SSDD – same shit, different day?

No change in symptoms, gee I wonder why
Maybe if you listened and tried you'd feel better

I/We can only do so much
Patients need to learn to care for themselves
If they can't
Don't come to me for help.

Poems that express this level of exasperation are rare, but this poem does accurately reflect a situational anger that many students experience with patients who they perceive as ungrateful or indifferent. For example, an exhausted medical student speaks harshly to the patient ("Just let me get through you"), suggesting that the patient is an obstacle to his survival. In the poem "After all we've done for you" (quoted in full in Chapter 12), the student blames the patient, who persists in dying, as if to spite the best efforts of the team to save his life. Yet another student compares the human body to a road system, and rather patronizingly cautions patients to "keep your streets clean," implying that otherwise chaos and messy traffic accidents lie ahead. In this restitution poem, good health is the responsibility of the patient, otherwise they bring accidents and chaos on themselves.

Journey stories

In a poem representing a journey from patient condemnation to acceptance, an alcoholic patient has his abdomen drained of fluid. The student is initially appalled, and in a series of derogatory and repellant images compares the patient to a termite queen, Jabba the Hut, and a pregnant woman. The student admits that it is just as likely that he is attempting to land an emotional punch as to make an "awkward connection" when he tells the patient that he knows he consumes vast quantities of alcohol no longer to get drunk, but simply to keep the delirium tremens at bay. Yet when the patient is "delivered" of his burden, the student realizes that the procedure, while alleviating discomfort, is ultimately futile in terms of addressing the underlying disease process, and his blame of the patient fades away. The expert medical team has successfully fulfilled its task, temporarily vanquishing the demon of alcoholism, but the truly wise guide is the patient, whose politeness, gratitude, and honesty teach the student an important lesson about the limits of medicine and the pitfalls of easy judgment.

Dark Star By: Brian McMichael
Originally appeared in Plexus, 2005, *p. 15, UC Irvine School of Medicine*

The unimaginable mass in his abdomen
Pushes mercilessly through his back
Passes instantly through the hospital bed
And sinks into the center of the earth
Pinning him in position
- a specimen in a collection
a great recumbent termite queen
a distended and humbled Jabba the Hut

Ballooning
Pregnant like a blister
Without shame or irony
He tells me, "I try to drink a 12-pack a day."
Do I hide my shock?
An awkward attempt at connection
Or is it that I'm trying to surprise him
fight back in the kisser
By predicting that he no longer gets a buzz
that some people drink like that
just to keep from getting the shakes
"Yep, and so I won't hallucinate like I did
last Wednesday."

In Labor-
    ed breathing
We deliver him by
    Caesarian invasion
Crossing the Rubicon into his homeland
by "tapping his belly"
Cause and Effect
    Ascites fluid is clear and golden

The stream shooting in through the needle
Produces a startlingly nice head
Inside the sterile vacuum bottles

He is polite and grateful
Chatting easily about his
Interesting and lost career
We fastidiously capture his
Disturbingly milky elixir
Easy blame slips away

7 liters later
he breathes easier
while at the same moment
the other person in the room
his dark star child
begins to grow again
inside his belly.

Witnessing stories

Many students are philosophical about the limitations that they encounter in their interactions with patients. A humorous poem refers to patients as "some of the quirkiest people I've ever met," but concludes sympathetically, "So many patients, so many issues/All of them new sensations, all of them eventually need tissues." This poem is an honest witnessing both of the frustrations inherent in patient care and of affection and compassion for patients. A similar poem also adopts a light-hearted tone that balances aggravation with warmth. One poem concludes nonjudgmentally that "convict or saint," all patients deserve optimal care. In another poem, the patient is "a nasty little man" who demands "a real doc," and is difficult, demanding, and uncooperative. However, when the student perceives the patient's suffering, their animosity towards this "difficult" patient evaporates. Witnessing the patient's distress overcomes the patient's annoying attributes, and defuses the student's dislike.

Another poem recognizes philosophically that some patients are cooperative, some are hostile, some are ignorant, some are well informed, some are drug-seeking, some are homeless, some are well off, some are from other countries, some are from jail, and some despise medical students. The student recognizes his limitations: "You can't force them to listen or take all their pills/Or even to care about all of their ills." However, he also recognizes that if you listen to the patient's point of view, they will always tell you something helpful. This poem witnesses the limitations of efficacy of healthcare – and of patients – but with a tolerant, patient attitude that still validates the patients.

The Clinic By: Frank Safar
UC Irvine

If you have time and feel so inclined
Come down to the clinic, there's people to see
All shapes and sizes just like you and me
Some are sick; some are well
Some have very little to tell

Some people have diabetes
And legs full of sores
Some people hear voices
And they're not mine or yours

Some people listen, others ignore
Some people get morphine and always want more
Some people know nothing about their condition
Some learn on the Net like a second volition

Some live on the street; some drive nice cars
Some don't speak English; some belong behind bars
Some haven't bathed and don't wash their clothes
Some hear "Med Student" and turn up their nose

You can't force them to listen or take all their pills
Or even to care about all of their ills
But if you can have them tell their point of view
They'll usually say something helpful to you.

In an adroit reversal of the concept of limitations, a student describes an encounter with a deaf patient. This poem, written from the patient's perspective, complains that her signs will fall on "deaf eyes," and that the student's hands are "speechless." It is the medical student who is perceived as inept, uncommunicative and "speechless." The deaf patient by contrast is full of potential for vibrant communication, but it cannot be activated because of the limitations of the student. The poem has implications beyond the specific clinical situation, and suggests to readers that it is often less a matter of the patient's "limitations" than of using one's imagination and creativity to overcome the inevitable barriers that arise between patients and students – or doctors.

Falling on Deaf Eyes By: Megan Jenkins
Originally appeared in Wild Onions, *Vol. VIII, 2004, p. 44*
Penn State University College of Medicine

While your hands sit idle in your lap
Speechless, with no intent
my hands sit quietly
anticipating . . .
Waiting for the moment when they can be understood.

Though the silence never ends
I can hear;
I can hear all the world's words . . .
the sound of sunlight
the sound of birds in flight
trees dancing without wind
All the laughter
The cries, and every sigh.

Though my silence never ends

You can see.
My hands are my voice, my ears, my eyes, and my ink for expression.
I crave to share my world of silence
and reaching out to you.

Language spoken through symbols;
Falling on deaf eyes
though listening to pacify
never comprehend the message.

I crave to share my world of silence
and am reaching out to you.

Transcendence stories

Sometimes the student's witnessing of the limitations of medicine achieves true transcendence. A student on pediatrics first describes the stresses of getting too little sleep and having too large a workload. His focus is on getting lunch, studying for the shelf exam, and getting a little more sleep. He expresses hostility to the parent of a pediatric patient who demands lab results. He feels like a secretary, a slave, and believes that his time is being wasted. Then the student begins to pay attention to the suffering of his young patients. He realizes the self-centeredness of his own preoccupations and how much more is at stake for these brave and long-suffering children. The narrator concludes that "Life is about perspective / Being grateful for what you have / Finding some shred of happiness in a sea of sorrow / Finding hope." This poem is an example of transformation – a change of perspective from self-pity to realizing that personal suffering is much less significant than the suffering of others. The poem ultimately adopts a position of humility and gratitude.

Another poem, which is organized around the cycle of inbreath and outbreath, portrays various patients in terrible states – gunshot wounds, stabbings, an overdose, psychosis. In the infinitesimal pause between inhale and exhale, the student experiences a moment of sanctity. Breathing out, she releases the darkness of hopeless lives as well as her own helplessness and sense of unworthiness. Breathing in, she affirms the sweetness of life and ". . . the dream of a / thousand healthy spirits / marching in unison." Breathing in and out, the student is able to maintain a kind of exalted joy in the presence of suffering. She realizes that doctors must "depend on brain but cling to heart." The poem culminates in a transcendent vision of the possibility of healing, even when confronted with horror.

A thousand healthy spirits By: Leila Sabet
Originally appeared in Panacea, *Summer, 2005 p. 27*
University of Florida College of Medicine

i allow you to make me feel
unworthy
i allow that
giving you permission
with my silent mediocre frame
while exploding inside
someday will explode outside

so i exhale and breathe the
darkness out of my mind
and inhale all sorts of sweet
head rush
and euphoric sense of oxygen
saturation

i pause
stand reflecting
on the moments of hurry
heated night flurry
of brownian bodies in sway-like
coordination
oneness
centered upon this cilia-filled
breath
flow of go no
go into crimson thoughts
robots with spirit
move about in artistic science
or scientific art
depend on brain but cling to
heart
to move the crimson ideas in
rhythm
with waves of rhythm
circadian style
up in the night
which lives full of forsaken beds
because of my euphoria
i can feel euphoric even
thinking about
the blood saturation in the shirt
of GSW
the vomit saturation of the
gown in tylenol OD
the urine saturation of sheets in
seizure #3
i can feel euphoric with
thoughts of
handcuffed jailed
schizophrenic voices inside his
head
telling him to cut his arm
to constantly harm himself
i can feel euphoric with
thoughts of
suture closing skin

and peroxide lysing cells
to wipe away the blood from
stabbed
drunk and
looking at me kind of funny
kind of scary
i wipe away blood spilling hate
wipe clean slate
with one act of washed feet
wipe away her crown of tears
with one kind motion of
sincerely
nurturing devotion
and exhaled is the darkness
of a hopeless life
in one great sob.
inhaled is the dream of a
thousand healthy spirits
marching in unison.

SUMMARY

Students realize that often they and their patients inhabit different worlds, and they sometimes have difficulty making connections with them. They notice separation from their patients, and experiment with emotional detachment, which they are often trained to believe is the correct professional attitude to pursue. As was suggested in Chapter 9, students struggle with anxiety and uncertainty in their encounters with patients. Occasionally they push patients away by defining them as irreducibly "other" and adopting a blaming, punitive tone. However, in contrast to studies which suggest that students' attitudes towards patients may become more negative as their training progresses, on the whole their poetry suggests that many students achieve a kind of bemused resolution, seeing the aggravating, anxiety-producing and downright inexplicable aspects of patient behavior, but simultaneously realizing that by extending a listening ear and a caring commitment to all patients they can usually achieve a satisfying and helpful interaction. They are prepared to acknowledge their mistakes vis-à-vis patients, especially interpersonal and psychosocial errors. Overall, these student-poets show themselves to be tolerant and nonjudgmental towards their patients. They are more than willing to stand with them, witness their suffering, question professional detachment as an inadequate emotional strategy, and occasionally, as a consequence, they are catapulted to a more elevated level of insight and faithfulness.

11 Tickling the Conscience: The Intersection of Medicine and Social Justice

Approximately 90 million Americans live on incomes at or below 200% of the minimum federal poverty standard. When they become sick, most of these individuals receive treatment in the public hospitals and clinics where medical students train, and whose patient populations are largely comprised of indigent, underserved, uninsured, poor white and minority patients and patients from non-dominant cultural backgrounds. Therefore it is reasonable to inquire about student attitudes towards such patients. There is some evidence that medical students are more aware than the general population that there is unfairness in the healthcare system, and that minority medical students and minority physicians are particularly aware of these discrepancies.[1]

Unfortunately, the available evidence, which is sparse, suggests that contact with underserved patients does not result in students developing greater understanding and empathy for the plight of the poor.[2] On the contrary, interaction with this patient population may result into an increase in negative attitudes towards the poor. One study found that as students became acculturated into the medical profession, their willingness to acknowledge healthcare disparities diminished.[1] Earlier studies concluded that, compared with first-year students, fourth-year students are less willing to provide care for indigent patients and have less positive attitudes towards these patients.[3,4] Ten years later, however, additional research confirms that these findings are essentially unchanged.[5] Generally speaking, medical students come from different educational and socioeconomic backgrounds to their patients. Yet they receive little education or training to help them to understand the kinds of constraints, stressors, and obstacles that confront the poor on a daily basis.[6] Recently, medical schools have attempted to develop curricula aimed at addressing this deficit.[7] These developments are welcome in view of findings which conclude that both the general and personal attitudes of students towards the underserved improve as a result of such curricular exposure.[8]

There is also growing interest and curricular initiatives to develop cultural competency in medical students.[9-11] As patient populations become increasingly diverse, it is evident that future physicians need better skills in practicing medicine across cultures. Research suggests that improving cross-cultural communication skills in healthcare providers is associated with better patient outcomes,[12,13] and that it has the potential to reduce health disparities[14] and improve access to care.[12]

The attitudes of students towards diversity training are equivocal, although survey-type methodologies tend to report positive attitudes.[15,16] One study of resident learners highlighted their concerns regarding insufficient "formal" education on this topic, and reported that they felt they were poorly prepared to deal with cross-cultural clinical encounters.[17] A different investigation concluded that much of learners' self-reported cross-cultural competency came from their own improvisational coping.[18] Yet learners were also concerned that formal cross-cultural education might result in stereotyping of different racial and ethnic groups, and that in any case it was excessively abstract and theoretical.[19]

Although some research has provided evidence that medical students' knowledge, attitudes, and skills can be positively changed as a result of participation in a cultural competency curriculum,[20,21] other studies suggest that exposure to a cross-cultural curriculum has little or no effect on student skill acquisition.[22,23] Furthermore, even when learners report having adequate cross-cultural communication skills and training, they feel that both systemic and patient factors inhibit their provision of quality care.[19]

Of further concern, research has documented medical learner attitudes of blame and negative judgment towards patients from different cultural and socioeconomic backgrounds.[19,24,25] In these studies, learners are likely to attribute cross-cultural difficulties to patient shortcomings. Some authors have also questioned inbuilt assumptions of power and arrogance in the whole concept of cultural competence, and instead have called for an emphasis on cultural humility in approaching cross-cultural medical encounters.[26]

Medical students also encounter major societal issues in the form of substance abuse, family violence (including child abuse and domestic violence), and abortion. Substance abuse, child abuse and neglect, and domestic (or intimate partner) violence are all major public health problems with significant morbidity and mortality. They are also issues that evoke strong emotions in many medical students. For example, negative attitudes towards patients with substance misuse disorders can interfere with optimal patient care.[27] Research has documented that from the medical school years through residency there are enhanced beliefs that alcohol- and drug-abusing patients overutilize healthcare resources and require care that is repetitive and which detracts from the care of other patients. Satisfaction achieved in caring for substance-abusing patients consistently diminishes over the years in training.[28] Studies also indicate that physicians often lack knowledge and confidence in addressing child abuse and neglect[29] as well as other family issues.

Medical education addresses all of these public health issues in didactic format, through special courses and workshops, and/or through clinical training. The quality and depth of such exposure vary widely, and it has been criticized for being insufficiently integrated with other curricular efforts.[30] For example, one survey found that although 91% of US medical students reported receiving at least some training in discussing intimate partner violence, only 20% reported extensive training, and only a little over 50% of senior students reported talking with general medicine patients at least sometimes about intimate partner violence.[31] Nevertheless, such training does generally improve both knowledge and attitudes. For example, students who had been exposed to training in substance abuse demonstrated significant positive changes in both attitudes and knowledge after such educational intervention.[32] In another study, attitudes towards patients with substance-abuse problems improved significantly after exposure to learning modules that included contact with actual patients. The level of dislike of problem drinkers also decreased significantly after teaching. Students in this study reported a greater sense of responsibility for providing intervention for substance-abusing patients and less anxiety about working with them.[27] One study of pregnant patients with substance-abuse disorders, who are often a target of student censure, found that students who attended an obstetrics-gynecology specialty clinic for such patients as part of their training reported that they became more comfortable in talking with these women and more nonjudgmental in treating them. Interestingly, over the period of the clerkship, students who did not participate in the specialty clinic became less comfortable in talking with these patients.[33]

Similar results are found in educational interventions directed towards various aspects of family violence. A survey of pediatric residencies concluded that 93% of respondents felt that their training in child abuse was useful or very useful, although only 66% felt very well or well prepared to deal with this issue in clinical situations.[29] It is also true that medical students will not receive this level of preparation during medical school, and will probably not experience comparable levels of comfort. One study of supplementary training for medical students with regard to domestic violence found that, after training, students demonstrated improved ease with and performance of relevant screening, and also felt more confident in addressing domestic violent issues with patients than those who did not receive the additional instruction.[34] Importantly, these improvements persisted over time. The value of direct clinical exposure, in contrast to didactic teaching alone, was demonstrated in a study which showed that students in an intimate partner violence didactic curriculum improved only in knowledge, whereas students who received didactic teaching plus clinical exposure increased in both knowledge and confidence in terms of recognizing problems and taking action.[35]

Abortion is a highly controversial societal issue that attracted the reflections of a few medical students. Medical school curricula generally do not spend much time on this topic. Student participation in abortion procedures is elective. However, some research exists which suggests that, in terms of attitudes towards abortion, a large majority of medical students believe that abortion education is appropriate in the preclinical and clinical curricula. The majority of students who do choose to participate in clinical abortion care rate it as a valuable experience,[36] and report that this exposure influences their view of a woman's right to access abortion services in a positive direction.[37]

Students occasionally use poetry to examine societal issues, as well as the interface between society and medicine. Most commonly, these "big picture" poems are intensely critical of social mores. They generally take the form of chaos stories or witnessing. Poems examining the underserved, immigrants, the poor, the underprivileged, and minority members of society and other disadvantaged people conclude that they are often treated badly – discriminated against, neglected, given second-class medical care, and discarded when possible. These poems are primarily works that witness to injustices perpetuated or reinforced by the healthcare system and wider society.

A Prayer upon the Passing of a Cambodian Gentleman in the ER
By: Curtis Nordstrom
Originally appeared in Yale Journal for Humanities in Medicine. *2004*

Yale University School of Medicine
Our Immigrant
Which art in heaven
How shall I pronounce Thy name?
Thy people come
Their will be ignored
on earth, as it could not possibly be in heaven.

Serve us this day our daily bread
And lead us not into temptation

by remaining in our presence
any longer than is absolutely necessary;
And deliver us from evil.

For Thine is the Kingdom and the Glory . . .
but the Power belongs to us.
Forever and ever
Amen.

This poem, prompted by the death of a Cambodian immigrant in an emergency room, pointedly uses the language and rhythms of the Lord's Prayer to examine the plight of marginalized, neglected patients. The poem is filled with ironic double entendres. The lowly immigrant who has just died is also "Our Immigrant," suggesting both the Son of God as the embodiment of the despised outsider, and the inevitability of the connection between those on the periphery of society and the rest of us. The narrator proceeds to note the difficulty of pronouncing the patient's name, the phrase reverberating with Old Testament prohibitions against uttering the name of God and thus reinforcing the sanctified nature of these discarded souls.

The religious overtones continue as the poem follows the patterns of perhaps the best-known Christian prayer, reminding us that those most cherished by Christ ("Thy people") are the poor, the forgotten, and the scorned. Instead of the Kingdom of God coming, however, it is masses of immigrants, seeking a better life, perhaps the kingdom of heaven on earth. And while, in the words of Jesus' parable, they will be "first" in heaven ("as it could not possibly be in heaven"), here on earth their will and needs are routinely ignored and demeaned. The poem goes on to beseech God for the traditional favors of "daily bread," generally interpreted as basic sustenance, although given the tenor of the poem, it is far from clear that this bread will be shared with the hungry poor, the immigrant or any other inconsequential people. Then, with the entitled arrogance of the privileged class, the narrator encourages the Lord not to remain here on earth any longer than is absolutely necessary. In the Lord's presence, the narrator might be led into "temptation," sometimes construed as a test of character. In yet another ironic twist, in the context of the poem, the narrator may be pleading not to have the virtues of our characters examined, as the results would surely be grossly lacking.

Just as we need the immigrant to rake our leaves and pick our fruit, we need the Lord to do our dirty work, to "deliver us from [the] evil" in which we are steeped – the evil of indifference, separation, and complacency. However, as the narrator recognizes, with both immigrant and the Lord, it is an uncomfortable relationship at best. Just as the immigrant's presence is an annoyance that hopefully will pass away quickly, like the patient, we prefer a safely demarcated zone between us and our God. The poem concludes with the smug intimation that although God may care for these people in heaven, in this world the power belongs to the ruling class, and will continue to belong to this class "forever." God is welcome to his Kingdom, so long as he leaves us alone on earth. This poem is a stark witnessing to the societal inequalities based on ethnicity, resources, and insurance status that persist in this country.

SOCIETAL PROBLEMS
Chaos stories

One student writes a tirade against the "cold, detached existence" that permeates society. Using a medical analogy, he wants to give an "antidote" to cure "this one disease / This plague . . ." The poem reflects the confusion of the narrator, who does not know whom to blame or hold responsible for all the social ills of indifference and callousness that he sees. He is overwhelmed by the uncaring attitude of society in the face of human suffering.

Witnessing stories

Witnessing poems tend to express resistance and protest. One poem criticizes the spread of the Wal-Mart culture, its impersonal vastness and single-focused profit orientation. It mocks a sign – "Jesus saves (when He shops at Wal-Mart!)" – and condemns capitalism as the new American religion. Another poem bemoans that what contemporary culture offers is simple, easy, worry-free, convenient, and rarely involves thinking. The student calls for inspiration, enlightenment, or revolution. In a similar poem, the narrator expresses disillusionment and disappointment at the failure of social revolutions. She condemns her generation, which seems to be filled with fear and anxiety, depressingly conformist and obedient. She dreams about "tear[ing] down the sky / and turn[ing] the world on its back." Another cultural critique targets the routinization of life. It describes a man walking during rush hour, as he goes about his business: "he marched on / jaw set . . . He did not care for the sky." The poem is suggestive of our inability to look beyond our immediate tasks and objectives. These are all examples of witnessing to, respectively, the limitations of consumerism, pop culture, and the mindless self-centeredness of most people's lives.

Interestingly, both Middle Eastern and American students occasionally reflected on the war that currently involves both regions. A poem by a student from Qatar probably describes the war in Iraq. It chronicles cycles of violence and destruction, while criticizing attitudes that ignore and turn away from the suffering. The poem enjoins people to care, to see, and says that they should ask "Why do the bombs fly south?" In another poem, the same student draws an implicit parallel between the US and the Roman conquerors, who seemed invincible, but who laid waste to all around them, eventually destroyed their own civilization, and became lost in turn. A poem by an American student contrasts the images of the war and destruction of Iraq on television with the comfort of his living-room. The poem suggests the unreality of very real images when viewed from a context of safety, and points to the incommensurability of the two worlds. Another poem by an American portrays a student studying biochemistry, memorizing biochemical building blocks. Himself a veteran from a family of veterans, he creates a mnemonic referring to American veterans who have died for no purpose. The poem intimates how the building blocks that construct humans end up as the detritus of war.

Other poems reflect a consciousness of issues such as poverty and hunger. In one poem, a homeless man who "carries his house" is waiting under an awning for the rain to stop. The poem presents a pathetic, isolated, cold image of two disconnected people – the man without a home and the narrator observing him. A poem from a Qatar student examines homelessness in the person of a cold, sick, hungry girl who has fallen asleep in the pouring rain. She lies completely exposed to the elements, which are "furious," "roaring," and "wailing." The child resists sleep, perhaps because it is too similar to death, but eventually she succumbs. No one notices or cares about the abandoned girl huddled on the "abandoned street." Here mercy is absent.

Midnight Strikes By: Hala Mint El Moctar Mohammed Moussa
Originally appeared in Paint the Walls, *2005, pp. 34–5*
Weill Cornell Medical College in Qatar.

Midnight strikes
And the furious rain
fills the darkness
with a damp silence

now broken with the thunder's roar
The wailing wind winds
the abandoned street
and the lampposts bend
in the bitter cold

As the girl shivers
until the thunder faints
and the storm is tamed
In that ghastly corner she lies

a corner whose darkness
is secured by a balcony
of an abandoned home
She starves for sleep

but resists
Is it the cold, the hunger
or maybe her feverish limbs
Yet the heavy lids surrender at last

to the dreariness of the night
She feebly clasps her lean hands
and lies on the drenched ground
exposed

Another poem also addresses the issue of hunger, this time describing a famished woman defying her fate, struggling, and shouting out "her sonorous wrath" "to strike down God." The woman, although despairing and in agony, is somehow simultaneously strong and unbowed. She defiantly shakes her carrot and cries out in a "hurricane voice." Her famished frame nevertheless gnashes its teeth with a mouthful of nails and bellows forth flames. The poet intimates that although this woman will pass away, and "will melt into the mud," she will leave behind "premonitions of a far-off earthquake." The poem taps into the anger of the poor around the globe and their potential to rise up and shake the established social order like an earthquake.

Hungry Woman By: Sheila Chan
UC Irvine, 2005

Mud clung to the fringes of her skirt tugging her to the ground.
She struggled, wielding her last carrot to strike down God for dinner.

Her hurricane voice, violent and strong, swept across the prairie.
The weeds shivered, cowering under her sonorous wrath.

Eyes polished bright
by the scouring of death pierced through wispy angels.

Withered arms parsed of tender flesh impervious bone
raw and ready to snap.

Her mouth of nails hammered at hunger.
Her gnashing stomach bellowed flames.

Intestines thrashing ether
hollow worms conduits suffused with agony.

Emptiness yanked on an idea
a whip lacerating space.
Hunger, that throbbing vacuum collapsed in spewing despair.

She will melt into the mud
her sinking fingers clawing at the clouds
leaving echoes, rumblings, premonitions of a far-off earthquake.

The plight of undocumented immigrants and their simultaneous rejection by and exploitation by society was also noted in several poems. In one representative example, the metaphor of building border fences suggests the barriers that are built into the social system to keep out the unwanted, nameless Others. However, as the author ironically notes, with money comes "good breeding," and then (how inconveniently) just the slightest tickle of compassion. We cannot turn away completely from their pain and misery. Reluctantly, "when the need is dire," one nail is removed to allow in the smallest seepage possible of those most frantic and most wounded. The desperate surge in, leaving only their bloody fingerprints as a sign that they have arrived.

Fences By: Sarah Blaschko
Originally appeared in Plexus, *2003, p. 24, UC Irvine School of Medicine*

Money
buys fences
to keep the Other out.

It buses them to the county line
and leaves exhaust
flung in faces without names.

And with money comes good
breeding (sometimes)

and good breeding
aches with conscience.

Maybe, tickles the conscience
if it was dire.

So to swat the conscience away
money
loosens the nail
of one board
in the fence.

They can swing it aside now
if they really need to.
If it is dire.

And it is dire
at first
tide of blood
blunt
force
trauma

They pushed through the
loose board in the fence
and left a smear of red fingers
on the whitewash.

INTERSECTION OF HEALTHCARE AND SOCIETAL PROBLEMS
Underserved, uninsured, and minority patients
Chaos stories

The issue of inadequate and inequitable healthcare coverage lurks around the edges of some students' awareness, with its implication that uninsured patients sometimes have appallingly poor access to care and sometimes receive less skilled care from less well-trained physicians. Such situations often provoke feelings of chaos and helplessness in student-authors. In one heartrending poem, a student confronts an uninsured patient in pain who needs an operation that he cannot afford. The poem concludes with his unanswered cry: "I feel so alone and crummy." Unable to work, he uses up his savings. The patient has become the victim of an indifferent healthcare system.

Another poem describes a middle-aged Latino patient with possible smoking-related tuberculosis or cancer who reminds the medical student of her father. He is "trusting, simple, solid/with rough hands stripped and broken by labor," defined by "simplicity, hard work, love of family and friends and God." However, of the entire medical team, only the student is able to see this "core." She wants to protect and befriend him, but she cannot solve his problems. The patient is finally discharged, without a clear understanding of his diagnosis or treatment plan, wondering "where was the healing he had sought." Although the patient persists in being thankful for the kindness of the student, she is left with a feeling of failure. The student is ashamed of the limitations of the healthcare system, of which she is now a part, vis-à-vis an uninsured, immigrant patient population, of whom she is also a part.

He reminded me of my father By: Mabel Romero
UC Irvine

He reminded me of my father
with his dark eyes and guttural laugh
trusting, simple, solid
with rough hands stripped and broken by labor
I had felt them years ago playing, guiding, and protecting.

Hemoptysis they said a smoker of many years
Purposefully the tube went in despite the struggles and plea
exhilarated, congratulated, content
Any questions, I said yet prepared my exit
The gentle roughness of his hands prevented my departures.

Hablas espanol? He hesitantly prodded
I explained the possibility of TB
scared, confused, trusting
I wanted to protect him and become a friend
to tell him it could be cancer when the others remained silent.

The blood kept coming speckled with his concerns
insurance, diagnosis, and his inability to pay
grateful, unsure, trusting
I returned each visit without an answer or solution
and left embarrassed by his sincere gratitude.

Scribbled on a napkin, a letter to his parents he shared
thankful for his blessed life, his ability to work, his loving wife
joyful, honest, fulfilled
Simplicity, hard work, love of family and friends and God
These defined him, were his core, but only I was lucky enough to know.

After the last lab test and procedure he was free to go
He barely protested but where was the healing he had sought
bewildered, confused, distrustful
There's nothing more to do for you here they said and left
I shrank from his dark questioning gaze.

I stayed, attempted to explain the assessment and the plan
He gathered his things, the letter was the only one of value
distrustful, confused, unsure
but still grateful for all I had done
I struggled to understand what "all" he meant
and left feeling I had failed this man
whose heart and hand and eyes I'd known before.

Other poems bitterly recall culturally insensitive, inadequate, and inappropriate health-care experienced by writers and their families as a result of cultural and language differences. One medical student catalogues family members who were treated without consideration for their limited funds, given outdated or incorrect medications, or allowed to die in pain. This student recognizes that the legacy of such treatment can be "a distrust that seems almost insurmountable," and doubts that she will be able to overcome it.

Witnessing stories

More often, however, when students pay attention to these issues, they choose to witness to injustice and align themselves with oppressed patients. They align themselves with the poor and immigrants who often do not have adequate access to the American healthcare system. Students who themselves are from minority and low socioeconomic status backgrounds are particularly passionate in their allegiance. For example, a medical student from Vietnam contrasts the poverty of his homeland and its associated diseases with the excesses of the USA that produce their own lifestyle-related medical conditions. This poem is a reminder to the student of why he is in medical school and what his responsibilities are to the poor and underserved.

Where I came from . . . By: Cory Bui
UC Irvine, 2002

Where I came from
Doctors make 30 dollars a month
Here my lunch costs 5 dollars . . .

Where I came from
Kids, myself included, sell scrap metal for a living
Here I learned that lead is poison . . .

Where I came from
Food is a scarcity
Here obesity is a disease . . .

Where I came from
A classmate of mine had polio
Here polio . . . what? . . . show me one case

Just a reminder to myself
Of where I came from
Very different . . .

Just a reminder to myself
Of where I came from
. . . and why I'm here.

In another poem, a Latina medical student forms a bond with a middle-aged Hispanic male patient who is HIV positive, and has lung cancer and a drug addiction. The staff dismiss his pain and label him pejoratively as "a big cry baby." The patient establishes a connection by telling the student that she reminds him of his daughter. In this poem, student and patient are clearly aligned against other healthcare providers, in part through bonds of culture. The student has discovered a depth and richness in the patient that have been overlooked by the other staff, and he becomes her teacher, mentor, and surrogate parent on the rotation, giving her advice about life and doctoring. This poem expresses resistance to "rules" of engagement with patients. It is a patient from a similar cultural background who becomes the student's most trusted teacher.

Mi Hija By: Sandy Ramos
UC Irvine

First time I met Mr. Vera
39 y.o. HIV positive, lung cancer
Lying flat on the surgery table
Chest open, two ribs removed
A lung lobe removed
The tumor too close to the Great Vessels

Second time I met Mr. Vera
SICU, a patient screaming
At 4:30 a.m. the nurses were too busy
He's a drug addict, morphine doesn't work
He's a big cry baby
Were the excuses

Third time I met Mr. Vera
Saturday morning on the surgical wards
Staring at the wall
When I introduced myself
Said I looked too young, reminded him of his daughter
Rude, made crass and inappropriate comments to the nurses, to me
When I answered back, he found his match

Fourth time I met Mr. Vera
Had to remove one of the two chest tubes
First time for both of us
Mi hija, just do like the doctors say
Pull it and don't worry about me
I'm a tough *viejo*
Don't hesitate, never hesitate

I met Mr. Vera
As I wheeled him down to X-ray
Down the long corridor of the silent VA
Mi hija, always look out for number one
Can't take care of number two without taking care of number one
Mi hija, don't worry too much
Don't care too much, about your patients

Although few non-minority students addressed the issue of treatment of minority patients within the healthcare system, when they did do so, they appeared to be strongly aware of inequities in access and care. One poem addresses issues of racism, sexism, and social mores by considering the life of an elderly female black patient, and all the ways in which her life has been limited by the racial barriers that she has encountered. The student, writing in the first person, expresses some guilt, some responsibility for all that the patient has endured, and thinks that she "must have expected more [from life] than a poem." Yet she notices that, despite her suffering, the patient is "oddly content." The student realizes that she must resist the easy refuge of pity.

A similar poem expresses empathy for the complexity of the myriad medical, social, and emotional problems that confront one African-American woman. The patient tells a chaos story, crying out to the doctor for help: "Oh doctor, doctor, what can I do?" Her husband has died, her brother is dying of AIDS, and she is all alone, grieving, depressed, on disability, suffering from obesity, high cholesterol, diabetes, and hypertension. The doctor is sympathetic, and pledges to help the patient. However, soon it is time for him to move on to the next patient. Without demonizing the compassionate but harried physician, the poem does not turn away from the multiply-layered suffering of the patient, and recognizes the limitations of the help available to her.

African American female patient By: Cyrus Khaledy

UC Irvine, 2002

Once upon an afternoon dreary
I walked in, and held my breath
I didn't know where to begin . . .
I lost my husband a year ago
I've been on disability for six months now
I realize that I am quite alone
No friends, no relatives to keep me warm.

I ask the physician, what can I do?
I feel so helpless and so weak too
I don't have the energy to walk
I've been sleeping randomly, in and out
I wake up in the early morning of dawn
I just lay there, crying in bed
I hug the pillow ever so tight
It shall be my only comfort tonight . . .
Oh doctor, doctor, what can I do?

My parents are not here, but in New York
My brother is dying of AIDS
I come to you for advice
But alas, you have only bad news to dispense
My cholesterol is skyrocketing
My weight has gone out of control
Eating has become my new obsession
To deal with this grief and despair
How can I make any concessions?
When life seems so unfair . . .
Oh doctor, doctor, what can I do?

It's been five months that I have been depressed
These medications don't help soothe my soul
I make a Prayer to God, ask him to help me through

I only get complete silence in return
Nothing seems to be answered
Nothing gets done
Silence is my only companion tonight
Oh doctor, doctor, what can I do?

My brother has AIDS, I have hypertension
I feel cheated by life
My husband was my only friend
I lost my companion, my mentor and my confidant
Only in the course of one summer night
I feel anger, despair, and loss.
I feel like he left me without saying goodbye . . .
I guess death really did tear us apart . . .
Oh doctor, doctor, what can I do?
Please help me through this somehow.

He solemnly looks at me and says
"I'm so sorry for everything you had to go through in life.
There is nothing I can do or say
that will bring your husband back from the dead
We have to take life, one day at a time.
Deal with each struggle one by one
No need to feel so overwhelmed
I'm here to help you, be there for you.

It's ok to vent and cry
Don't keep it all inside
If you exercise, now and then
Your hypertension will be kept in check.
And take these medications
for your cholesterol.
And these for your depression
And these for your diabetes.
Take them all and you shall be fine."

But doctor, what about the grief?
I no longer have a confidant
I have no friends to talk and walk about
What about a job, to pay these bills
What about my health insurance?
Surely, my only solution isn't just pills?

"Ma'am, I'm so sorry, I wish I could help you some more.
Unfortunately, your fifteen minutes are up.
I have to go and see the next patient now
I will hopefully see you in a month . . ."

Sometimes students adopted the voice of a patient from a culturally different background, writing in the first person. This approach has the effect of both imagining the perspective of that patient, and of creating a sense of emotional immediacy. In a typical poem, a Spanish-speaking pediatric patient expresses distress at being in the hospital. His lack of comprehension of what is happening to him seems to be underlined by the language differences. In contrast to other poems without a cross-cultural component, in which the medical student is perceived as a friend, in this poem the child rejects this idea, and continues to repeat an anguished refrain, "No me pique!" ("Don't stick me"), and it is not clear whether the student understands this. A heartbreakingly poignant poem written in the voice of a 13-year-old pregnant Latina girl prays to the Holy Virgin of Miracles to send her either a man who will marry her, or her period. This poem conveys the voice of a child poised on the brink of womanhood, at once naive and worldly-wise. The isolation and hopelessness of her situation permeate the writing.

In yet another poem, the author writes warmly and understandingly in the first-person voice about the conflict between a diabetic diet and traditional Mexican foods, which become symbolic of familial/communal sharing and connection. Although in this poem the doctor is not portrayed unsympathetically – she worries about the patient and sends reminders of her appointment – her primary focus is the dietary violations, whereas the patient is aware of the many ways in which foods tie her to her culture. The poem witnesses the physician's basic lack of cultural understanding and sensitivity. All of these poems are examples of witnessing the confusion and isolation from the perspective of the culturally different patient.

Language discordance
Chaos stories

Several poems tackle the specific issue of language discordance between patient and provider. These situations can be exhausting and confusing to students from the dominant culture who have little or no Spanish or other language skills, and are the topic that they wrote about most often when considering cultural differences. One student encounters a parent who speaks only Spanish, and her first thought is "God, I hope this won't be a mess," as she fears that between her own limited medical skills and her inability to understand the mother, the patient's care will be compromised.

In a similarly frustrated poem, the focus is on the student's struggle with a second language during a pelvic examination. The student deplores her linguistic clumsiness and is overwhelmed by the patient's rapid flow of incomprehensible words. An examination that would inevitably be awkward is made infinitely more distressing by the lack of a shared language. The imagery of a child's puppet show, in which the patient's head appears "onstage" above her drape covering her bent knees, adds a note of absurd incongruity. The patient's attempts to describe the birth of her last child seem to require as much linguistic contortion and labor as the actual delivery. The encounter ends unsatisfactorily, with the student only able to "hope" that the patient understands the key aspects of her care.

Catching Comprehension By: Meghann Kaiser
UC Irvine, 2003

I am referring to her in the masculine
Too late to catch myself
I can't remember the words to apologize
Nor explain why I need to. I hope she understands

Legs slouched spread-eagle, feet propped up
Knees bent awkward at eye level with me
And the drape strung out between them
Fluttering in time with the air conditioner
Like the makeshift blanket stage of a second-grade puppet show
While I cower in the corner opposite
Beneath a burden of unrelenting English.
Not the flu, not a head-ache, nor a cough, lower back pain
I know the words for head and back, but
Pap Smear?
*Como se dice la cosa de que viene los bebes?**

I am sifting through expressions
Trying to catch comprehension
As she cranes her head forward
Her face wobbles into view onstage
I look up from my notes in time to see
Words blurting, bobbing, bubbling, all transparently, erratically
I go flailing after
While doors slam overhead, people talking elsewhere pop them
Just outside my grasp.
She is re-enacting her youngest son's birth.
I can't tell what happened when, or why, but
Her face squints and pooches in the pains of communication.
My interpretation insufficient for medical advice
My hand comes to rest on her right ankle
The sticky residue of fractured phrases
And sweat, invests my palm.
No se, Senora.†

Am I the sole witness before the line-up
Each contortion a suspect of meaning
I offer her phrases from my dictionary
And await recognition
The evidence of convicting diagnosis
An explanation of my thoughts, myself
I hope she understands.

In another poem, although the patient speaks English as a second language, he is soon lost in the medical-speak of the doctors, and worries that he is missing important nuances and implications. He ends up isolated and alone. These poems are both examples of the chaos that is produced and the limitations and inadequacies that occur as a result of language barriers in healthcare.

---

* Literally, *"What do you call the things that babies come out of?"*
† *"I don't know, Senora."*

Restitution stories

These poems tend to present good intentions on the part of students. In the following poem, a dialogue takes place between a Spanish-speaking patient and the medical student, who has limited Spanish-language skills. The patient presents his symptoms, but worries that the "doctora" does not understand him. The student grasps all that she can, paying careful attention to the patient's words and nonverbal signs. Then she takes the initiative to bring in an interpreter, and the result is a satisfied, grateful patient, secure in the knowledge that he has a doctor who cares enough to want to accurately understand what he is saying.

I don't speak Spanish very well By: Laleh Gharahbaghian
UC Irvine, 2004

Tengo un problema. Doctora
Yo no veo bien
Y tambien tengo cansado
Yo no se que hacer
Comprende lo que yo digo?

> Hola senor. Hablo un poquito espanol
> I understand you have "a problem"
> You seem to be tired.
> What you said after I couldn't tell
> I'm sorry senor. I don't speak Spanish very well.

Tengo dolor en mi cabeza
Y mis musculos no sienten bien
Y mi espalda, no puedo mover mucho
Creo que necesita un antibiotico
Comprende lo que yo digo?

> I see that you have pain
> From the expression on your face
> I see you pointing to your neck and back as if they ache
> I want to understand why: I will get someone to help
> I'm sorry senor, I don't speak Spanish very well.

Si, una persona que habla espanol
Gracias que viene
Ahora puedo hablar contigo
y gracias la doctora
Que usted quiere comprender lo que yo digo

> I'm glad you came in today
> You seem to be in pain
> I want to give you the best care that we have here now
> I understand what you are telling about
> There is no need to thank us
> It's my job to figure these things out.

Witnessing stories
Occasionally, themes about language differences include the isolation and poor health-care that result for patients with limited or no English. One student considers the issue of physicians inappropriately using family members as interpreters – often children, who are more likely either to speak English well or at least to be more fluent than their parents. The narrator challenges the usual rationalizations for relying on family members for translation services, including the workload, the lack of trained interpreters, and the "simplicity" of the medical/discharge instructions. The student goes on to point out the potential inaccuracies, absurdity, and awkwardness of this approach by imagining an equivalent English-speaking child put in the position of having to translate for his mother. With the rhetorical lament "Can someone please make this stop?", this poem hints at the larger problematic societal context that allows such inappropriate and discriminatory behavior.

Excuses By: Stephanie Dittmer
UC Irvine, 2003

Five-year-old Latino boy . . . going to turn six soon.
Eighteen-month-old sister . . . recovering from an asthma exacerbation.
Thirty-five-year-old mother . . . speaking to her son in Spanish, "*Calmate!*"

The red-headed doctor walks in . . .

"Hello there! You are certainly a big guy!"
"Can you do me a favor?"
"Can you tell your mother that Teresa will be able to go home today?"
"Can you tell your mother that the nurse will be in to give her
the prescription and instructions?"

Can someone please make this stop?

No time to get a translator?
Eight other patients to see?
The instructions are simple?
Not giving her a prognosis/diagnosis/therapy?

Would it be acceptable if . . .

Five-year-old Caucasian boy going to turn six soon.
Eighteen-month-old sister . . . recovering from an asthma exacerbation.
Thirty-five-year-old mother . . . speaking to her son in English
"Would you please calm down!"

The red-headed doctor walks in . . .

"Hello there! You are certainly a big guy!"
Can you do me a favor?"
"Can you tell your mother that Cindy will be able to go home today?"
"Can you tell your mother that the nurse will be in to give her
the prescription and instructions?"

Drug and alcohol abuse
Chaos stories
Students frequently deal with the health effects of substance abuse in their patient encounters, and occasionally choose to memorialize these experiences through a poem. These patients, and their circumstances, can evoke chaos stories that reflect the student's own helplessness and futility. In one poem the student writes about a female drug user in the third person. She recognizes that the patient may be saved for tonight, but tomorrow "she'll squeeze this night into a new syringe." The poem suggests the futility of treatment. The ultimate outcome for this patient is death. Another poem reflects on a friend's drug addiction. The narrator offers his understanding, warmth, and reaching out to the friend's rationalizing "crying soul," "shrouded heart," and "unshed tears," and finds that his efforts are insufficient. The narrator is helpless to save his friend.

Journey stories
One student initially refers to himself as a skeptic who doubts his drug- and alcohol-addicted patient's protestation that he wants to reform and make a new start. However, by the end of the poem the student realizes that he, like much of society, has made a snap judgment about the patient based on cursory observations, and he feels ashamed that he made the mistake of not looking deeply enough at the patient's situation. The poem ends on a hopeful note, in that the homeless man has "killed" the student's doubts and judgmental attitude. In this poetic journey, the student moves from stereotypic negative judgment and condemnation to appreciation and respect, his unlikely guide being an alcoholic patient. The student's own doubt and skepticism must be dealt with if he is to overcome his prejudices.

Witnessing stories
In another poem, the medical team keeps a homeless, alcoholic patient going: "Roll on a little while longer, Bill / While our physical heart keeps firing / Our medical status is still alive." However, their compassion is qualified. The team blames the patient for being "Just Not Strong Enough / For when long ago he fell, he stayed fallen." "We say it's his own weak fault." The team saves the patient, but simultaneously blames him. This poem witnesses both the team's efforts to save an alcoholic patient, and their attitude of blame and condemnation towards him for not having enough will-power to change his life.

Child abuse
Witnessing stories
A pediatric rotation is a required part of third-year clerkships, and students almost always encounter child victims of physical, emotional, and sexual abuse, as well as of maternal–fetal drug and alcohol addiction. These instances of innocent suffering, often inflicted by the very people who are supposed to protect and safeguard children, are deeply troubling to students. During reflection sessions, students on pediatric clerkships at my home institution consistently report feelings of anger, rage, and heartbreak at the plight of these innocent victims. However, their poems tend to be witnessing rather than chaos narratives, showing greater perspective and insight than they often demonstrate in discussions. Many of these poems urge society to take greater responsibility for this problem. For example, one poem asserts that each child deserves joy and happiness. The writer concludes that society needs to protect children from abuse and abandonment.

In a similar poem, a student reflects on a drug-addicted baby. She highlights the infant's innocence, its "pristine condition," and eulogizes it as "a precious treasure" that should have "a future full of opportunity and hope." However, the student fears that although medicine can heal the child's external wounds, the internal wounds "will be reborn for generations to come." Then the author proceeds to catalog the likely future problems of this child, and concludes with the forlorn hope that the baby will "beat the odds." Another poem describes the life of an abused child from her accidental conception to her being beaten by her drunken father. This poem also explores the generational effects of child abuse, suggesting that it is a vicious cycle that tends to repeat itself. The poem asks "Who will save this child's life?", implying that although medicine can repair her broken bones, society needs to address the deeper roots of the problem.

Domestic violence and rape
Witnessing stories
When students write about domestic violence, they are surprisingly nuanced in their interpretations. One poem denounces this "whorish crime," yet recognizes that change is difficult for both abuser and victim, thus witnessing the complexities of an abusive relationship. Another poem describes the narrator's mother, who was abused. The mother takes Prozac, which calms her, to deal with the psychological aftermath but ". . . She/is less herself, less ferocious." The title of the poem, "Floral Remedies," refers both to the flowers that the mother would place on her nightstand to soothe her hurt away, and the "bouquet of psychiatry" that has made her "still and beautiful." This poem witnesses the tragedy of domestic violence, and the imperfect healing powers of medical intervention. Another poem about a woman who survives being shot by her husband is a testimony to the tragedy of domestic violence and the courage of the victim.

Yet another poem tackles the effects of witnessing domestic violence inflicted on a child. A little girl tells the truth about domestic violence in her family, consoles her little sister, and admits her fear to the police. She remembers that she used to get stickers from her doctors for being brave during routine procedures such as immunizations, but where are the rewards for her courage in this horrific situation? This poem challenges medicine's ability to address, rather than paper over, real social problems. In another poem about witnessing domestic violence, a poem notes the child's regressive behaviors and laments the destruction of her innocence. The student-author wants to restore the child's innocence by "giving back wings" to her, but she recognizes that there is a long "line of broken angels behind you/Waiting for their 15-minute appointments." In this witnessing poem, the narrator rejects a simple find-it-and-fix-it approach. There is no easy way to restore these "broken angels."

In the following poem about date rape, told in the victim's voice, the poet provides important insights into the power dynamics of sexuality and rape. Initially, the narrator describes her desire for sexual power and control, and dresses and acts in a way that attracts the attention she craves. But then things go horribly wrong, as the balance of power shifts to the unidentified rapist, who deprives the narrator of her power as easily as he removes her clothes. Suddenly she is consumed and vulnerable, and in shame she conceals the injuries that her assailant has inflicted.

Power By: Akiva Kahn

Originally appeared in Plexus, *2006, UC Irvine School of Medicine*

I crave the sense.
I dress the part.
I am. I fake.
I lie. I act.

I walk my head
held high my breasts
exposed under a black bra
and white unbuttoned shirt.

You ate it up.
I controlled your lust
And then, in your
dark cold black room

You stripped my clothes
You stripped my power
You ate me up.
My act is flawed.

My heart is racing
As I push my
breasts back into the white
bra which shows

through under the thin
pale blue sweater
I use to hide the marks
you left on me.

Abortion

Journey stories

Very few students grappled with the extraordinarily divisive and polarizing issue of abortion. In one poem, a pregnant woman considering an abortion looks for abnormalities in her fetus as a way of justifying her decision. Initially surprised, the medical student realizes that the father is "emotionally unavailable," the patient already has two children, and the family has no money. She understands the patient's dilemma, and sees her as full of "fear/sadness/strength." At first the student sees only the stereotype of an irresponsible abortion-seeking woman. However, as she listens to the patient's story, she is able to see the patient herself more clearly, rather than merely her idea about the patient. This poem represents a journey on the part of the student from judging the patient's wish for an abortion to understanding her perspective and respecting her situation.

Is baby okay? By: Lena Schulz
UC Irvine, 2003

Is baby okay?
Abnormalities?
How big?
No problems?
Anything?
Anything at all?

"sigh"

Strange.
Unexpected.
Patient wants pictures.
Smiles.
Loves.
But
So many questions.
Unusually intense.

Strange.

Father.
"Emotionally unavailable."
Catch word.
Two small children.
No money.
How to cope?

I understand.
"Abnormalities"
Make the choice easier.
She is torn.

She smiles.
Behind her smile —
Fear.
Sadness.
Strength!

Witnessing stories

A poem entitled "Pride . . . Prejudice" shows the author's willingness to wrestle with the complexities of the abortion issue in a nuanced, empathic manner. "Pride" describes the act of conception, and the hope and promise that it brings. The fetus represents the truth, the future. "Prejudice" refers to abortion. This part of the poem explores the ethics of abortion, and points out that a life (that of the baby) is always exchanged for a life (that of the mother). In this case, death is the outcome of love. The poem protests against the societal regulation of personal and private matters. It struggles with how to reconcile justice and religion, whose intersection becomes a two-headed beast, a destructive monster.

SUMMARY

Only a handful of students used their poetry to protest against social injustice, or to tackle the intersection of larger societal issues and medicine, such as homelessness, hunger, lack of health insurance, poverty, minority status, alcohol and drug abuse, child abuse, domestic violence, and abortion. Those who did so positioned themselves to express solidarity of marginalized patients and other members of society, and expressed strong critiques of societal indifference and moral culpability. The students who chose to address these issues through poetry may not have been typical of medical students in general. Certainly they demonstrated little or none of the negative, judgmental, and patient-blaming attitudes that are documented in the research literature. On the contrary, they were sensitive to healthcare inequities, aware of the necessity of cultural competence in healthcare providers, and sympathetic to the plight and dilemmas of marginalized patients.

In writing about cross-cultural encounters, students generally express compassion and concern for these patients. Students from minority backgrounds speak with added authority, and also express particular empathy, identification, and outrage. Students from dominant-culture backgrounds often focused on language difficulties, and wrote about their frustration and helplessness in trying to communicate with linguistically and culturally different patients. In general, the physicians in these encounters are portrayed fairly negatively – either concerned but detached, or patronizing, stereotyping, and superficial in their relationships with patients. The commitment of these student-poets is steadfastly with the patients.

REFERENCES

1 Wilson E, Grumbach K, Huebner J, *et al.* Medical student, physician, and public perceptions of health care disparities. *Family Medicine* 2004; **36**: 715–21.

2 Wear D, Kuczewski MG. Perspective: medical students' perceptions of the poor: what impact can medical education have? *Academic Medicine* 2008; **83**: 639–45.

3 Crandall SJ, Volk RJ, Loemker V. Medical students' attitudes toward providing care for the underserved: are we training socially responsible physicians? *JAMA* 1993; **269**: 2519–23.

4 Crandall SJ, Volk RJ, Cacy D. A longitudinal investigation of medical student attitudes toward the medically indigent. *Teaching and Learning in Medicine* 1997; **9**: 254–60.

5 Crandall SJ, Reboussin BA, Michielutte R, *et al.* Medical students' attitudes toward underserved patients: a longitudinal comparison of problem-based and traditional medical curricula. *Advances in Health Sciences Education: Theory and Practice* 2007; **12**: 71–86.

6 Leacock E. *Culture of Poverty: A critique.* New York: Simon & Schuster; 1971.

7 Doran KM, Kirley K, Barnosky AR, *et al.* Developing a novel Poverty in Healthcare curriculum for medical students at the University of Michigan Medical School. *Academic Medicine* 2008; **83**: 5–13.

8 Cox ED, Koscik RL, Olson CA, *et al.* Caring for the underserved: blending service learning and a web-based curriculum. *American Journal of Preventive Medicine* 2006; **31**: 342–9.

9 Beach MC, Cooper L, Robinson KA, *et al.* Strategies for improving minority healthcare quality. *Evidence Report Technology Assessment (Summary)* 2004; **Issue 90**: 1–8.

10 Special theme issue on cultural competence. *Academic Medicine* 2003; **78**: 560–87.

11 Skelton JR, Kai J, London RF. Cross-cultural communication in medicine: questions for educators. *Medical Education* 2001; **35**: 257–61.

12 Smedley BD, Stith AY, Nelson AR (eds). *Unequal Treatment: Confronting racial and ethnic*

disparities in health care. Washington, DC: Board on Health Sciences Policy, Institute of Medicine of the National Academies; 2003.

13 American Medical Student Association. *Achieving Diversity in Dentistry and Medicine (ADDM)*; www.amsa.org/addm/#cult

14 Alexander M, Grumbach K, Remy L, *et al.* Congestive heart failure hospitalizations and survival in California: patterns according to race/ethnicity. *American Heart Journal* 1999; 137: 919–27.

15 Dogra N, Karnik N. First-year medical students' attitudes toward diversity and its teaching: an investigation at one U.S. medical school. *Academic Medicine* 2003; 78: 1191–200.

16 Dogra N, Karnik N. A comparison between UK and US medical student attitudes towards cultural diversity. *Medical Teacher* 2004; 26: 703–8.

17 Weissman JS, Betancourt J, Campbell EG, *et al.* Resident physicians' preparedness to provide cross-cultural care. *JAMA* 2005; 294: 1058–67.

18 Park ER, Betancourt JR, Kim MK, *et al.* Mixed messages: residents' experiences learning cross-cultural care. *Academic Medicine* 2005; 80: 874–80.

19 Shapiro J, Hollingshead J, Morrison EH. Primary care resident, faculty, and patient views of barriers to cultural competence, and the skills needed to overcome them. *Medical Education* 2002; 36: 749–59.

20 Crosson JC, Deng W, Brazeau C, *et al.* Evaluating the effect of cultural competency training on medical student attitudes. *Family Medicine* 2004; 36: 199–203.

21 Crandall SJ, George G, Marion GS, Davis S. Applying theory to the design of cultural competency training for medical students: a case study. *Academic Medicine* 2003; 78: 588–94.

22 Beagan BL. Teaching social and cultural awareness to medical students: "it's all very nice to talk about it in theory, but ultimately it makes no difference." *Academic Medicine* 2003; 78: 605–14.

23 Kai J, Bridgewater R, Spencer J. "'Just think of TB and Asians', that's all I ever hear": medical learners' views about training to work in an ethnically diverse society. *Medical Education* 2001; 35: 250–6.

24 Shapiro J, Hollingshead J, Morrison E. Self-perceived attitudes and skills of cultural competence: a comparison of family medicine and internal medicine residents. *Medical Teacher* 2003; 25: 327–9.

25 Culhane-Pera KA, Reif C, Egli E, *et al.* A curriculum for multicultural education in family medicine. *Family Medicine* 1997; 29: 719–23.

26 Tervalon M, Murray-Garcia J. Cultural humility versus cultural competence: a critical distinction in defining physician training outcomes in multicultural education. *Journal of Health Care for the Poor and Underserved* 1998; 9: 117–25.

27 Silins E, Conigrave KM, Rakvin C, *et al.* The influence of structured education and clinical experience on the attitudes of medical students towards substance misusers. *Drug and Alcohol Review* 2007; 26: 191–200.

28 Lindberg M, Vergara C, Wild-Wesley R, Gruman C. Physicians-in-training attitudes toward caring for and working with patients with alcohol and drug abuse diagnoses. *Southern Medical Journal* 2006; 99: 28–35.

29 Narayan AP, Socolar RR, St Claire K. Pediatric residency training in child abuse and neglect in the United States. *Pediatrics* 2006; 117: 2215–21.

30 Hill JR. Teaching about family violence: a proposed model curriculum. *Teaching and Learning in Medicine* 2005; 17: 169–78.

31 Frank E, Elon L, Saltzman LE, *et al.* Clinical and personal intimate partner violence training experiences of U.S. medical students. *Journal of Women's Health* 2006; 15: 1071–9.

32 Matthews J, Kadish W, Barrett SV, *et al.* The impact of a brief interclerkship about substance abuse on medical students' skills. *Academic Medicine* 2002; 77: 419–26.

33 Ramirez-Cacho WA, Strickland L, Beraun C, *et al.* Medical students' attitudes toward

pregnant women with substance use disorders. *American Journal of Obstetrics and Gynecology* 2007; **196**: 86.e1–5.

34 Jonassen JA, Pugnaire MP, Mazor K, *et al.* The effect of a domestic violence interclerkship on the knowledge, attitudes, and skills of third-year medical students. *Academic Medicine* 1999; **74**: 821–8.

35 Moskovic CS, Guiton G, Chirra A, *et al.* Impact of participation in a community-based intimate partner violence prevention program on medical students: a multi-center study. *Journal of General Internal Medicine* 2008; **23**: 1043–7.

36 Espey E, Ogburn T, Leeman L, *et al.* Abortion education in the medical curriculum: a survey of student attitudes. *Contraception* 2008; **77**: 205–8.

37 Espey E, Ogburn T, Dorman F. Student attitudes about a clinical experience in abortion care during the obstetrics and gynecology clerkship. *Academic Medicine* 2004; **79**: 96–100.

12   I am Afraid as I Ponder That Inevitable End: Death and Dying

In the last decade or so, awareness that medical students were often ill-prepared for dealing with terminally ill and dying patients led to the systematic introduction of palliative care, death and dying, and end-of-life care (EOLC) curricula in all US medical schools. These curricula tend to focus on the clinical management of dying patients – for example, pain control. Psychosocial aspects of these curricula are often operationalized as specific tasks, such as "breaking bad news."[1] Encouragingly, one study reported that, since 1998, student perceptions of the adequacy of the end-of-life curriculum have improved noticeably.[2] Furthermore, some research suggests that students' attitudes towards terminally ill patients, especially older patients, are generally favorable.[3] Another study found that contact with dying patients helped students to put their own lives and priorities into better perspective, and demonstrated the importance of the therapeutic relationship at the end of life.[4]

However, many students still do not feel well prepared or supported as they care for dying patients.[5] In one study, although students valued preclinical end-of-life courses, they emphasized the importance of training during actual inpatient care experiences in which teams could openly acknowledge impending death, role-model humane end-of-life care, and respect students' participation in patient care.[6] In fact, however, these ideal circumstances do not always materialize, and students often experience significant role confusion in EOLC.[7] Another study comparing student satisfaction with EOLC curricula in the UK and the USA found that students in the latter country evaluated the culture of medicine and the attitudes of physicians as significantly less supportive of the importance of such training.[8]

Here, too, the hidden curriculum exerts a considerable influence. One study documents discordance between what is taught about EOLC in formal coursework and what actually happens on the wards.[9] Students frequently complain of an absence of appropriate role-modeling and guidance from residents and attending physicians. An earlier study of third-year students found that 41% had not observed a physician talking to a dying patient, 35% had never discussed care of a dying patient with their attending physicians, and a large majority had never witnessed a surgeon telling a family that someone had died.[10] In a more recent small study,[11] 25% of students who experienced a patient's death as highly emotionally charged rated the amount of support they received from supervisors as extremely inadequate. There was no discussion of the death in 63% of the cases in which the patient was cared for by the student's team. Based on their attending physicians' responses, students concluded that death and emotions were regarded as negative aspects of medicine.

The extent to which students feel an emotional readiness to confront end-of-life issues in patients and to actually put into practice critical moral attitudes[12] is debatable. Some evidence suggests that it may be easier to teach students specific knowledge and skills relating to management of dying patients than to influence their emotional responses to these same patients. For example, after a brief EOLC intervention, students showed significant improvements in competence and knowledge, but not in attitudes towards death and dying.[13] Students themselves express a great deal of worry and uncertainty about EOLC,[5] and recognize the importance of receiving guidance in terms of managing their own strong emotions in response to death and dying,[6] and developing appropriate coping strategies.[14]

Like most people, medical students are susceptible to fear of death, and identify their greatest concerns as fear for significant others, fear of the dying process, and fear of the unknown.[15] They also experience many other complex emotions in the course of caring for dying patients. Although one study found that student attitudes towards dying patients are typically characterized by attachment, empathy, and advocacy,[6] another study reported a variety of student emotions, ranging from feeling connected and joyful to being sad, anxious, and frustrated, and struggling to balance emotional connection and distance.[4] Students may also experience feelings of guilt, fear, blame, and impotence in the presence of dying patients.[9–14] Another paper noted students' tendency to avoid or deny the sadness, hopelessness, and helplessness that they associated with dying individuals.[16]

One project[17] asked students to visualize their own death and to write reflective essays about their experiences with regard to death. Analysis of this work revealed that students were concerned about appropriately expressing emotions, dealing with personal grief and emotional detachment, communicating effectively with patients and family members (including listening to patients and respecting their decisions), spending enough time with patients and families, and shifting the emphasis from curing to caring. Another study that used a range of arts-based reflection modalities showed that students used these tools to explore their own fears of death, their helplessness in the face of the dying process, and at times their discomfort with the medical heroics that are engaged in with a view to extending life. They often searched for meaning in how patients died.[18]

When medical students write poetry about death and dying, they focus on many of these same issues. They are especially concerned with examining their emotions and how to be in relationship with dying patients.

After All By: Pierangelo Renella and Matthew Donnelly
Originally appeared in Plexus, *2001, p. 24, UC Irvine School of Medicine*

In a darkened room now you gasp for air
All that's left is your fading sight.
You never thought that you could be this scared
Your final day becomes your first night.

This faded struggle crept into my world
Burrowed deep beneath my skin.
Have these hands failed their most sacred trust?
Why go on fighting when no one wins?

CHORUS
(After all) After all you've done for them where are they now?
(After all) After all you've given them they should be here!
(After all) After all we've done for you all hope is gone.
(After all) After all . . .

This haunting memory lay soaked with fear
Hours saved were fraught with pain.
The thought hangs heavy on this guilty heart
Release this sorrow, keep me sane.

You search for meaning in the window pane
Friends and lovers roll across your eyes.
Your shortened time helps to keep us sane
While broken wings take you to the sky.

CHORUS
(After all) After all you've done for them where are they now?
(After all) After all you've given them they should be here!
(After all) After all we've done for you all hope is gone.
(After all) After all . . .

In this co-authored poem, two students describe their own feelings of helplessness when, "after all we've done for you," the patient is still dying. The poem touches on many aspects of death and dying that are reflected in other students' writing as well. The first stanza empathically focuses on the patient, addressing him* directly in the second person. In so doing, the narrator(s) acknowledge the closeness of the relationship. Here, the narrator honestly imagines the suffering and fear of the patient, who is face to face with his own death. The predominant image is one of darkness closing in – a darkened room, sight diminishing, and perpetual night imminent. The other image is fear – a recognition of overwhelming dread.

In the next stanza, the focus shifts to the narrator. He turns from the patient's predicament to his own. The patient is now referred to in the third person ("this faded struggle") as the student becomes conscious that the patient's dying process has permeated him as well. The boundaries between the living and the dead, the sick and the well are suddenly perceived to be frighteningly porous and penetrable, as the world of the patient blends with the student's world and creeps under his very skin. This sense of contamination leads to further distancing – the narrator proceeds to talk about "these hands" as opposed to "my hands", and wonders whether "they" have failed the "most sacred trust" of preserving life. Guilt, however, is quickly replaced by cynicism and bitterness: "Why go on fighting when no one wins?" This line also suggests the level of investment that the student has made in the patient's recovery. Not only is the patient "not winning" by dying, but also the student is losing a cherished role as healer, hero, and savior.

The chorus that follows mentions both "you" and "them" and "we" and "you." The first set of pronouns is without clear referents. They could refer to the patient ("you," returning to the second person), and to friends and family members ("they") who were the recipients of the patient's care and concern, but who have abandoned him now that he is dying. However, another interpretation is possible. The pronoun "you" might also refer to doctors who have done so much, and sacrificed so much for their patients ("they"), yet after all this effort, all these resources of time, energy, and caring spent, the poem asks, "Where are they now?" Where are those patients? The implication is that they are all dead and gone. This interpretation receives support from the following two

---

* I have arbitrarily designated the patient in this poem as "he."

lines, which seem to refer more clearly to the students and the healthcare team ("we"), and petulantly laments that "After all we've done for you," instead of a restitution story and a happy outcome, "all hope is gone."

While the chorus represents a resentful crying out against the unfairness of the universe, the following stanza returns to the theme of foreboding. The narrator's memory of this patient's dying is "soaked in fear." This phrase may convey the patient's fear, which has already been established. However, it may also describe the student's own fear in recalling his patient's death, perhaps as he wakes from a nightmare soaked in sweat. Again the boundaries have blurred. Patient and student share the fear. Similarly, the next line suggests that the "hours saved" – perhaps the brief prolongation of the patient's life through aggressive medical intervention – were "fraught with pain." It is not clear in this case who was suffering, and it is quite likely that, like the fear, the pain in this case belongs to both patient and student. Next, the student returns to his feelings of guilt ("this guilty heart"), still unable to approach his own feelings directly and continuing to refer to himself in the third person. The thought of the patient's suffering is a heavy responsibility; and the narrator implores someone (the doctors, perhaps, or God?) to "release this suffering" (an example of synecdoche, in which suffering stands in for the patient), not only for the sake of the patient, but also to preserve the *student's* sanity!

In the final stanza, the narrator once again adopts a position of intimacy with the patient, now addressing him directly as "you." Yet there is only imperfect resolution at best. The patient is "searching" for meaning, but there is no indication that he has found it. A window-pane reflects only the patient's own face, nothing more. Friends and lovers pass before the dying man's eyes, but the word "roll" connotes a casual insignificance. Even at this critical juncture, the narrator cannot maintain focus on the patient. Again the narrator reverts to the importance of keeping "us" (perhaps the medical team, or the two medical students writing the poem?) sane, even if it is at the price of the patient's "shortened time." True, the spirit of the deceased patient ascends heavenward, but it is on "broken wings." In dying, the patient has been damaged, and so has the student. It is not too much of a stretch of the imagination to suggest that the student also feels that *his* wings – perhaps the wings on which he intended to ascend to physicianhood – have been irreparably harmed.

DEATH OF LOVED ONES
Chaos stories

Sometimes students meditated on the death of loved ones, usually grandparents or parents, in their poetry. Often these poems are a cry for help. Death is portrayed as the end of a futile struggle and, in many cases, as long overdue. The emotions expressed in these poems include sorrow, grief, loneliness, separation, and loss. One student writes of missing the smells and hugs of a friend who died of leukemia, and states that when she died she "took my soul." Many of these poems focus on the suffering of family members who survive. The authors long for peace, but cannot find it. One poem employs the metaphor of night as the narrator's jailer and bed as her prison as each night she tries to break free from her grief.

In another poem, bearing the title "Forces," the narrator learns of the death of a loved one. This poem explores the many meanings of force, including the double entendre of a "grave force" – at once both serious and fatal. When the narrator hears the news, "All at once, the world is too heavy / For me to stand / . . . No strength against gravity." The play on words continues: "I carry flowers to your grave / But I cannot stand / The paucity of you / Here I am prone / To wish for your return." The author begs: "I seek the strength / To fight these grave forces." An analogy is drawn between the force of gravity and the force of loss, which weighs down the narrator. The poem explores the contrast between "prone" and "standing" – laid low and erect. The force of the grave is "powerful, heavy, enduring." The poem is an embodiment of the overwhelming impact of death.

Restitution stories
Occasionally students tell a restitution story about the death of a loved one. These poems suggest that death brings not loss but release. In one such poem, the death of the narrator's loved one is peaceful, natural, and "just as I'd want it to be." In another poem, the narrator's encounters with nature evoke memories of the deceased, and she hopes that for her loved one the vista now is "even more beautiful."

One student writes about the death of a physician-relative – someone dear to the student, as she has inherited his stethoscope. The poem memorializes the loss of a good physician (his "healing hands") who has now returned to dust. The tone is melancholy, fragmented, and forlorn, yet there is a sense of continuity, a passing of a revered profession from one generation to another. The poem has an air of restitution through its focus on systemic continuity and restoration of normalcy.

Transcendence stories
Once in a while, personal losses are linked to patient deaths. In one such example, a student writes about the death of his grandmother. He uses this loss to consider that every patient who dies is someone's mother, grandmother, son, or father. This poem is an example of transcendence in which the student's own tragedy triggers a sudden awareness and empathy.

DYING PATIENTS
Students encounter dying patients through hospice programs, and on hospital wards. Students' narrative choices in reflecting on these patients run the gamut from chaos and helplessness to journey, witnessing, and transcendence. Notably in the minority are restitution stories, since death has vanquished the ability of medicine to restore. Student poetry examines the patient's helplessness and fear, the student's own disappointment at the limits and futility of medicine and the need to act in the face of death, the normalcy of death (and rejection of that normalcy), connecting with patients, and particularly the need to support a humane death with dignity, and larger speculations about death.

Chaos stories
Patient futility and helplessness
In contemplating the dying process, students can concentrate on the patients' sense of being trapped, their helplessness and their hopelessness. This perspective tends to produce chaos stories. One such poem, written in the voice of a patient with lung cancer, focuses on the "genetic programming" that led her to develop this disease, like music written on a page or like "being dipped / in a water I will never dry off." Here the dominant metaphor is a sense of being ensnared, unable to escape or be rid of her disease.

Another patient is described in the language of the medical chart as a "65 yo white male" with end-stage cirrhosis, hypertension, multiple small strokes, divorced, estranged from his children, and in an unstable living situation. Although he tries to put his affairs in order, especially with his children, it is too little, too late. The poem uses a poignant analogy to the Cubs baseball team (the patient is a Cubs fan) who "make it to the National League play-offs / and lose the pennant 3 games to 4." The patient is overtaken by death just at the point when he is making his life mean something. In this poem there is no tidy, happy ending. Everything is crumbling, even the patient's efforts to put his life in order.

Student futility and helplessness

Many students wrestle with a personal sense of helplessness that arises when they realize that medicine cannot always cure or otherwise save gravely ill patients. In this scenario, students are devastated when confronted with the limits of what medicine can do for the patient. These students seem to be operating within a narrative which states that, with sufficient knowledge, physicians can reliably forestall death. When this becomes impossible, their poems are filled with chaos. For example, one student is appalled when an 18-year-old patient dies. Nothing can be done to save her, and nothing can even be said to comfort the family. She addresses the deceased girl directly: "But [no words] would come / What could be said? / So I got on with the day / And you were still dead." The restitution story of heroic medicine has been shattered, but there is nothing to replace it.

Several of these poems describe Code Blues (resuscitation of a patient who has gone into cardiac arrest). A Code Blue can generate excitement, even panic in a lowly third-year student. The student's initial assumption is that this is the ultimate assertion of medical power in the face of death. As one student describes his response, he was "flying like a jet that is stealth", his goal being "to prevent death." However, when the patient is pronounced dead, he feels helpless and doesn't know what to do. Another medical student is wracked with helplessness when a DNR patient codes: "I am screaming for us to do something." In both of these poems, the students are confronted with the limits of the restitution story and the limits of medicine. They have no alternative stories that are satisfying.

In another poem about a code, the student describes his initial exhilaration. At first the patient, an 82-year-old man with aspiration pneumonia, looks as if he is going to survive. Then he becomes unresponsive. The resident asks for "suggestions," then "objections," and finally calls the code. The student is shocked, disbelieving, dumbfounded, and numb. The residents begin to joke about the patient, and the chief resident counsels the medical student not to be offended. Paradoxically, the student is not offended, but relieved: "I don't mind / It's a relief to hear them do it / Because I cannot." The student struggles with his feelings of surprise, sorrow, awe, and "unaccountable loss." His initial exhilaration has been replaced by emptiness.

The chorus of another poem reiterates the theme of "mourning" because medicine cannot help the woman who dies of a myocardial infarction, the young woman who loses her sight in an accident, or the child diagnosed with leukemia. Seeing all this suffering, the student concludes: "What can I do? Watching their plight / Mourning am I tonight."

One student begins by listening to a patient's physical signs, motivated by curiosity, "anxious to learn of your condition." However, when she realizes that the patient is terminally ill, the student listens for something that will provide hope, a better answer. Finally, unable to face the devastating implications, she refuses to listen at all to the doctor's grave pronouncement, delivered in harsh, painful language, because it means the end of any possibility of survival.

In another chaos poem, the medical student must convey the diagnosis of a terminal illness to her patient. The student's words transform the patient into something hopeless, but the student herself cannot feel their sting and hurt. She sees the effect of her news in the collapse of the patient's shoulders, the pain that pools around the patient's eyes, in the patient's trembling hands, and the beating of the patient's heart. The student, however, feels only "numb, nothingness" when she has to say goodbye. She both literally leaves the room and figuratively abandons the dying patient. This poem is a cry for help. Confronted by the futility of action, the student is unable to comfort or provide solace. She is in as much despair as is the patient.

Another student must break bad news to a patient with cancer. The student feels helpless. She is able to tell the patient only that she will have surgery tomorrow, but she is unable to discuss the difficult prognosis, or present the complete picture to the patient. At first the student is unable even to wake the patient. She whispers reassurance, but does not believe her own words: "How can I comfort your crumbling body?" Medicine can intervene, but it cannot always save. In this chaos story, the student is at a loss as to how to approach the patient when she cannot tell a restitution story. In a similar chaos poem, a student delivers the bad news of a terminal diagnosis to a patient, an old World War Two veteran. The student is overwhelmed because, unlike the patient, who "knew nothing of limitations," and was counting on his "new doctor" as his last hope, he knows that there would be no Yanks coming to rescue this "old soldier," he knows how little medicine can offer him.

One poem describes a patient undergoing surgery for advanced-stage ovarian cancer. Everyone knows that this procedure can postpone but not prevent her inevitable death. The patient is a sweet-natured, pleasant woman, and the poem implies that such a death is unfair and wrong. This cry for help protests that there is no meaning or fairness in death. In another poem, set in the room of a dying patient, the attending physician says, "there is nothing that can be done." The medical student is incredulous, and wonders how this is possible in view of all the amazing advances of modern medicine. These poems are cries for help because the students feel strongly that something should be done in these scenarios of death and dying, and yet there seems to be nothing to do. Unlike witnessing, these poems are not able to take a position (for example, to side with the patient), but instead focus on the student's own anxiety and frustration.

Students rarely find meaning or "naturalness" in the deaths of children. These poems offer no answers, and express anguish at the perceived senselessness of these deaths. For example, one such poem is in the form of a eulogy for a child who has died from cancer. The poem focuses on the following: "an outing to the beach/brings eternity seemingly within reach . . . /we believe we can/Take it, keep it in our pockets along with M&M's and satin ribbons." "They [the mother and child] both suppress/and hold the torture" of pain and impending death. This poem acknowledges that dying cannot be held at bay, but only postponed by a passing moment of normalcy. One poem adopts the viewpoint of the mother of an infant who dies at 27 days. It is a hopeless situation from the start. There is no comfort, "there is only pain from the/sounds of dying at 26 days", and there is no celebration, "there is only anticipation of/unknown tragedy before day 27."

The following poem is a lament about both the limits of medicine and the tragedy of a child's death. The narrative line of this poem starts off with a bone-weary but dedicated team of physicians rushing to the rescue of a dying child, priming the reader's expectations for a heroic restitution tale. We are apprised of the severity of the situation by the images glimpsed in passing – a pediatric cancer patient surrounded by the signs of his disease and its treatment, as well as his "preoccupied mother," foreshadowing the dying boy and stoic mother who are the team's ultimate destination. The team quickly arrives at the child's room, where yet more medical personnel are assembled, guided by their leader who has situated them strategically "to ward off evil spirits." The boy behind the curtain (number 3?) is actively dying, bleeding from multiple causes that the narrator carefully enumerates, each phrase a reaffirmation of medical helplessness. In a further ironic twist, the narrator adds a refrain from a child's song about the wiggling, jiggling spider, to describe the cancer devouring the boy. In the concluding lines, we learn that although the team worked valiantly throughout the night, in the end they were unable to ward off death. The narrator adopts a passive, medicalized voice to describe "everything else tried" (by whom?) that ultimately proved futile. The pervading tone is one of helplessness and failure.

Peds Onc Consult By: Brian McMichael
Originally appeared in Plexus, 2006, UC Irvine School of Medicine

It's late, on-call-tired
we dash into a third-floor room
for a cross-cover page
as always both ceiling-mounted TVs are on
tuned to separate channels.

we whisk past a preoccupied mother
the boy standing there with those foreboding
sparse wisps of hair
infused with too many lines
running from as many IV bags
hanging starkly on a wheeled pole

we round a curtain to find
a squad of posed action-figures
resolutely standing guard
strategically placed by their leader
to ward off evil spirits

slumped rag-doll sideways
a pale, pale, thin boy
with dark-crusted, cracked lips
blood slowly seeping from purple little bumps
here and there

The shiner he sports
you wish
was from getting punched
but it's not, it's

from the rock-bottom platelet count
from the cancer
from the treatment
from the chromosome
from the mutation
from the virus
that wriggled and jiggled and wiggled inside him

the mom calmly consents to the platelet transfusion
which along with everything else tried through the night
will not save him from bleeding out
even till morning.

Restitution stories

Religious beliefs are the most common way in which students find some kind of restitution when confronting death and dying. Here the tragedy of death is superceded or annihilated by one's belief in God and the promise of heaven. In one poem, the patient dies on a Sunday, "almost time for church/As if she knew, or possibly God was ready, to take her home." Others rationalize that "it must have been her time to go." Some students accept that life "at any moment . . . could be His [God's]."

In the following poem, the student feels helpless about his inability to save or even help "severely sick" elderly patients. In an encounter in which the narrator must confront death across a cultural divide, he initially feels a similar uselessness. However, when he prays with the patient's son, his sense of meaning is restored.

Spirit of Medicine   By: Jaime Rosa-Duque
UC Irvine, 2003

I was only a volunteer, a volunteer who knew nothing about prescribing medicine
a volunteer seeing severely sick geriatric patients again and again
a volunteer with emotions I wished I could jettison.
Then, one day, an Egyptian lad sat by his dad
He told me about his life and his eyes were sad
I wished I were a doctor who could write him a cure on a notepad
And even though I lacked this skill he didn't care
Because all he asked of me was to help him in prayer
And together we spoke to God for his father whose fate
      in imminent death we are naysayers
Thereafter, both he and his father felt much better through our shared ritual
That from that day on, I became convinced the power to cure
      is much more spiritual.

A different poem contains chaos elements, but ultimately attempts to tell a restitution story through the idea of the soul going to heaven. The student is distressed by the patient's terminal condition, the callousness of his residents, and the fact that "nothing can be done" to save the patient's life. The student attempts to balance his feeling of helplessness, and his sense that "kind words" have little real value, by rationalizing that the patient is bound for "a better place."

Yet another student is deeply troubled when he encounters in one ER cubicle the child victim of a drunk driver, and in another cubicle the driver herself. The poem hints at the unfairness of the outcome. The driver is already recovering, while the innocent child's fate remains uncertain. Confronted with the medical system's inability to correct this injustice, the student "says a prayer" and vows to "drive more carefully." In this poem, the narrator attempts to regain a sense of control over the random nature of suffering both through an appeal to a higher power and through his own efforts. The title may allude not only to the (hoped-for) recovery of those involved in the accident, but also to the student's belief in the fairness and rightness of the world.

Recovering from a Trauma By: Roy Nambudripad
UC Irvine, 2003

Into the emergency room, I enter with great excitement.
At the bedside, I stand with much amazement.
On the gurney, a little victim calls out for her mother.
In the adjacent trauma room, a drunken woman shouts with anger.
By the side of the girl, a calm resident begins to examine her eyes.
Next to the junction of the two rooms, my mind suddenly begins to realize.
Out on the roads, an accident took place.
From my own thoughts, redness began to fill my face.
Before the final minute of my shift, the older woman begins to recuperate.
For the future of the little girl, I can only contemplate.
During my exit, I complete a prayer
Towards the outside world, I drive with care.

In a somewhat atypical poem, a dying child reflects on the patches of her grandmother's quilt, each one being different, but when assembled together telling a story. The patches are like the pieces of her life. She feels as if she has "discovered a pattern / And wonders why it makes me smile, and others cry." She looks forward to being reunited with her grandmother in death, and being free of pain. She hopes that the quilt will be a reminder and a comfort "for those I leave behind." The poem reflects an acceptance and even positive anticipation of death. It is unusual in that it tells a restitution story in which the child's death is a blessing.

Witnessing stories
A few poems that address the futility of medicine in the face of death adopt a more witnessing attitude. The title of another poem, "a little short of breath," refers to the apparently innocuous symptom of a patient who is discovered to have widely metastasized and untreatable cancer. The medical team is helpless in the face of this devastating development that has sneaked up on both patient and doctors in a quiet, almost quotidian way. The poem uses the metaphor of bicycling to suggest the wheel of life and the inevitability and power of death. The tone of this poem is not as desperate as a cry for help, and is closer to a witnessing of the inevitable cycles of life and death, and how all too often even physicians must stand as observers of this process, rather than healers.

a little short of breath By: Lorena Hillman

Originally appeared in Plexus, *2001, p. 38, UC Irvine School of Medicine*

a little short of breath
you told the resident
that's how you felt a
couple days ago
on your usual
daily five-mile
bicycle ride

fine before then, no problem at all

you hadn't had any
trouble breathing no
chest pain or other
pain no wheezing or
fever or racing heart
or swollen ankles

quit smoking 10 years ago

realized you didn't have
to continue your
20-year habit
girlfriend didn't like it

stupid waste of
money anyway

    saw some blood when I went to pee

never saw that before
so after a couple
days decided you
might as well come
in to see the doctor

anyone you'd like us to call

we asked after seeing
the report of a
grapefruit-sized tumor
overtaking your bladder
mets to the lungs and
not just a few

    one day cycling
        one more two more
            three more turns
                of the wheel
                next day gone.

In another poem, a patient is dying of cancer, and the team repairs a defective rectal tube which has allowed the patient's feces to leak all over the bed. The poem focuses on the futility of this intervention: "And we held her on this earth one more night / And we signed out, proud we did our job, / a Victory, no one died on our shift." The poem mocks the unstated norm that it is a "failure" for a patient to die while one's team is on, but if the patient dies on the next shift, the earlier team is exonerated of responsibility. This poem demonstrates the limitations of medicine in that the medical team cannot save the patient's life – they can only save their own reputation. It also ridicules the insularity of their worldview because, despite the tragic outcome, they are "proud we did our job." The tone of this poem is one of resistance. The student refuses to accept that the futile actions of the medical team are meaningful.

CALLS FOR MORE LIMITS TO MEDICAL INTERVENTION
Witnessing stories

Although many students are dismayed by the inability of medicine to always ward off death, many other students have the opposite reaction, calling for *more* restraint in the treatment of dying patients. Students in this position ask the ethical question, in the title words of one poem, "Just because we can, should we?" These poems describe terminally ill patients who are ready to die, but who are being kept alive by extraordinary technology. These poems most often take the position of witnessing to the patient's distress, and align themselves with the patient against the medical establishment. In one such poem, "They told her" (already discussed in Chapter 8), a young woman who is dying of lymphoma does not respond to treatment. Her physicians are unwilling to stop the treatment, but the patient says that she has had enough: "She told them that she had to keep her body in one piece, or she would lose her soul." The doctors tell her that she is "giving in, and then they begged her to fight." What the patient craves is to die peacefully and with dignity. What the doctors demand is a prolongation of the patient's fighting spirit. In a poem with a similar message, an elderly patient with leukemia is ready to die, but is upset that his doctors are not empathetic and do not seem to want to honor his wishes. Although he did not want chemotherapy, his family insisted, and now the patient feels that he was forced by his doctors to undergo a useless and grueling treatment. In another poem, a drug addict with multiple medical problems, including AIDS, is also "ready for the fall [ready to die]", but challenges the medical team by asking whether *they* are ready for his death.

A similar poem adopts the voice of a dying patient, a Korean War veteran, who longs for the freedom of death, but his doctors won't let him go: "The white coats bully me into doing what they believe is best." He pleads to deaf ears, "Let me be that warrior you once saluted/ . . . let me be free in my dreams." The patient sees his dignity being progressively taken away from him. This poem witnesses the helplessness and despair of the patient, and his sense of being trapped by the healthcare system. It is an act of resistance against the established protocols of hospitalized death.

Dream By: Antonio Duran
UC Irvine, 1999

I wake to the thrust of metal fangs
that bleed me for information.
I try to scream

but nothing comes out. I try to cry
but the tears are already dry
My voice is parched for the blessed swab of water
My lips are cracked
but I can no longer taste the blood.
Each breath I take
is a new summit for me to conquer
Each image that passes by
is a blur of white coats and green uniforms.
     All I feel is pain
but all I want is freedom to feel it on my own.
They try to keep me
but I want to go.
They try to feed me
but I want to starve.
Starve me of this attention
for I no longer want it.
let me be free
let me be free
let me be free to dream
They try to live for me
but I already lived.
Let me go
Let me be free
Let me accept my life as it already is
The white coats bully me
into doing what they believe is best
let me live the way I want to live
I may breathe with challenge
but it still is my breath
not this tube strapped to my throat.
I try to move but you lock me down.
I try to make my life clean
but you tie my hands.
As I lie in what was once a clean bed
I witness my proud life whittle away.
Let me be that warrior you once saluted
let me sheathe my blade this last time
I want to return to my home
let me go home
let me go home
let me be free in my dreams.

Another student writes a poem about his elderly grandmother, whose lingering death in a nursing home is depriving her family of precious resources, yet medical technology persists in prolonging her life. In the particulars of his family's situation he finds universal dimensions of a larger issue, namely what are, and what should be, the limits of healthcare. In another poem, a 51-year-old patient with spina bifida has a cardiac arrest leading to a persistent vegetative state. The family wants to say goodbye, but the team keeps the patient alive. The student pleads, "Let her go," but no one listens. These poems align themselves with patients who are ready to die, but who are being kept alive by their doctors and by technology.

DEATH AS A NORMAL PART OF LIFE
Restitution stories

Patients are often seen as being ready to die, satisfied that they have lived a good and full life and can pass away with peace of mind. In some cases, the student is reassured by the patient's humor, confidence, acceptance, and fulfillment. These poems most often resemble restitution stories. Some, but not all, of these poems have a religious component. Death is normal, acceptable, and not to be feared. It is the appropriate, peaceful conclusion of life. In one such poem, the patient is ready to die. He appreciates the doctor's efforts, but now just wants the doctor to stay near "and see me through." The patient asks the doctor to hold his hand. He is no longer afraid, and he feels that he has accomplished all that he wanted to in life: "I've ran and laughed and cried and loved – now it's time to move on." If they meet in the afterlife, he will greet the doctor as his friend: "I will come to you with open arms."

Many of these patients are elderly, and are represented as having led long and meaningful lives, and as having no fear of death. One student writes of an elderly dying patient, "Ma'am, you make growing old look damn good." Another says to a similarly elderly female patient, "You are so calm/and filled with peace/No regrets/No fears/Just ready for the next phase of the journey." In another example, a 92-year-old woman prepares herself for death. She asks only to "die with dignity/To be without any discomfort, suffering, and hurt," and to have someone listen to her story. The student believes that the patient had a good death: "It is however a wonderful thing to know/That she died without any pain at all, and that her wishes had been fulfilled." In another poem with restitution overtones, a dying patient is "sent home to die." The student admires the patient's strength, hopes, and dreams, and believes that the patient's "soul lives on, a treasured memory." Although the poem witnesses to the patient's courage, it also has an element of restitution because the patient's courage seems to "balance out" the unfairness of her early death, as does her soul living on, and her memory being treasured. The attitude of students towards such patients is both admiring and grateful. These patients help to ease some of the students' own fears about death.

Witnessing stories

Some poems adopt a stance of resistance towards this comforting view. In one such poem, a patient has just received the news that he is going to die. The physician's bad news contrasts with the dying patient's vivid appreciation of each last moment of life. Ordinary activities, such as eating an ice-cream cone, hugging a baby, listening to someone playing the cello, or lingering outside with friends, become invested with great preciousness. The patient cannot resolve whether life has meaning ("To hell with what it all means"), but recognizes that "This [life and love] is so good." This poem witnesses the patient's reality – the preciousness of each concrete detail of his life – and refuses to hide behind a simplistic acceptance of death.

ACCOMPANYING THE PATIENT ON THE JOURNEY TOWARDS DEATH

Many students demonstrate great courage in their poetry when they choose to "accompany" the patient in the dying process. Rather than focusing primarily on their own helplessness and terror, or trying to restore the patient to life, they seek to stay with the experience of the patient. Some of these poems literally tell a journey narrative with their dying patients. These poems emphasize the challenges and difficulties that the student faces, as well as what they can learn and how they can grow as a result of this experience. The most common conclusion seems to be the importance of appreciating life and living as fully as possible: "Thus we have to live the best we can / and cherish and love every moment."

In a classic journey poem, a medical student chronicles the journey of a 50-year-old woman who is dying from ovarian cancer, and in the process documents her own journey from an initial negative assessment of the patient to perceiving the patient as a teacher and role model. At first the student sees the patient as angry, defensive, impatient, fearing loss of control, in denial, and with a litany of physical complaints. She relies on active planning and aggressive fighting in her stance against her disease. This patient has a strong spirit and is not afraid to express her opinion. Despite the challenges that she poses, the student is sympathetic because she realizes that the patient is "losing her place in the world . . . / unsure where to focus her energy." The "demon" patient is recognized as a profound teacher. Later the patient simultaneously resists loss of order and tries to make sense of what is happening to her. She is honest about her fear of loss of relationships and loss of self. In the end, she holds fast to her beliefs, focuses on the lessons that she has learned, and accepts death. The student concludes that it was an honor to have known this patient, and feels gratitude for the patient's sharing this last phase of her life with her. The medical student sees her patient as an example of grace, strength, and dignity, and feels that she was changed for the better as a result of knowing her. The patient has taught her about friendship, the importance of touch, not postponing life, learning from losses, and working to accept all parts of life.

Another student has a similarly intimate experience with a dying patient. In this poem, a naive medical student becomes a regular visitor of the dying patient Ben. Yet Ben is not miserable or despairing – rather, he is "spunky" and full of life. When he starts to decline, the student is forced to confront his own powerlessness and despair. Yet in the wake of Ben's death, the student realizes that he has learned a crucial lesson about the brevity of life and the importance of not taking it for granted. The format of this poem is a journey, in which death is the enemy, the dying patient acts as the guide and teacher, and the student becomes a better, wiser person (and hopefully a better future physician) as a result of the encounter.

Ben By: Danny Botros
Originally appeared in Plexus, *2003, p. 32. UC Irvine School of Medicine*

For the last few weeks I've been visiting a person I never knew
And for the last few weeks I've realized that I've learned something new
I used to take life for granted and thought that everyone around me
    was never going to pass
But now I understand that life, in essence, is short and I
    never know how long it will last

Ever since I've been visiting a person named Benjamin
It's been one of the first times where a stranger has gladly said, "Come in"
That first week I saw him, I almost felt he was unlucky
But when asked what he'd like and Ben answered, "I would love to have
    wild sex"
I knew he was feelin' spunky

In his situation, Ben as I called him, was in good spirits and uplifting
However, during the weeks, he became quieter, and I almost felt like
    he was drifting

I remember the second time I saw him in his chair, looking a little quieter, and
    paler only after a week.
I felt like I was helpless and to me things looked bleak

But, realizing that no matter how quiet Ben was over the weeks, he was always
    there listening to my voice
I knew that it was only a few days ago when he opened his door and welcomed
    me in by his own choice

At this point, there was absolutely nothing I could do
Except for trying to comfort him, and maybe whispering in his ear "Thank you"

Because I thought, this may be the last time I'll see Ben
I thought this was it, and I would never be able to say bye again

But at the point where Ben was so somber that he said nothing for the entire hour
I thought that this was the point where I had lost all power

So realizing that life may soon be coming to an end
I knew that I could be close to losing a person I'd finally considered a friend

So I bid him a farewell and told him I would be back to visit him in the
    coming days
Although I knew he was too weak and frail to even breathe out a phrase

So, on the next visit, I pulled up to the terrace and walked to the front door
Where I buzzed in my code and the caregiver asked me, "Who are you here for?"

As she opened the door for me, I told her Mr. George, and she went back to her
    desk and looked through some piles
Where she found a folder with what looked like someone's files

"Mr. George passed away on Thursday evening," she said
"Was not doing so well over the last few days," as she finished what she read

Sometimes it almost takes someone you know or befriend
To make you realize that life, as you know it, can come to an end

So when we see others we care about, including our family and friends
We have to remember to look at them in a whole different lens

In a viewpoint that helps us appreciate others in a whole new way
Because it is the memories we have of them that will never go astray.

Witnessing stories

Some of the poems that choose not to turn away from the dying patient witness to the situation of the patient, deciding to join with the patient against the other physicians and health professionals, who are perceived as uncaring and detached. In one poem previously discussed, a dying patient's eyes look "far away/To a place where nothing hurts/And rectal cancer doesn't exist." The poem describes the patient's loss of dignity – lying naked, full of tubes, leaking yellow-brown feces "for all the white coats to see." Her "sickly, pale body violated/By mutated cells and human hands both." Not only has her disease insulted her, but so have her doctors and caregivers. Her eyes represented "the last part of her life/The cancer could not reach/Because they're gone, already moved on." The student witnesses with painful clarity the price that cancer exacts from this patient, and does not attempt to whitewash the terrible nature of her dying. Nevertheless, the student remains firmly "on the side of" the patient, "against" the callous physicians, in an act of resistance. Her resistance mirrors the patient's resistance against her cancer by "moving on" to an unreachable place.

Transcendence stories

Sometimes we catch glimpses of transcendence in such poems. In one typical poem, the student is initially caught up in the excitement of resuscitation efforts. He describes in rapid succession CPR, epi injections, and cardiac charge to bring back a coding patient. Despite these efforts, the patient succumbs. An unknown person on the team mentions that the patient's son is waiting in the lobby. All of a sudden, the narrator realizes, "She has a son/She is a mom." In this moment, the previously unknown patient becomes a human being, and the student's awareness of death becomes not just an abstract concept, but reality. The last lines of the poem, in which the narrator ponders his own death, finally place the medical student and the patient on the same vulnerable, mortal, human level. The poem shows an evolution in the student from callous excitement to a more human and therefore vulnerable plane.

In another poem discussed previously, a very old woman is dying, and calling for her mother. The student realizes that the patient is following "the steps all feet will tread/the linear decay of the body." The student marvels at the capacity of the mind to "circle back" in time, "flying back" to the past, but too late. There is no mother there for the patient, only the medical student who mourns that "I am not her mother." However, in a final act of maternal nurturance, the student meets the patient's need: "I hold the downy head in my hands." This poem has a strongly transcendent quality. The student first witnesses the isolation and loneliness of the dying patient. After initial resistance, at the last moment, the student consents to boundary-crossing to hold the patient in a maternal, tender posture.

In another poem, a female patient, a former dancer, used the self-discipline of her profession to fuel her fight against death. Dying, she never spoke, but cried out her pain in a kind of "silent music." On the night when she died, the student imagines her dancing "with whispers of bittersweet peace/so exquisite . . ." Her "final bow" coincides with "the monotone wail from the EKG machine." This narrative contains elements of restitution because it represents a kind of final triumph over death, and runs the risk of romanticizing the dying process. However, it also restores an element of dignity and beauty to the patient, allowing her to reclaim her essence as a dancer in death, and it transforms the student's understanding of what death is all about.

PHILOSOPHIZING ABOUT THE NATURE OF DEATH
Restitution stories

Sometimes the encounter with death leads to wider philosophical reflections. In a metaphorical poem, life is portrayed as a comfortable but stuffy house that no one wants to leave. No one knows what awaits outside, and the narrator and everyone in the house do everything possible to stay put. However, when the narrator finally must leave, he discovers the beauty and companionship that are found "outside the house." This poem is a restitution story in that "Home" is restored to the inhabitants, and is even better and more companionable than it was before.

Coming Home By: Barry Beutler
Originally appeared in Wild Onions, *Vol. VIII, 2004, p. 29*
Penn State University College of Medicine

A HOME Safe
warm, comfortable, I think.

Light shines through the window.
Still, I feel complacent to remain in this abode.
Everyone seems to agree.
We like our little home.

Occasionally some gather eagerly around the window
peer out and discuss in trembling, anxious voices.
What would it be like to travel out there?
But we quickly turn inside
pushing the thoughts out of our minds.

Frequently
though less eagerly
some gather around the door.
Usually after someone has exited.

"Why did they go?" we regret.
"They will be happier," we comfort
though none wish to make this *happy* journey.

But what is this warmth?
And these beautiful sounds of the outside?
I've never heard such music.
Children playing on the streets, laughter
sunshine unfiltered by glass
so bright.
And so many old friends —
I've scarcely forgotten how stuffy it was
in that little house.

Witnessing stories

One poem considers the concept of time in relation to death, observing that both patients and doctors want more of it, while "Too much of it creates an uncertain dying/

Too little of it creates death." In a similar vein, another student writes about the passage of the seasons, and is consoled by the thought that although time inevitably marches on, nature is governed by a master plan. The poem uses the seasons as a metaphor for life – although it seems unfairly brief, there is a guiding plan, and life leads to life. Stepping even further back, "Ode to a Dying Bumblebee" considers the death of one small insect within the vastness of the universe, and implies that human beings aren't much more important. Reflecting on his father's death, a student struggles to come to terms with the meaning of life and death. Watching a falling star, he says goodbye to his father, and concludes "how the world loves to change / when it thinks you are no longer looking." Another poem reflects on life as beginning with birth – a miraculous, joyful, memorable event, filled with endless possibilities and hope, but inevitably concluding with sorrow, suffering, dementia, and death.

SUMMARY

Sometimes students write about the death of beloved family members or friends. These poems typically exhibit a lack of resolution, and are elegiac in tone. As the research literature suggests, the death of loved ones is a particularly fraught subject for medical students who encounter death on a regular basis. Students also frequently write about dying patients, seemingly trying to penetrate the mystery of death from the vantage point of a profession whose raison d'être is the preservation of life. In the presence of death, students often express helplessness and a sense of futility, confirming certain findings of research studies that have examined medical students' attitudes towards patient death. They have entered medicine thinking that, with sufficient knowledge, death can always be turned aside. They expect some action to be taken, and are shocked and disillusioned when this is not possible. Deaths of children are especially disturbing and hard for students to accept.

Restitution stories about the dying process often have a religious orientation, or a belief in the normalcy of death as part of life. These narratives are most likely when the patient is elderly and seems to be reconciled to death. Such poems mirror research findings that medical students have a generally positive attitude towards older dying patients. In a related vein, terminally ill patients also bring into students' awareness the need for moral limits on medical intervention, a concern that has also been documented in the research literature. However, these narratives generally take the form of witnessing, advocating for the futilely suffering patient in the face of medical heroics.

Sometimes students' poetry tries to join with the patients even as they move towards death. Research shows that, when confronted with dying patients, students recognize the importance of the therapeutic relationship, and the need to shift from curing to caring. This awareness is often represented in their poetry. For some, the patient's dying becomes a shared journey, full of life lessons. This reflects research which shows that, in the presence of dying patients, medical students often use the experience to examine their own life priorities. For others, participating in the care of a dying patient offers the opportunity to witness, to express solidarity with an event that they cannot fully understand. For a few student-poets there is a sense of transcendence, in that the initial meaning of the patient's death has become changed and elevated for the student. This may be similar to the findings of the study cited at the beginning of this chapter, which identified joy and connection as emotions experienced by students in the face of death and dying. Students also reflect generally about death and its meaning and implications, expressing variously curiosity, fear, and hope.

REFERENCES

1 Garg A, Buckman R, Kason Y. Teaching medical students how to break bad news. *Canadian Medical Association Journal* 1997; **156:** 1159–64.

2 Sulmasy DP, Cimino JE, He MK, Frishman WH. U.S. medical students' perceptions of the adequacy of their schools' curricular attention to care at the end of life: 1998–2006. *Journal of Palliative Medicine* 2008; **11:** 707–16.

3 Lloyd-Williams M, Dogra N. Caring for dying patients – what are the attitudes of medical students? *Support Care Cancer* 2003; **11:** 696–9.

4 Ellman MS, Rosenbaum JR, Bia M. Development and implementation of an innovative ward-based program to help medical students acquire end-of-life care experience. *Academic Medicine* 2007; **82:** 723–7.

5 Wear D. "Face-to-face with It": medical students' narratives about their end-of-life education. *Academic Medicine* 2002; **77:** 271–7.

6 Ratanawongsa N, Teherani A, Hauer KE. Third-year medical students' experiences with dying patients during the internal medicine clerkship: a qualitative study of the informal curriculum. *Academic Medicine* 2005; **80:** 641–7.

7 Fernandes R, Shore W, Muller JH, Rabow MW. What it's really like: the complex role of medical students in end-of-life care. *Teaching and Learning in Medicine* 2008; **20:** 69–72.

8 Hammel JF, Sullivan AM, Block SD, Twycross R. End-of-life and palliative care education for final-year medical students: a comparison of Britain and the United States. *Journal of Palliative Medicine* 2007; **10:** 1356–66.

9 Rabow M, Gargani J, Cooke M. Do as I say: curricular discordance in medical school end-of-life care education. *Journal of Palliative Medicine* 2007; **10:** 759–69.

10 Rappaport W, Witzke D. Education about death and dying during clinical years of medical school. *Surgery* 1993; **113:** 163–5.

11 Rhodes-Kropf J, Carmody SS, Seltzer D, *et al.* "This is just too awful; I just can't believe I experienced that . . .": medical students' reactions to their "most memorable" patient death. *Academic Medicine* 2005; **80:** 634–40.

12 Olthuis G, Dekkers W. Medical education, palliative care and moral attitude: some objectives and future perspectives. *Medical Education* 2003; **37:** 928–33.

13 Porter-Williamson K, von Gunten CF, Garman K, *et al.* Improving knowledge in palliative medicine with a required hospice rotation for third-year medical students. *Academic Medicine* 2004; **79:** 777–82.

14 Williams CM, Wilson CC, Olsen CH. Dying, death, and medical education: student voices. *Journal of Palliative Medicine* 2005; **8:** 372–81.

15 Hegedus K, Zana A, Szabó G. Effect of end of life education on medical students' and health care workers' death attitude. *Palliative Medicine* 2008; **22:** 264–9.

16 Block SD, Billings JA. Learning from the dying. *NEJM* 2005; **353:** 1313–15.

17 Rosenbaum ME, Lobas J, Ferguson K. Using reflection activities to enhance teaching about end-of-life care. *Journal of Palliative Medicine* 2005; **8:** 1186–95.

18 Rucker L, Shapiro J. Becoming a physician: students' creative projects in a third-year IM clerkship. *Academic Medicine* 2003; **78:** 391–7.

13 Is This the Way of Life? Reflections on Love and Life

Although medical students are interested in who they are becoming as doctors, and how their relationships with patients develop, they also write many poems that are more personal in nature, and unrelated to medicine. Students' reflections on love lost and gained and meditations on life in general are examined below.

Revelation Road By: Hala Mint El Moctar Mohammed Moussa
Originally appeared in Paint the Walls. 2005. p. 5
Weill Cornell Medical College in Qatar

When the night spreads its dark wings
And the wind allows the soft breeze to dance
Then revelation road in front of me sings
And you catch me in an unexpected trance

My eyes flicker in the sudden contentment
Of being softly kissed by the breeze
My spirit skips into one gait excitement
As the stars titter at the brush of the palm trees

A mosaic of passions tampers with my emotion
A multitude of tunes plays with my voice
My soul ascends with the swinging motion
Of a desire to feel a renewed sense of rejoice

I yearn to carve every moment's inspiration
On the scales of every passing palm tree
I wish to enclose every heartfelt sensation
For I'm me no more, or is this really me?

In this poem, the narrator experiences a moment of "revelation" – a sense of at-oneness with the night, the breeze, the stars, and the palm trees, all of which are enlivened and personified through a kind of synesthesia. The night spreads its wings, the breeze is dancing, and the road is singing. The narrator is kissed by the wind, and her spirit skips in response. The sibilant, alliterative "s" sounds soothing and comforting, as the stars giggle at the soft touch of the palm trees. Like the road, her soul itself lifts its voice as it rises with "desire," the élan vital that motivates and fills our existence. She is filled with contentment, excitement, passion, rejoicing, and inspiration. In losing herself, she finds her essence: "For I'm me no more, or is this really me?" It is a memorable moment of mystical union in which the narrator becomes one with the natural world around her, a transcendent expression of the poet's conviction of the interconnection and interrelationship of all life.

THE ANGUISH OF LOST LOVE
Chaos stories

When contemplating the end of love, many poems express anger. A narrator wants a lover, yet resents the inevitable risks and vulnerability that he must assume. The poem uses the metaphor of putting his "heart on a fork," and anticipates that the process necessarily leads to broken-heartedness and tears. One poem refers to "pretty girls" who "make you feel like nothing," who play with young men, excite them, "make us idealists," and then drop them "while we moan and die." Another poem describes a couple engaged in a destructive romantic relationship. The woman has a false façade, and is devious and manic. She "disarms and disables." Their dream, "a chancy dance of romance," has become a nightmare. In yet another example, the narrator compares his lover to a rose, but also acknowledges her beauty as a dangerous flame which burns with both love and deceit. The narrator takes pleasure in the lover's pain and disappointment, which are as sweet as sugar to him. He enjoys his revenge because her beauty wounded him deeply. Another poem describes a decidedly unromantic interlude in a prison-like motel room where the shade jams open onto the interstate, providing a "drive-by peep show." They have sex like "captured animals" – she "never came faster." The scene is bleak and unfeeling. Whatever love had once existed has vanished.

In a poem entitled "Ode to the Peach," patterned after a poem by Pablo Neruda, the narrator celebrates the delights of a peach, while simultaneously using it as a metaphor to extol the pleasures of a sexy, desirable woman. However, like a woman, the fruit can betray him by becoming overripe, then "stinking and attracting flies / then I can't stand you." At the core, the disappointed poet finds not a heart, but only "your hard little brain."

Ode to the Peach By: Brian McMichael
Originally appeared in Plexus, 2006, UC Irvine School of Medicine

You are called by your color
but during the summer
you become sun-tinted
taking on to yourself
the prerogative of the redhead
and on the inside too –
the deeper you go the redder you get
intensifying to the color of blood

My soft, fuzzy love
you fill my hand
with your yielding
rounded density
you invite me with
your voluptuous curves
your feminine little cleft

Your succulent sweetness
evokes in me the desire to
delve into you
to eat you

to eat you until your juice
runs down my chin
I will not want to stop
once I start

Even when I sink my teeth
into your luscious flesh
you make only the sound
of a heart between two beats
tasting nearly like nothing
delicate with a hint of fragrant sharpness

In the late summer
your overripeness
falls to the ground
becoming oozy, squishy masses
like dung —
stinking and attracting flies
then I can't stand you

Even into the autumn
You are inescapable
your slices unexpectedly peek at me
from my bowl of milk
you cruelly snuggle
into my ice cream
and usurp every dessert —
shamelessly splayed
atop the tarts, the cobblers
the pies for all to see

Fruit of the Deep South
alone in the dark winter
I break down
tormented by
your one solid defect
that when I had finally
arrived at your core
I found your hard
little brain
where your heart
should have been.

Witnessing stories

Other poems about lost love have elements of both chaos and witnessing. These poems are sad and mournful rather than angry. A representative poem addresses a former lover. Now that the lover has gone, the narrator is filled with grief. The poem uses the metaphor of a bleeding heart that sheds "rose-colored tear drops" that fall into a lake the size of the narrator's sadness.

Another poem also mourns lost intimacy, and expresses the narrator's yearning and need. He acknowledges that "now is after" – he is stuck in a present that will always be defined as "after" love and companionship. Consumed by memories at once beautiful and painful, he savors what is irrevocably lost to him.

Ghost By: Stefan Samuelson

Originally appeared in Reflexions, *Vol. XII, Spring 2005, p. 69*
Columbia University College of Physicians and Surgeons

I loved someone completely then
But now is after
Standing in the shower with the water slipping over my shoulders
Soft-scented candlelight whispering through the curtain
I remember the simple intimacy of you washing me
I press my eyelids together to brighten the memory
And savor what it was like to need so unhesitatingly

One student complains of being alone for too long, and hungers for human touch, the warmth of another, the passion of intimacy. She knows that often the pleasures of the flesh do not contain much truth. Still, she is willing to settle for lies, "shadows of what's real," if only, through these lies, she can reclaim some feeling. A woman describes a failed love affair. Although she made many sacrifices for her lover, she could not relinquish her religion. She feels "older than beach and sea . . ." She knows that she will one day be "the hollow apparition of a whisper at sunrise." Another poem sadly recognizes that the object of the narrator's devotion does not reciprocate his feeling, but instead casts a "withering breath" on his burning desire.

A poem to a former lover laments that this person cannot sustain a "friendship built on mutual trust, respect." The narrator remembers "the wonder of the love we shared," but regretfully recognizes that "It was just not enough." The poem uses images of a "rift" opening up, and parallel tracks that have "started to digress" which create a sense of distance and separation. Another poem documenting the death of love acknowledges that the narrator cannot pretend to something that is no longer there. The ex-lover wants reconciliation, but it is too late to recall their dreams. To renew the relationship would be "so absurd." This poem is a witnessing of the death of a relationship. A similarly themed witnessing poem describes a fight between a couple when their old car breaks down in the desert. The image of a souvenir Navajo jar shattering on the pavement is a metaphor for the shattering of this relationship.

Another witnessing poem about a lost love sees the features of the former lover in various random encounters. The narrator recalls that, in physics, it is possible to "calculate the end of motion." The poem, of course, is filled with ordinary motions – paying for whiskey, looking in a rearview mirror, loading groceries into a bag, pouring coffee. Each of these motions has a beginning and an end. Finding the features of her lover on these random faces, the narrator recognizes the end of the emotion that she once felt for this man.

I found your nose By: Sarah Mourra
UC Irvine, 2005

I found your nose
In an Oakland bar
On a homeless man who paid for whiskey
with
three speckled green pears

I found your eyebrows
In a Barstow gas station
On a teenager who stared
Through the shattered glass of his rearview
mirror

I found your hands
At the market yesterday
On the clerk who asked me
Paper
or
Plastic?

I found your mouth
Down the street
On the dark-haired man who bites his lip
As he pours my coffee

My physics teacher said
We can calculate
The end of a motion

I looked down at my notes
And saw
The end of emotion.

THE MIRACLE OF LOVE GAINED
Chaos stories
Many student poems are paeans to the joy of love, and usually tell witnessing, journeying, or transcendent stories. Occasionally love, although positive, is so overwhelming that it produces an experience of chaos. In one such poem, in the presence of her lover a young woman wants to laugh to express her joy, but only small lip twitches and tears come. She babbles mindlessly with her lover, but never says the words that she needs to say. Language is inadequate in the presence of love.

Restitution stories
The fear of loss of love can produce the bliss of restitution. In one such example, the narrator dreams turbulently of her lover's death, only to wake and realize that he is still alive. The simple sound of the water running in the bathroom fills her with giddy joy. When she discovers that she has not really lost him, she rejoices in his physicality and aliveness, and recognizes that "I have meant to tell you things." Like encounters with actual death, the nightmare motivates her to tell her love.

Dreaming Your Death By: Karen Wong

Originally appeared in Reflexions, *Vol. XII, Spring 2005, p. 42*
Columbia University College of Physicians and Surgeons

I.

The footsteps and whispers in this old deaf house
are not mine.
I am searching
for the point your gaze is holding.

Yesterday, you still tossed
and caught your heartbeat in your hand
as soundly as I now breathe.

When I believe your wax hands and your sunken blood
my breath punches its way out
to settle over your lips.

2.

Light buzzes.
My knots unravel in a shudder of laughter
and I'm still shaking.

The faucet in another room
is all I want to hear.
Each drip reminds me:
this is what it is to be awake, this is what it is to be alive.
I think I have meant to tell you things.

3.

I have wanted
to turn your palm with both hands
find your pulse
and kiss it beneath the skin.

Journey stories

Many students perceive themselves to be on a relational journey, facing and overcoming challenges in partnership with the beloved in order to achieve the reward of love and commitment. In an example of a journey poem, one student struggles with fear and desire, but believes that it is only by standing together with his romantic interest that "another day" will arrive. In a poem that reaches a similar conclusion, the author draws an analogy between a personal relationship and the glass cotton used in the chemistry lab, which is both supple and delicate, but is also capable of cutting and drawing blood. The poet realizes that although a relationship is risky and hard to handle, self-protective strategies that are appropriate in the lab can destroy the mysterious connection of love. One poem draws a parallel between the necessary maturing in the educational process and the equally necessary maturing in an intimate personal relationship. Both involve a journey full of sweat, blood, and tears. But there is an emergence, a coming together on the other side that is rewarding and uplifting. A female student writes a humorous poem about marriage from the perspective of the husband. In this poem the narrator lists all of the challenges and limitations of marriage – it's like a job, full of sacrifice and inequity, but all of that is more than balanced out by love. In the concluding stanza, the narrator becomes serious, and admits that he could not exist without his being in love with his beloved, and her being in love with him. In these and similar poems, love involves trial by fire, but the narrator comes away with greater wisdom and commitment.

Transcendence stories

There are many examples of transcendent poems that emphasize the unity of self and other that can be found in love. In one such poem, the lovers are separated geographically, but are "never alone / United in spirit, we remain one." A similar poem speaks about the souls of lovers being imprinted one on the other. Although physically separated, they are absolutely devoted: "I don't love you because you're beautiful / You're beautiful because I love you."

Another poem describes two soul-mates who have been restored to each other. The author complains that the lack of each other "erodes holes in my soul." The souls of these lovers walk in matched strides, have "interlocking daydreams," "shared thoughts . . . / reflecting faces / knowing our minds are in precisely the same place." They are perfect complements.

Restitution By: Elizabeth Ballard
Originally appeared in Panacea. *Summer 2005. p. 2*
University of Florida College of Medicine

Longing for indulgences whose lacking erodes
holes in my soul
eyes scanning, ears straining, hands searching
hearts draining
pouring out silent thoughts splitting
running out lost
saving for the drops that land
just right
on the senses of the soul whose stride matches mine
interlocking daydreams like fingers clasped tight
together we sit as if in our own
solitude
heavy silence of shared thoughts
smiles creep across reflecting faces
eyes dancing, heartbeats racing
knowing our minds are in precisely the same place, space
without form or dimension
the greatest thought knowing its complement is.

In another transformative poem, love opens the poet to "a world of dreams," new feelings and desires. At the end of the day all she wants is to hold hands with her lover and say "I love you." A different poem reflects on the narrator's intimate relationship, and realizes that the two of them are filled with love and trust. They are intertwined, their relationship electric, "real." The narrator admits that "I am remade in your gaze." With this lover, she becomes all that she can be. The narrator of another poem calls his lover Eve, to suggest the Garden of Eden nature of their love. Their love transcends life and death: "we were ready to go afar / Beyond the limits of life and death . . . / Ready to make our hearts ignite."

In another example of a transcendent narrative, the narrator describes her lover floating in water. The narrator joins her lover, and their union is described as both beautiful and overwhelming. They "sink and drown, dissolving / into little fragments of sea." Love dissolves entity, even the separateness of selves. The poem also suggests the inevitable cycle of love and death. The final stanza describes fish shaking the dust of the lovers' disintegrated bodies from their scales. In this poem, love survives and transcends their death and dissolution, diffusing throughout the water.

Love and the Lake By: Sheila Chan
UC Irvine, 2005

You, cradled in waves
that fill your crevices, embrace your hairs
stroke your scabs.
Water delicately encircling their edges
easing them off
smooth.

You, bob gently so as not to disturb
the spaces between the surface and your body.
I wade in carefully
softly turn you over
brush my fingers, leaving
gentle trails of warmth in your skin.

Beauty, floating fragile on the surface.
The quiet precision of lips coming together
eyes gently closed.
As the water opens up, revealing
unveiling an enormous black expanse.

Water, a huge liquid envelope
folds of water surround us, raise foam
gulp us whole.
And wrapped in each other we
sink and drown, dissolving
into little fragments of sea.

The fishes, covered in emulsion
shake the dust of us off their scales.
Little orange lights, yellow pearls.
And again, calm water
undulating like layers of fresh silk, glowing
full of love.

In a final example of love as transformation, the narrator uses the insistent repetition of the title line to emphasize the themes of desire, sensuality, and ultimately transcendence. The poem mixes tropes and metaphors to create imagery of vivid passion. However, mere passion is insufficient to represent the narrator's feelings. The lovers will be transformed into seasons, into tempestuous weather, and even into insanity. Through her lover, the narrator is not only enlivened, but also connects with her life force, "the energy of [her] soul." In the presence of her beloved, she becomes most fully herself.

It's you that I want to come see By: Pouneh Nasseri
Originally appeared in Plexus, 2008. *UC Irvine School of Medicine*

It's you that I want to come see
I will wear cherries as earrings
Color my lips with velvet red roses
It's the scent of jasmines that I will wear as my perfume
And flames of fire as my garment

It's you that I want to come see

I will come and take you with me
As we become fall
Fill up the streets with a harvest of love
Be the storm, become the rain
And slowly, become insane

It's you that I want to come see
So I could breathe in your scent
Taste your nectar
Become alive a thousand times with your touch
And feel in harmony with the energy of my soul

It's you that I want to come see

So you could remind me of the woman that I am
So you could show me the beauty and secrets of love
So you could make me feel good
So you could let me trust

It's you that I want to come see

You are the secret of hope
You are the glory of the morning
You are mysterious like the ocean
You are fulfillment of all my sensations

It's you that makes me feel life's vibrations
It's you that has made me forget all my temptations
It's you that lets me be me
It's you that I want to come see.

HOW TO LIVE LIFE
Chaos stories

Other poems ask larger questions about the meaning of life. Occasionally, these are chaos narratives. A young man is poised "on the edge of life/ready to jump out." He appeals to a supposedly wise guide (none other than Sigmund Freud), but the help that this individual can offer is limited. Although the narrator's thoughts have been analyzed and he understands all of their symbolism, he is still afraid. Symbolically, his penis is "limp." He is afraid to take the next significant step in his life.

Restitution stories

Other poems tell heroic restitution stories. One student-poet refuses to accept Hemingway's conclusion that life breaks even the strong. He has survived the death of his parents, and asserts "That in the end I'll always soldier on/That I will always fight to feel alive . . . /So when you say life even breaks the strong/I hope that in the end I'll prove you wrong." This student believes that he will be able to overcome even the most adverse circumstances.

Journey stories

Sometimes students use an explicit journey metaphor to reflect on the meaning of life. A representative poem is a meditation on the nature of humankind from a developmental perspective, from birth through to maturity. The poet reflects that we are delicate and frail, "fearfully and wonderfully made." As we grow and learn, we "gain knowledge of the good and evil around us/Within us", and "With much knowledge, comes much grief." Humans are both good and evil, generous and selfish. They exhibit sacrifice and devotion as well as anger and rage. They are capable of love, but it is "fragile, delicate and frail." Our life exists within the context of the hope and promise of faith, an enduring love that sustains us through life and keeps us "when this journey comes to an end." In this case, religious belief is the "wise guide" that gently teaches and corrects as the individual confronts the challenges of life. Another poem tells the story of Icarus and Daedalus. In the author's view, the soaring of the son on his wings of wax is worth the inevitable descent. In this telling, the myth becomes a confirming metaphor for how to live life, with daring and openness to experience, because death is inevitable.

Witnessing stories

In asking these larger questions, students often sound a cautionary note, or express resistance to "established" views. These poems warn that all too often we are on the wrong path, misconstruing our priorities in life. One poem criticizes people for always rushing, for not stopping to appreciate the beauties of nature, for pursuing success, and for playing "this [stupid] game." The student-poet emphasises the importance of making the most of our short time on earth – not by making money, or surrounding ourselves with material things, but by valuing the qualities of love, respect, and appreciation of beauty.

Another poem speculates about the indifference of most people to seeking the larger meaning (if any) of life. They are oblivious to its inexorable ebb and flow, the endless cycle of birth and death that surrounds them, and seem completely absorbed by their quotidien routines. The narrator cannot decide whether life is a question, a test, an experiment, an illusion, or simply a meaningless struggle.

I wonder . . .   By: Sajeda Lamia Azad
Originally appeared in Paint the Walls, *2005, p. 36*
Weill Cornell Medical College in Qatar

The sun shines every day
No matter what happens
Life goes on (as usual)
Everyone goes their own way.

It's like an odd omen
Life ebbs and flows, like the water
Never-ending, merely appearing to stop
Only to deceive the human.

But, can it be perceived
That within this stream
Births take place and deaths do happen
But to those unconcerned, this idea is never conceived.

Is this the way of life?
Or is this merely a test?
A question, an experiment, which leads to some final result?
Or just an illusion, reality being an ongoing strife?

In another poem, the narrator describes the cycle of life in terse first-person subject/ simple past-tense verb rhyming phrases. Each developmental milestone and phase of life is contained in a single straightforward verb. The poem suggests the mundane ordinariness, insignificance, and impermanence of life, and the inevitability of its ending. The poem is not a despairing cry for help, as it contains an element of gratitude ("I thank / I sigh"). Although the structure of the poem can be seen as the form of a journey, its absence of mentors and valuable lessons makes this poem closest to witnessing. It expresses appreciation for life's experiences, but also admits to their randomness and ultimate meaninglessness.

Life (56) By: John Grace
Originally appeared in Scope, *Vol. VII, Spring 2000*
Southern Illinois University School of Medicine

I swam
I birthed
I came
I nursed.

I cried
I saw
I learned
I crawled.

I stood
I walked
I played

I talked.

I schooled
I cared
I jumped
I shared.

I drove
I kissed
I fell
I missed.

I left
I dormed
I grew
I formed.

I loved
I wed
I worked
I bred.

I changed
I burped
I watched
I heard.

I helped
I taught
I threw
I caught.

I left
I strayed
I wept
I stayed.

I sold
I aged
I moved
I ached.

I lost
I quit
I mourned
I sit.

I look
I think
I breathe
I stink.

I thank
I sigh
I close
I die.

Other poems also reflect on the arbitrariness and potential meaninglessness of life. In a typical example, a poem meditates on the haphazard nature of interpersonal connection and opportunities that are lost forever. Another poem is a philosophical witnessing of the random way in which life "switches" (with the rapidity of a light switch?) from light to dark, from friendship to hatred, from peace to war, and from good to evil. Love is here one day and gone tomorrow. At the point of conception, future life contains infinite possibility and promise. However, once the haphazard determinations of gender, race, and (future) victim or aggressor are made, much of what will follow suddenly becomes predestined. The narrator is conscious that even right and wrong can change with the flip of a switch that alters the point of view from which it is considered. In the end, she wonders whether reality is only a matter of perspective.

Switches By: Roya Saisan
Originally appeared in Plexus, *2005, p. 37. UC Irvine School of Medicine*

It's dark inside
Just in my head?
In my room, the building?
Or has the world
lost sunshine altogether?

Switch

Now I see light
But where does the light end
and Darkness begin?

We laugh together today
We walk, talk, hold hands
We love and cherish.

And then there is
Tomorrow
How to know
What tomorrow will bring

Turn

Perhaps an enemy who was
the friend
To despise, hate and
Obliterate
A country with the push of a
button
A friend with the trigger of
a gun

Or a glance from the corner
of your eye

Before the baby
There is no one
A seed, a hope
perhaps

Birth
and the world is here

Flip a coin —
Black or White
Male or Female
Victim or Aggressor

Right or wrong?

To me
or to you?
Everything changes
Depending on your view

Through a microscope
Or a telescope
Or 20/20 human eyes
Are these just the evils of
time and space
Or our own deficiencies

To
Stop
To think and to feel
Before the switch is made to

Real

Or is it
Real only to you?

Sometimes these philosophical reflections acknowledge the oneness of humanity, but find it to be a broken and flawed unity, as imperfect as the individual him- or herself. In the following poem, which is narrated in the first-person voice, the speaker presents himself as proud and invincible. He is the "spirit of life" that impels us all forward, the embodiment of desire that motivates him towards peace, harmony, and contribution to the world. However, as the narrator looks deeper, the tone becomes more modest. He admits that he is only "normal" and "human." He still speaks for the world, but now he speaks for ordinary humanity as well. In fact, he is just like us. Like everyone, he has struggles and difficulties. Doubts and obstacles complicate his life. Although he is filled with desire and élan, he also knows boredom, sadness, and a sense of worthlessness. When we truly "look from the inside," being human is composed of all these elements.

Look from the inside By: Jon Kea
UC Irvine, 2003

I am the world.
I am infallible.
I am the conqueror.
And I am the spirit of life.

I Desire to be content.
I Desire to be at peace.
I Desire to be in tune.
And I Desire to be productive.

Indecisive describes me.
Normal describes me.
Human describes me.
"Like you" describes me.

I have struggles.
I have difficulties.
I have doubt.
And I have barriers.

Boredom consumes me.
Sadness consumes me.
Sleepless night consumes me.
And Worthlessness consumes me.
I am the world.

Another witnessing poem describes the sculpture of a god without hands. It has an "immortal, impoverished/Beauty" that is a symbol of his frailty. The sculpture represents a perfect body worn away by time. The poem implies that time and life will inevitably wear us down and reveal the brokenness behind our perfect facades.

Transcendence stories

Some students' reflections express what their narrators experience as the mystery and oneness of life. In a poem titled "Snapshot from the Clouds," the narrator sees life as full of contradictions and mystery. The universe, no matter how thoroughly it is analyzed by scientific methods, remains ultimately impenetrable. Following a similar theme, another poem addresses a "rationalist" who believes only in facts, the laws of nature, and predictable patterns. To this person, the universe is "pure, simple, sensible, and true," describable and knowable. The narrator, by contrast, appreciates trust, mystery, and what is unknown.

In a light-hearted poem titled "Flow," the narrator invites the reader to join "the flow," get "cool and mellow." She advises that when you can recognize that "all is one," "You'll find yourself inspired/Refreshed, at ease, fecund." By relaxing into the oneness of life, you are renewed. In a poem with a similar theme, a sunset triggers one student-poet's plea to consider reaching beyond our limited self to the oneness of all things. The poem advises the reader to acknowledge the sorrow and anguish, pain and guilt within them, and then to look beyond this suffering to the "bright purity of joy." The student realizes that "the beauty of a sky with sunset" lies within, and counsels the reader to "peer inside."

SUMMARY

Like poets throughout the centuries, these medical students wrote poems that expressed the anguish of love lost, and the transformational, transcendent possibilities of love found. When students contemplate the nature of life, occasionally they express fear or see themselves on a heroic trajectory. More often they choose to witness to the absurdity and randomness of life, or to be in awe of its mystery and connection.

14 *Strangers in a Strange Land: What Matters to Medical Students on Their Journey and How They Tell About It*

Medical students tell stories through their poetry. They use these stories to try to make sense of the new world in which they find themselves, and the new relationships they must learn to navigate. They interrogate significant rite-of-passage experiences, such as the anatomy course, their first patient, death and dying, patients from different socioeconomic and cultural backgrounds, and how issues of social justice intersect with the practice of medicine. They try to figure out who they are, what they are losing of who they were, and who they might be becoming. They pay attention to both negative and positive physician role models in terms of what they should be learning and what they should be avoiding. They are not afraid to directly examine their own experience with patients, and often see patients as their teachers and guides, as well as their companions on an often-challenging journey, and even occasionally as their enemies. Although student poetry focuses on the experience of becoming a doctor, for these students it is part of a larger project of understanding themselves as people, reflected in their exploration of their most intimate relationships and on occasion the meaning of life itself.

Within every content theme, I found evidence of a range of different narrative typologies. Regardless of whether students were focusing on their experience in anatomy, their treatment at the hands of their supervisors and teachers, or their own patient encounters, they wrote many chaos poems that were essentially cries for help. These poems gave voice to students' shock, bewilderment, confusion, and fear at the gap between their idealized expectations and the realities of medicine and medical training. These students offered their raw struggles without resolution. Students were most likely to tell chaos stories when they were reflecting on their own personal experiences (whether as a person or as a medical learner) or those of family members and loved ones. In particular, students' experience of *being* medical students evoked a sense of chaos. However, it is important to note that, *through the very act of writing about chaos*, this work necessarily assumed an element of witnessing. In effect, one could argue that students writing chaos poems, at least in part, were witnessing to their own chaos. Thus it is important to attend to chaos stories for at least two reasons. First, medical educators should take note of the prevalence and intensity of distress that medical students experience – distress that is often minimized or normalized. Secondly, either spontaneously or when offered the opportunity, medical students have the capacity to productively reflect on their own disorientation and wretchedness. Such awareness is an important first step towards healing.

Many poems also took the form of restitution stories. In response to chaos, a natural impulse is to restore order – to demonstrate, at least to oneself, that everything is under control and makes sense after all. It must be noted that restitution stories in and of themselves are not "bad" or misguided. In fact, a case could easily be made that most people desire restitution stories if they can get them. In the absence of any independent, contextual information about the situations that students described in these poems, it is impossible to know whether a given restitution poem is an accurate representation of the student's experience, or a psychological defense mechanism fulfilling a hoped-for fantasy. Both can be true, even at times within the same poem reporting the same event. All that can be concluded is that the authors of these poems wanted the following: cadavers to be at peace with dissection and mutilation; the painful, stressful, and pressured demands of medical school to be meaningful and ultimately rewarding; patients to be grateful and happy; dying patients to have lived good lives and be reconciled to their deaths; and doctors to be benevolent experts who could usually put the damaged patient back together again.

Although the meta-context for most of these poems was the overarching metaphor of students embarked on a journey of acculturation into medicine and a discovery of self-as-doctor, poems depicting particular journey stories were not too prevalent, perhaps because these types of narratives generally take an overview perspective over time, and most student poems focused on a particular discrete event. Journey poems asked "What can I learn?", and acknowledged that the student is embarked on an inevitable process of growth and change. Most of these poems included some or all of the classic elements of the journey narrative – the reluctant every-person hero (usually themselves), challenges and obstacles (in the form of stresses and pressures), monsters and demons (ranging from insensitive attending physicians to death itself), wise guides and mentors (sometimes physicians and residents, more often patients), trials and testing, and eventually important lessons learned that enable the student to return to society better equipped to provide succor and service.

Students writing journey poems accepted, at least implicitly, that part of the medical education experience is identity formation, and saw themselves as growing in both knowledge and wisdom. The focus of a journey story ultimately tended to be on the hero (usually the medical student) and how this individual had suffered, grown, and risen to the challenge. Thus journey stories, although containing companionship and group identity, remained above all stories of the self. Journey poems often had elements of triumphalism in that they generally intimated that whatever collateral suffering occurred along the way was made worthwhile by the achievement of their increased knowledge and understanding.

Not every student experience is a restitution story, nor can it always be framed as a triumphant journey. It is greatly to students' credit that they so often told witnessing stories, in which the focus was not primarily on their own distress, or their own growth, but on a clear-sighted and honest seeing of experiences that were complex, ambiguous, and could be understood differently from multiple perspectives. Whether students are witnessing to their own experiences as learners, to interactions between doctors and patients, to their own relationships with patients, or to injustices in the healthcare system or wider society, they often adopted a position of resistance. They rejected the dominant narrative and, in an act of courage, adopted countervailing positions. These sometimes involved questioning the nature of medical education, challenging the ideal of professional detachment, choosing to identify with and advocate for the subjugated patient rather than the high-status physician, and acknowledging rather than covering over the suffering and isolation of some patients. When students concentrated on their own difficulties and treatment, they often seemed unable to move beyond chaos. However, when their attention shifted to the suffering of patients, in a surprising number of poems they chose not to turn away, and not to support what they perceived to be moral limitations in the status quo. Rather, their decision was to give voice to those who often were voiceless.

Finally, occasional poems assumed a transcendent tone. These differed from journey stories in that they were epiphanic, the result of a moment of grace, and they involved less specific lessons learned than a sudden transformational shift in the way that the narrator understood the world and him- or herself. In this type of poem there was a kind of alteration in consciousness. These poems sometimes expressed a sense of common humanity in which divisions of "doctor" and "patient" were less important than their shared predicament of the human condition. Such poems often contained a healing element as well, sometimes for the patient, but most prominently for the student. They were often imbued with a sense of awe and wonder.

Below I shall discuss the intertwining of content themes and narrative typologies in more detail.

ANATOMY

Restitution emerged as an important narrative for exploring the anatomy experience. Students were aware that they were creating an imbalance in life, doing something "forbidden" in ordinary society. They were anxious to right this balance, to reclaim order and stability. They looked for permission, encouragement, and forgiveness, and in their writing they often imagined the cadavers supplying these attitudes. Restitution was also achieved on the student's part by promising to be respectful and to make use of the knowledge they gained for the benefit of others. Another variation of the restitution story was the dehumanization of the cadaver, which reinforced the sense of clear boundaries and reduced the cadaver to a teaching tool or object. Although students hoped for restitution, when they contemplated the act of donation in particular, their poems often assumed an element of chaos because they had difficulty accepting that, despite having given informed consent, the donors would really have agreed if they had known what would happen to their corpses. However, even these poems usually took a restitution turn, imagining the cadaver as ultimately happy with his or her choice.

Other poems, in which the cadaver served as guide and teacher, a benevolent and wise companion along the path, were more like journey stories. They possessed the defining elements of a reluctant hero (the student), brave and generous companions (usually the cadaver, but sometimes their peers), challenges and obstacles to be overcome (sometimes exams and knowledge acquisition, and sometimes the sense of violation and brutality), mentors and guides (again, sometimes the cadaver, but occasionally the instructor). These poems also had the requisite archetypal ending in which the hero, having learned and grown, was now able to contribute their greater knowledge to improve the larger world.

When students imagined the life of the cadaver, the poems were closer to witnessing because the focus was less solipsistic and the students were not so much trying to resolve something as trying to honor and move closer to the life that had passed. A number of poems expressed identification with the cadaver. These were poems of resistance and witnessing in the sense that they rejected the hegemonic view of clear separation between living and dead, student and cadaver, and instead attested to the blurriness of these boundaries.

When students explored their emotional reactions to dissection, their starting point was often a cry for help. However, the directions that the poems then took were various. Some continued to reflect lack of resolution, and remained in a state of chaos, especially those who experienced unremitting guilt about the act of dissection and those who sought resolution through emotional detachment. Others evolved into a restitution mode. Still others seemed to find a kind of grace in the experience of dissection that surpassed restitution and moved into a transcendent narrative of awe and wonder.

As the symbolic introduction to the profession of medicine, anatomy poems showed students struggling to maintain a sense of normalcy, rationalizing the disturbing aspects of their experience. Yet particularly when they shifted focus from self to cadaver, I found students beginning to witness to the experience of others and to express solidarity with them. Even at this point of beginning, students sometimes expressed awareness of a transformative, transcendent dimension to the practice of medicine.

BECOMING A DOCTOR

Poems exploring this theme often reflected on the stresses of medicine, the suffocating environment, the negative ways in which the student was changing as a person, and feelings of loneliness, self-sacrifice, fear, exhaustion, and being overwhelmed, exploited, and at times humiliated. In the title of one poem, medical school became "the end of innocence" – an all-consuming process that stripped the student of their previous identity. Especially when the student was the target of uncaring or demeaning behavior by residents and attending physicians, the most typical response was a cry for help containing confusion, hurt, and anger. At times the movement of the poem was either towards restitution (stress rationalized because the student was learning important information, or was being inducted into the secret society of the profession) or more occasionally towards transcendence (for example, when the student was able to place their own suffering within the context of the greater suffering of patients).

Knowledge acquisition itself was often perceived as a problematic issue. Most students found the quantity of learning to be overwhelming, and they responded variously with cries for help, restitution, and resistance. Towards the end of the third year, students often wrote restitution stories that acknowledged their growing knowledge, competence, and self-confidence. There were also journey stories that embodied the sense of the student acquiring special, privileged knowledge, developing new perspectives and ways of seeing as a result of the process of becoming a doctor. Some of these journey poems evolved into narratives of transcendence, which involved experiencing transformative insights into life, death, and medicine. Other poems, which were in the minority, represented resistant counter-narratives in the sense that they rejected the dominant story of an upward path to success and competence. These students recognized that the complexity of physicianhood included pretense, limitations, and actual error. Their poems expressed doubts about their training, and even questioned their decision to pursue medicine as a career.

In contemplating the process of becoming a doctor, student poets sometimes recognized explicit journey elements, particularly in terms of passing the torch from parent or mentor and fulfilling obligations to family and culture. As their understanding of medicine expanded and deepened, student narratives become more of a witnessing to the complexity and multi-dimensional nature of the experience. At times, students invoked spiritual and religious support to assist them on their path. These poems usually took the form of either restitution (faith compensating for their doubts) or transcendence (grasping larger meanings beyond their own lives and difficulties).

BECOMING A PATIENT

When students probed the patient experience, their stories took many forms. Students heard patients' pleas for compassion, and acknowledged their fear, pain, and suffering. Sometimes in the process the students themselves sank into chaos, overwhelmed by the tragedies around them. Sometimes they resorted to restitution stories as a way to counteract the patient's suffering and despair. However, often they were able to simply serve as a witness, in the sense of opening themselves to the experiences of their patients. These poems attempted to record the patient's experience while preserving the patient's dignity. Many of them combined chaos from the patient's perspective with the act of witnessing, which students seemed to feel as a kind of moral obligation when confronted with the patient's suffering. These poems uniformly demonstrated deep understanding of and empathy with the patient's perspective, and willingness on the student's part to see their patient's situation, and not to rationalize or shy away from it. Some of these witnessing poems took a position of resistance, in that they rejected labels and stereotypes often applied to certain categories of patients (such as "noncompliant," overweight, or drug-abusing patients), and looked for the patient's humanity. These poems unabashedly aligned the student with the othered, unacceptable patient, even at the risk of separating from the high-status representatives of the medical establishment.

Many of the poems that considered the experience of child patients (and occasionally their parents) told stories of restitution, and these works were particularly likely to cast the pediatrician in a heroic, curative role. However, the predominant narratives that were told about sick children and their families were in the form of witnessing. Despite, or perhaps because of, the innocence of children and the injustice of their suffering, students rarely told chaos stories in these situations, but instead expressed solidarity with child patients, affirmed their worth, and paid tribute to the strength of the parent–child bond. However, when the student became the patient, the poems often descended into chaos (reflecting the student's feelings of being out of control, isolated, and abandoned) or restitution poems (in which an omnipotent physician restored the frightened student to health).

DOCTOR–PATIENT RELATIONSHIPS

Student poems acknowledged both positive and negative physician role models as they observed the way that their resident and attending teachers interacted with patients. Many of the poems written from a positive perspective told restitution stories, in portraying a competent and caring doctor who restored health and wellbeing to grateful patients. It seemed from the student viewpoint that there was a strong appeal for a positive role model to be associated with a happy, curative ending. Occasionally these positive renditions of the doctor–patient relationship adopted a journey typology, in which a journey towards either recovery or at least understanding was taken by the patient under the wise and compassionate guidance of the physician. Other journey poems involved growth and transformation for the physician. Poems about positive role models also favored witnessing, acknowledging moments of connection and commitment between doctor and patient, and the healing power of relationship. These variations showed students' flexibility in defining "good" role models, in that they recognized that being a successful role model was not completely dependent on positive (in the sense of curative) outcome.

Overall, there were many more poems about negative physician behavior than about positive behavior (with the exception of descriptions of pediatricians). When the relationship between doctor and patient was perceived as a negative one, the poems used the form of either chaos or witnessing. In other words, students either lost their reference points in the face of negative role modeling by physicians, or more commonly felt compelled to bear witness to such behavior, rather than simply allow it to disappear unacknowledged. Witnessing poems gave voice to the patient's pain exacerbated by an uncaring physician, and also at times witnessed the patient's resistance, or that of the student, to such behavior. Overall, these poems represented the student's decision not to ignore or turn away from inappropriate, unprofessional, and insensitive behavior, even when it was manifested by a superior. They condemned the physician and often instead chose to identify with the patient, who was in some way ethically or emotionally harmed by the behavior in question.

STUDENT–PATIENT RELATIONSHIPS

Students engaged with conviction in examining their relationships with patients. When students wrote about their connections with patients, they wrote some chaos poems, but mostly their narratives described journeys or witnessing. Journey poems described fighting off the demons of disease or uncaring residents, and the student growing in wisdom, insight, and maturity. These poems often cast the patient in the role of wise teacher, and in this sense were similar to certain anatomy poems with a restitution slant, in that the patients' bravery and acceptance helped to reconcile and reassure the student in the face of suffering, pain, disability, and death.

Probably the most common narrative type used to explore connection with patients was witnessing, in which students were unafraid to identify similarities between themselves and their patients, and also admitted to seeing family members and loved ones in the faces of their patients. These poems of witnessing recognized and even embraced parallels between patients and students. Often the witnessing opposed the student and patient to the institutional hospital culture that seemed to oppress and victimize them both. When students transmuted feelings of solidarity with patients into becoming patient advocates, their poems veered more strongly into restitution narratives. In these poems, it was through the student's heroic interventions that the patient was restored to dignity and significance, or conversely, the student was restored to a meaningful and valuable role. However, students who adopted an advocacy role also told stories of journeying, witnessing, and transcendence, as they discovered the moral rewards of speaking on behalf of a disenfranchised other.

Occasionally, students wrote poems about their immersion in the triangle of patient, family members, and medical team. These poems could be cries for help, in which the student was overwhelmed by the complexity of the dynamics. A rare poem adopted an anti-restitution tone in blaming the parents of pediatric patients for standing in the way of treatment. Other poems simply bore witness to the collateral suffering of parents, spouses, and family. Occasionally, these poems expressed a moment of transcendence, in that the student experienced a transformation in consciousness as a result of contact with the patient and/or family.

A critical issue for students was where they chose to position themselves on the continuum of emotional detachment and emotional involvement in relation to patients. Emotional connection was perceived as essential, but also as frightening in its ability to overwhelm and consume students. Students feared that becoming involved with patients would damage not only their objectivity but also their ability to function emotionally. For this reason, this issue generated many chaos stories, as students struggled to perceive clearly what they needed to do for themselves and for their patients. At the opposite end of the spectrum, emotional connection with patients also led students to moments of transcendence, and sometimes catapulted them into a deeply felt experience of true doctoring.

However, other witnessing poems recognized that the connection between student and patient was complex and imperfect, and acknowledged that the self can never fully comprehend the other, and that at many points the student's and the patient's priorities, agendas, and paths diverge. Students were aware that as many, perhaps more, facets of life separated them from as connected them to their patients. At times they felt trapped by their patients, yet guilty about their ability to escape from the hospital when their patients could not. These contradictory feelings often led to poems of chaos. At the opposite end of the emotional continuum, students observed their emotional detachment from patients, mostly in a form that witnessed their encroaching lack of feeling, and worried about valuable parts of themselves being lost, much as they had during anatomy. Student mistakes vis-à-vis patients (generally errors of attitude rather than skill) were generally reported through witnessing poems. Students seemed to be able to reflect nondefensively on these errors, perhaps because at this stage of their training there was not too much at stake (i.e. they did not have the level of responsibility that would literally endanger patients' lives).

When students were frustrated or annoyed with patients, they tended to frame their emotions in terms of chaos, "anti-restitution" stories. In these poems, restitution of health and wellbeing seemed just beyond grasp because of the "willful" resistance of the patient, who was portrayed as their own worst enemy, paradoxically the primary obstacle to the student (and medical team) delivering good medical care. However, students also frequently witnessed to the limitations of their patients, and approached their imperfections more philosophically. In these poems, acknowledgment of patient flaws did not interfere with commitments to compassion and providing quality care. Occasionally such poems had a transcendent quality because the students were graced with an epiphanic insight through contact with a patient that enabled them to put their personal troubles and trials into perspective.

MEDICINE AND SOCIAL JUSTICE

When students contemplated the injustices of wider society, which overall happened infrequently, they generally adopted a perspective of witnessing, expressing resistance to materialism, poverty, hunger, the dilemma of undocumented immigrants, and war. At times, students also considered the intersection of social issues and healthcare, describing the health consequences of inequitable access to care, alcohol and drug addiction, various aspects of family violence, and unwanted pregnancy that they observed on a daily basis. These stories were occasionally chaos narratives, when pervasive, systematic suffering overwhelmed the student's sensibilities, but more commonly they were witnessing narratives, in which students called attention to the relationship between social wrongs and their job as student-physicians. Generally speaking, students identified with the poor, the underserved, and minority and immigrant patients who are often penalized by the inequities of the healthcare system. However, students from outside the dominant culture tended to speak with greater authority and passion. Students who were members of the dominant culture were more likely to express frustration and irritation with regard to the additional difficulties created by lack of a shared language with certain patients.

DEATH AND DYING

As students struggled with death, both of their own loved ones and of their patients, they tried out various narrative styles. Some students resolved their anxieties through restitution, either by describing the medical team's heroic actions in (temporarily) forestalling a patient's death, or by endorsing the belief that death itself is natural, or a prelude to a better life. Some wrote poems that were chaos stories, cries for help. These students were frightened, helpless, and confused, and had a sense of futility as a result of confronting the reality that medicine cannot ultimately triumph over death. They expressed despair not only at the biomedical limitations, but also at the emotional limitations of physicians who seemed to abandon or withdraw from chronically ill and dying patients.

Other students demonstrated an attitude of acceptance towards the limitations of medicine. Their poems tended to take the form of witnessing, and suggested that physicians can compensate for limitations through compassion and presence. In an interesting twist, some students wrote about the need for the profession of medicine to impose limitations on itself – to ask not what it *can* do, but what it *should* do. These poems sided with terminally ill patients who did not want further treatment, and often expressed resistance to medical models that continued to pursue apparently futile interventions which deprived patients of dignity and control.

Still others viewed their involvement in the patient's dying process as a kind of journey that they undertook with the patient, in which the student learned important lessons about the value of life from their patient. Others chose to take a position of witnessing, acknowledging the tremendous pain, helplessness, and suffering of patients and their families, without attempting to rationalize or restore dignity. The deaths of children in particular provoked a response of witnessing. These deaths seemed impossible for students to rationalize or to normalize – all the student could do was stand with the child's and family's suffering. Sometimes, in the presence of death, students were able to write poems of transcendence in which they were inexplicably moved to awe in the presence of the tragedy and unexpected moments of grace at the end of life.

LOVE AND LIFE

Students, like poets throughout time, wrote about love, sometimes expressing the chaos and despair of love lost or failed, and sometimes celebrating its transformative power. At times students also asked themselves the "big" questions about how to live life, and whether it is a random or meaningful process. They explored many narrative approaches for reflecting these imponderables, sometimes through giving voice to feelings of chaos, sometimes seeing life in journey terms, sometimes portraying restitution in the sense of triumphing over difficult life events, and sometimes in improbable moments of wonder that created glimpses of a larger coherence and meaning.

CONCLUSION

Medical students are indeed strangers in a strange land, and this is at once their vulnerability and their strength. Like all people, they try to make sense of their new, awe-inspiring, sometimes frightening and always bewildering lives through storytelling. They show remarkable good sense and fortitude in identifying what really matters in their training – the remarkable event of anatomy that is their "no-looking-back" initiation into a weird and wonderful world, the mysterious and poorly explicated process of becoming a doctor, how to adapt to losing parts of themselves even as they grow into other parts, determining which kinds of knowledge are important and which are not, deciding which individuals are worthy to be their role models and who are the residents and doctors they must not become, and the multiple, ever-changing, amorphous experiences of people who are actually sick, suffering, and dying, and whose lives, like theirs, may well be changing for ever. Perhaps most importantly, in surprising numbers, students have the courage to look long and hard at their own relationships with patients, trying to sort out complex and nuanced dimensions of emotional proximity and distance, connection, detachment, advocacy, solidarity, and even rejection. Students grapple with the core inequities of the healthcare system and go toe to toe with death. They even find time to write about love, society, and the meaning of life.

In wrestling with these core issues, medical students explore various narrative typologies that probably both reflect and shape their understanding of their experiences. Not surprisingly, when the issues that they examine strike closest to home and their anxieties are highest, such as when they are talking about their own stress, confusion, and despair, students often resort to chaos stories. Medical educators may underestimate the suffering and distress of medical students, or rationalize it as normative. Chaos poems help us to confront this dimension of student life, and perhaps take more responsibility for ameliorating it when possible. Students can also look for quick fixes in restitution stories, trying to speedily put back together worlds that have, Humpty Dumpty-like, shattered into fragments. These neatly constituted realities are populated with exhausted but heroic medical students, wise, beneficent cadavers, and grateful patients who are cured under the hands of competent and in-control physicians. Such narratives make perfect sense amidst the many and often intense challenges that confront medical students. Restitution stories are by no means inappropriate. However, they may create emotional dysjunction when they are told inappropriately, in a way that does not authentically support the truth of a situation, or when they are told in a way that skims over important complexities and lack of resolution.

As a medical educator, I believe that what may be most noteworthy about the analysis of these poems is that, amidst their own difficulties and fears, time and again these students reported engaging deeply with their patients (more often than not in the absence of role models demonstrating how to do this), undertaking arduous and uncertain journeys with them, or simply committing not to turn away from them, and to do their best to record and witness to their suffering. Students were also receptive to moments of "grace" in medicine, when they allowed their profession to touch their soul. This potential for journeying, witnessing, and transformation in students' pursuit of becoming physicians is at once inspiring and humbling. At the very least, it reminds those responsible for educating and guiding these students not to get in the way of their searching intellects and open hearts. And at best, these insights into students' authentic grappling with their socialization into medicine should encourage medical educators in turn not to shy away from their ethical and moral obligations to these young doctors, but rather to step forward in solidarity with the idealism and high aspirations that they express.

Postscript: Writing Rings Around Death

It would make an interesting calculation for some graduate student in English literature to figure out how many poems have been written about death since the introduction of the written word. Even without a definitive answer to this question, it is obvious that poetry and death have a long shared history. Perhaps it is because when we have nothing else left, when we have run out of remedies and medicines and interventions, we still have words. They offer only an imperfect resistance to the inevitability of our own annihilation, but since they are all we have, we wield them as best we may.

I came to writing poetry in middle age, or perhaps it is more accurate to say that I came back to it. I had compulsively scribbled poems since childhood, only to abandon this pastime in college, when what I conceived to be real life overtook me. However, when various illnesses beset my children and my parents, and my body gave the first twinges of the aches and pains common to midlife, I turned again to the written word for clarity of understanding and also for comfort. I wrote about my own illness episodes, and those of my family. When my best friend died of breast and ovarian cancer, I wrote about that, too.

After I discovered for myself the healing properties of writing (how you can be miserable and in pain, write a poem about that pain, and afterwards still have exactly the same amount of pain but feel surprisingly better), and found these verified to some extent by the research literature,[1,2] I began to introduce writing into my own professional work with medical students. Building on existing models of reflective and point-of-view writing in medical school,[3,4] I encouraged my medical students to write about their patients, in poetry as well as in prose. I thought that writing poetry might help students to understand their patients – and themselves – from an entirely different perspective, through metaphor, image, symbolism, allusion, and indirection,[5] as well as liberating them from more conventional narrative forms of self-expression. On the whole, the students responded enthusiastically, and wrote movingly about their patients and their own lives. As they are surrounded daily by illness, death, and dying, perhaps it is not surprising that one topic that preoccupies their writing is death.

Medical students are mostly annoyingly healthy, energetic, smart, and capable young adults who like order, structure, and control. Death and dying tend to violate all of these positivist constructs about the nature of reality, and therefore often appear in student poetry as unruly, transgressive phenomena that do not fit their neat formulation of health and disease. Such poems conceptualize death as the ultimate enemy, the foe that students hope to defeat many times before at last yielding the field. Yet medical students also realize through their poems that somehow they must learn to become the facilitators and midwives of the dying process. In their writing, they wonder what death demands from them as physicians in training. They gaze hungrily at their dying patients, hoping that in their moment of transition they will reveal what is needed. What they seek is a way to affirm that although they are well on their way to becoming objective professionals, apparently incapable of shock or fear, they are still caring, compassionate human beings who can grieve the loss of a life.[6]

When I was diagnosed with a rare form of uterine cancer, in the time it takes to read a pathology slide, my life was expanded from teacher (and wife, mother, grandmother, daughter, sister, and friend – but that is another tale) to include that of patient. My recuperation from surgery and commencement of treatment was accompanied by an outbreak of generative energy, almost as painful as a case of shingles, because it forced me to attend carefully and unrelentingly to emotions and thoughts that consciously I would have much preferred to have avoided. Nevertheless, as artists have complained for centuries, the creative urge cannot be denied. In my case, it eventually took the form of a series of poems about cancer and death. These poems imagined me from the perspective of the grave (with a nod to Emily Dickinson), they cast death as an unwanted but omnipresent companion in every aspect of my life, and they tried to wriggle out from under the fear of death, if not death itself. Many of these poems emerged during an elective medical student creative writing group for which I served as faculty advisor, that serendipitously started up when I returned to work.

In my poems, I am still a teacher even as I became a patient. My poems are written in equal parts of pain and hope. I write them partly to begin to connect with other people who are experiencing the same unwanted intimacy with death that I am developing, and partly to stay connected with my students, whom I know are also often frightened, uncertain, and overwhelmed in the presence of mortality. Although they seek a guide, someone to show them the relevant landmarks along the journey, all I can be is a fellow traveler. In my writing I want to strip myself bare, to become as transparent as water, so that the line between patient and doctor, between professor and student blurs, until their doubts and ambivalence are reflected in me, and mine in theirs. I want to say only this: we are all suffering mortals. Let us help each other to move towards this final mystery with grace, dignity, and courage.

Of all the people who have written about death, none has ever discovered a way to use language to evade its grasp. No one has postponed the grim reaper's arrival by dedicating a sonnet to him. Yet in writing about death, from differing and shared perspectives, my students and I have moved closer to dying. Death remains inscrutable, but through writing poetry that names it, we have in some strange way befriended it, or if not that, then at least we have familiarized ourselves with its many guises and come to recognize its varied approaches. In this strange intimacy, achieved word by painfully crafted word, there may be found resolution, and beyond that, even consolation.

REFERENCES

1 Smyth JM, Stone AA, Hurewitz A, Kaell A. Effects of writing about stressful experiences on symptom reduction in patients with asthma or rheumatoid arthritis. *JAMA* 1999; **281**: 1304–9.
2 Pennebaker JW. Telling stories: the health benefits of narrative. *Literature and Medicine* 2000; **19**: 3–18.
3 Branch WT, Pololi L, Frankel RM, *et al.* Small-group teaching emphasizing reflection can positively influence medical students' values. *Academic Medicine* 2001; **76**: 1171–2.
4 Charon R. Reading, writing, and doctoring: literature and medicine. *American Journal of the Medical Sciences* 2000; **319**: 285–91.
5 Campo R. *The Healing Art: A doctor's black bag of poetry.* New York: WW Norton; 2003.
6 Henderson SW. Medical student elegies: the poetics of caring. *Journal of Medical Humanities* 2002; **23**: 119–32.

Index